Major Theories of
Personality Disorder

■ ■ ■

SECOND EDITION

edited by
Mark F. Lenzenweger
John F. Clarkin

THE GUILFORD PRESS
New York   London

© 2005 The Guilford Press
A Division of Guilford Publications, Inc.
72 Spring Street, New York, NY 10012
www.guilford.com

Printed in the United States of America

This book is printed on acid-free paper.

Last digit is print number: 9 8 7 6 5 4 3 2 1

Library of Congress Cataloging-in-Publication Data

Major theories of personality disorder / edited by Mark F. Lenzenweger, John
F. Clarkin.—2nd ed.
    p. cm.
  Includes bibliographical references and index.
  ISBN 1-59385-108-1 (hardcover: alk. paper)
  1. Personality disorders. I. Lenzenweger, Mark F. II. Clarkin, John F.
  RC554.M24 2005
  616.85′81–dc22

                                                    2004019448

About the Editors

Mark F. Lenzenweger, PhD, is Professor of Clinical Science, Cognitive Psychology, and Behavioral Neuroscience in the Department of Psychology at the State University of New York (SUNY) at Binghamton and Adjunct Professor of Psychology in Psychiatry at the Weill Medical College of Cornell University, New York City. He also directs the Laboratory of Experimental Psychopathology at SUNY–Binghamton, where he conducts research and teaches on personality disorders, schizophrenia, schizotypy, and statistical methods.

John F. Clarkin, PhD, is Professor of Clinical Psychology in Psychiatry at the Weill Medical College of Cornell University and Director of Psychology and Co-Director of the Personality Disorders Institute at New York–Presbyterian Hospital. His academic writing and research have focused on the phenomenology of the personality disorders and the treatment of patients with borderline personality disorder.

Contributors

Aaron T. Beck, MD, Department of Psychiatry, University of Pennsylvania, Philadelphia, Pennsylvania; Beck Center for Cognitive Therapy, Bala Cynwyd, Pennsylvania

Lorna Smith Benjamin, PhD, Department of Psychology, University of Utah Neuropsychiatric Institute, Salt Lake City, Utah

Eve Caligor, MD, Department of Psychiatry, Columbia University College of Physicians and Surgeons, New York, New York; Columbia University Center for Psychoanalytic Training and Research, New York, New York

John F. Clarkin, PhD, Department of Psychiatry, Weill College of Medicine of Cornell University, New York, New York; Personality Disorders Institute, New York–Presbyterian Hospital, White Plains, New York

Richard A. Depue, PhD, Laboratory of Neurobiology of Temperament and Personality, Cornell University, Ithaca, New York

Seth D. Grossman, PhD, Institute for Advanced Studies in Personology and Psychopathology, Miami, Florida

Otto F. Kernberg, MD, Department of Psychiatry, Weill College of Medicine of Cornell University, New York, New York; Personality Disorders Institute, New York–Presbyterian Hospital, White Plains, New York; Columbia University Center for Psychoanalytic Training and Research, New York, New York

Mark F. Lenzenweger, PhD, Department of Psychology, State University of New York at Binghamton, Binghamton, New York; Department of Psychiatry, Weill College of Medicine of Cornell University, New York, New York

Björn Meyer, PhD, School of Psychology and Therapeutic Studies, University of Surrey Roehampton, Whitelands College, London, England

Theodore Millon, PhD, DSc, Institute for Advanced Studies in Personology and Psychopathology, Miami, Florida; Department of Psychology, University of Miami, Miami, Florida; Department of Psychiatry, Harvard Medical School/McLean Hospital, Belmont, Massachusetts

Paul A. Pilkonis, PhD, Department of Psychiatry, Western Psychiatric Institute and Clinic, Pittsburgh, Pennsylvania; Department of Psychiatry, University of Pittsburgh School of Medicine, Pittsburgh, Pennsylvania

Aaron L. Pincus, PhD, Department of Psychology, The Pennsylvania State University, University Park, Pennsylvania

James L. Pretzer, PhD, Department of Psychiatry, Case Western Reserve University, Cleveland, Ohio; Cleveland Center for Cognitive Therapy, Beachwood, Ohio

Preface

Nearly 10 years have passed since we published the first edition of *Major Theories of Personality Disorder*. The ensuing decade has been an exciting one indeed with respect to the advances that have occurred in our understanding of the fundamental nature of personality disorders as well as their treatment. In assembling the second edition of *Major Theories*, as many of our colleagues refer to this volume, we invited all our original contributors to revise, amend, and extend their original position pieces in light of the advancing empirical literature in personality disorders research. We also invited them to offer their most recent thoughts and creative ideas with respect to their own theories of personality disorder. We encouraged all of our contributors to "take risks," as it were, and to again advance novel propositions within the context of their models as they saw fit. We are excited to note that all of the chapters that were included in the first edition of *Major Theories* have been substantially revised and updated for this edition; some chapters were nearly completely rewritten. Thus, the second edition contains much that is new and intellectually stimulating. Moreover, we have added two new chapters to the second edition, namely, an additional chapter on interpersonal theory by Aaron Pincus and a chapter on an attachment model of personality disorders by Björn Meyer and Paul Pilkonis. These chapters were added to further expand the richness of the interpersonal perspective that is quite central to the basic nature of personality disorders.

As we did earlier, we continue to view each of the theoretical models in this volume as a research heuristic, a stimulus for both further theory/model development and empirical research. No comprehensive and integrated model of personality disorder exists; however, we believe the fertile models presented in this volume along with recent advances in research strategy will move the field closer to such a model in the coming years.

Indeed, the past 10 years have witnessed great strides in basic research strategies in psychopathology. For example, there is a growing and informative neuroimaging literature; one sees increasingly sophisticated application of genomic research strategies; the relevance of advanced statistical procedures (e.g., taxometrics, finite mixture modeling) for resolving important questions has become evident; neurobiological and behavioral neuroscience findings are frequently being incorporated into models of particular disorders; longitudinal studies of psychopathology have begun to bear long anticipated fruit with the passage of time; and, importantly, clinical treatment trials have improved in quality. Clearly, this is and promises to continue to be an exciting time in psychopathology research in general, and we believe many of these methodological and substantive advances will continue to find their way into personality disorders research. It is also our hope that the area of personality disorders research will see an increase in support, from many venues, for the basic research endeavors of those energetically seeking to unravel the complexities and fundamental nature of personality pathology.

As we noted in the first edition, personality has long held the attention not only of psychologists and clinical psychiatrists but also of theologians, philosophers, and novelists. This fascination lies in the notion that an understanding of the human personality will yield insights into the fundamental nature of humankind. Understanding personality will tell us "what makes us tick," so to speak. All students of personality are reincarnations of this age-old desire to understand the motivations and wiles of the human psyche.

Since the introduction of DSM-III in 1980, 25 years ago, and its creation of a separate diagnostic axis (i.e., Axis II) for the personality disorders, interest in the description and classification of the personality disorders has expanded dramatically. The growing empirical research base, driven in part by the introduction of Axis II, continues to illuminate a variety of fundamental issues in our understanding of the personality disorders. Moreover, this rapidly accumulating body of empirical data clearly indicates that the personality disorders remain of great interest to research clinicians and psychopathologists, confirming the long-standing interest of the practicing clinician who has always noted the prevalence and disruptive nature of personality pathology. Clinicians know all too well that the treatment of personality disorders is difficult, and that these disorders greatly diminish the quality of life for those who suffer from them.

An increased and continuing research effort in the personality disorders area remains welcome and is to be encouraged. However, as we noted in 1996 in the first edition, there remains a profound need for theoretical clarity about the nature and causes of personality disorders. This impression has indeed lingered as the empirical literature appears, at times, to grasp for a sophisticated theoretical footing. This volume continues to attempt to fill that theoretical void with an explication of several rich major contemporary theories of the personality disorders. Our vision for this volume is as before, namely, to assemble a number of position statements from creative senior theoreticians, each reflecting a distinctly different vantage point in his or her model. We continue to see ourselves as extremely fortunate to be able to call on our outstanding colleagues in the personality disorder field, who responded enthusiastically to our idea of a second edition of *Major Theories*, all with the same enthusiasm with which they greeted the initial effort. Our new contributors were also eager to join this effort and the ranks of our prior contributors. We believe we have assembled a truly exceptional group of individuals who have each thrown theoretical light on the personality disorders from their respective viewpoints of cognitive-behavioral, psychodynamic, interpersonal, attachment, ecological, psychometric, and neurobiological perspectives. Once again, we have opened this volume with our own chapter that lays the groundwork for those that follow, highlighting a variety of historical issues in this area as well as junctures in the research approaches to personality pathology that require greater clarity. It is our firm belief that personality disorders research is continuing in its "second phase of development," one that has a crisper focus on etiology and pathogenesis, and we argue that sound theoretical models will continue to be essential tools in helping us map this new and exciting uncharted territory.

An effort such as this does not stand alone. It is embedded in a rich professional, clinical, and academic matrix. Therefore, we would like to take this opportunity to thank our chairman of psychiatry at the Weill College of Medicine of Cornell University, Dr. Jack D. Barchas, for his scholarly advice, administrative support, and continued enthusiasm in connection with this specific undertaking. His breadth of view about the human condition is inspiring and his generative support has proven essential to our research in personality disorders. Finally, we should also like to thank the many colleagues who offered us useful feedback on the first edition of *Major Theories* as well as students at Harvard, Cornell, the State University of New York at Binghamton, and other universities for their valuable insights into the ways in which each chapter in this volume could be improved from their vantage points.

M. F. L.
Ithaca, New York

J. F. C.
White Plains, New York

Contents

Major Theories of Personality Disorder

■ ■ ■

CHAPTER 1

■ ■ ■

The Personality Disorders
History, Classification, and Research Issues

MARK F. LENZENWEGER
JOHN F. CLARKIN

> In the dialogue between theory and experience, theory always has the
> first word. It determines the form of the question and thus sets limits
> to the answer.
> — FRANÇOIS JACOB (1982, p. 15)

Theory without data runs the risk of ungrounded philosophizing, but data
without theory lead to confusion and incomprehension. The definition of
the personality disorders in DSM-III (and its successors, DSM-III-R, DSM-
IV, and DSM-IV-TR) as well as their separation from other clinical syndromes (Axis I disorders) greatly enhanced the legitimacy of this class of
psychopathology as an area for research and personality disorder research
has shown unprecedented and exciting expansion over the past 25 years. It
was the thesis of first edition this volume (in the spirit of the quote from
François Jacob) that the time had come to articulate contrasting and competing (at times, partially overlapping) theories of personality disorder in
order to stimulate some intellectual clarity within the growing body of
empirical data on the personality disorders. We remain convinced that personality disorder research will only move forward appreciably when guided
by rich and sophisticated models. With the second edition of this volume, it
remains our hope that the models and theories of personality pathology

1

presented here will continue to serve not only as an organizing function but, perhaps more important, as useful heuristics for continuing empirical research on the personality disorders.

A BRIEF HISTORICAL OVERVIEW
OF PERSONALITY DISORDER THEORIES

One can trace the conceptualization and articulation of personality and related personality pathology in the history of psychiatry and clinical psychology, and in the development of personality theory and research in the tradition of academic psychology. Whereas there has traditionally been considerable interaction between psychiatry and clinical psychology, the writings and research generated by the field of academic psychology have been focused mainly on normal personality and had little relationship to the clinical traditions. This separation was promoted not only by the physical locale of many clinicians (i.e., hospitals and medical centers vs. university departments of psychology) as well as the reasonable aims of both groups (clinicians diagnose and treat the impaired and dysfunctional, whereas academic personality psychologists view normative functioning and normal personality organization as the object of study). Our goal here is not to review the history of personality theory and related personality disorder theory. Rather, our major focus here is to briefly summarize the conceptualizations of those personality theorists who have ventured into the area of personality disorders or the relationship of personality to pathology. Our overview is, therefore, necessarily selective and makes no claim to be exhaustive; we provide references which the interested reader can pursue.

Vaillant and Perry (1985) trace the articulation in the history of clinical psychiatry of the notion that personality itself can be disordered back to work in the 19th century on "moral insanity." By 1907, Kraepelin had described four types of psychopathic personalities. The psychoanalytic study of character pathology began in 1908 with Freud's *Character and Anal Erotism* (1980/1959) followed by Franz Alexander's (1930) distinction between neurotic character and symptom neuroses and by Reich's (1945) psychoanalytic treatment of personality disorders.

Clinical Psychology and the Assessment
of Personality Pathology

The most unique contribution of clinical psychology to the history of personality and personality pathology was the development and application of psychological testing instruments for the assessment of personality pathology in clinical settings. The flowering of the traditional "full battery" approach to personality assessment in clinical settings is exemplified in the writings of Rappaport, Gill, and Schafer (1968). According to these authors, diagnostic testing of personality and ideational content was concerned with "different types of organizations of the subject's spontaneous thought processes, and attempts to infer from their course and characteristics the nature of his personality and maladjustment" (p. 222). The focus of this traditional approach was shaped by the environment of the day—that is, by the psychiatric diagnostic system in vogue (officially and unofficially) and the predominantly psychodynamic treatment approaches.

In contrast to the full-battery traditional approach, the Minnesota Multiphasic Personality Inventory (MMPI), the well-known self-report inventory, was first published in 1943 by Starke Hathaway, PhD, and J. Charnley McKinley, MD (Hathaway & McKinley, 1943/1983), with scales measuring salient clinical syndromes of the day such as depression, hypochondrias, schizophrenia, and others. The fact that the MMPI was called a personality test is itself a manifestation of the intertwining of concepts of clinical syndromes and personality/personality pathology. Interestingly, however, only two (Scale 4: Psychopathic deviate and Scale 5: Masculinity/Femininity) of the original nine clinical scales actually assessed constructs akin to personality traits or attributes; Scale 0, developed later, was designed to assess social introversion.

In more recent times, there has been less emphasis in clinical assessment in psychiatric settings on projective tests used to assess personality defined in a global sense (owing to concerns about validity, see Lilienfeld, Wood, & Garb, 2000), and more focus on the development of successors to the MMPI that have used advances in psychometric development and are more closely tied to a diagnostic system that makes a distinction between Axis I syndromes and Axis II personality pathology. Illustrative of these instruments are the Millon Clinical Multiaxial Inventory (MCMI; and its successors, the MCMI-II and MCMI-III) and the Personality Assessment Inventory (PAI; Morey, 1991). Given the historical role and importance attached to the clinical interview procedure in psychiatry as well as the advances achieved in the design of structured interviews for the major mood disorders and psychoses (e.g., the Present State Examination [PSE] and Schedule for Affective Disorders and Schizophrenia [SADS]) through the 1970s, it was a natural development to see the careful development of semistructured interviews (e.g., the Structured Clinical Interview for DSM-III-R [SCID-II; Spitzer, Williams, & Gibbon, 1987] and the PDE [Loranger, 1988]) that reliably assess personality disorders as described in the DSM system. Today the standard and most well-accepted approach to the diagnosis of personality disorders remains the structured interview approach with a number of excellent interviews to choose from (International Personality Disorders Examination [IPDE; Loranger, 1999]; Structured Interview for DSM-IV Personality [SIDP-IV; Pfohl, Blum, & Zimmerman, 1997]; Structured Clinical Interview for DSM-IV Axis II Personality Disorders [SCID-II; First, Spitzer, gibbon, & Williams, 1997]). It is worth noting that unlike its peers, the IPDE is configured to assess *both* DSM-IV and ICD-10 diagnostic criteria for personality disorders (Loranger et al., 1994). Axis II structured interviews still remain primarily used in research settings, their integration into training program curricula has increased, and their application in clinical work is encouraged. The interested reader is referred to Zimmerman (1994) for an excellent review of the many critical issues that surround the diagnosis of personality disorders (see also Livesley, 2003; Loranger, 1991a; Loranger, 2000).

Other self-report personality questionnaires have been developed to capture the dimensions thought to be related to the diagnostic criteria on Axis II. This would include the work of Livesely and colleagues (e.g., Schroeder, Wormworth, & Livesley, 1994, 2002) and Clark (1993). Some would speculate that the personality disorders involve maladaptive and inflexible expressions of the basic dimensions of personality as captured in the popular five-factor model of personality (see Costa & McCrae, 1990; John, 1990) or the interpersonal circumplex model of personality (e.g., Wiggins & Pincus, 1989, 2002). Energetic efforts have been made to describe the personality disorders on Axis II in terms of the five-factor model from a conceptual point of view (Costa & Widiger, 2002; Morey, Gunderson, Quigley, & Lyons, 2000), with some measure of consistent empirical support (Saulsman & Page, 2004; Schroeder et al., 1994, 2002) (see below). An alternative dimensional model that is firmly rooted in underlying neurobehavioral systems conceptualizations (e.g., Depue & Lenzenweger, 2001, and Chapter 8, this volume) is also now available as an alternative to the nonbiological lexically based five-factor approach. Finally, a comprehensive self-report instrument, developed within a clinical setting, now exists that is designed to capture both the putative dimensions underlying normal personality as well as those domains relevant to the assessment of DSM-IV-defined Axis II disorders (i.e., the OMNI Personality Inventory and OMNI-IV Personality Disorder Inventory, Loranger [2002]).

Academic Psychology

The field of personality within the larger academic world of psychology has been a time-honored tradition that has suffered its ups and downs (see Hogan, Johnson, & Briggs, 1997; Pervin & John, 1999). An examination of the reviews of the field of personality in the *Annual Review of Psychology* provides an historical sense of the academic debates in the field and the issues that were passionately fought over in the past (e.g., do traits exist?) (e.g., Funder, 2001). In 1990, Pervin, a senior observer of the field, enumerated the recurrent issues in personality research and theory, some of which are relevant to and may be rethought (and fought) in the field of personality disorders: (1) definition of personality; (2) relation of personality theory to psychology and other subdisciplines, including clinical psychology; (3) view of science; (4) views of the person; (5) the idiographic–nomothetic issue; (6) the internal–external issue; (7) the nature–nurture issue; (8) the developmental dimension; (9) persistence and change in personality; and (10) emphasis on conscious versus unconscious processes.

Traditionally, academic personality psychologists studied nonclinical populations, they were more interested in the "normal" personality and consequently gave little attention in their theories to abnormal personality or personality pathology. For example, Gordon Allport (1937) one of the early leaders of normative personality theory, criticized Freud for suggesting a continuum of personality pathology; instead he postulated a division in personality processes between the normal personality and the neurotic personality. The tendency on the part of academic personologists to theorize about and research normative personality most probably reflects not only their substantive area of interest (i.e., normalcy) but also their training (i.e., absence of training in clinical methods and lack of exposure to psychopathological populations) and place of work (the university psychology department as opposed to the clinic and/or psychopathology laboratory). Until relatively recently, there were few academic personologists who extended their theorizing or empirical work to the pathological personality realm, exceptions such as Henry Murray (1938) and Timothy Leary (1957) are well known. This is a theme that will reverberate through the second edition of this volume: In what setting does the theoretician of personality disorders work, and how does that affect the resulting theory?

THE NEO-KRAEPELINIAN REVOLUTION, DSM-III, AND THE BIRTH OF AXIS II

Just as the academic personologists have focused on the normative personality and its structure and development, those in the clinical area (clinical psychologists, psychopathologists, psychiatrists, psychoanalysts) focused their attention and efforts on the pathological variations seen in human personality functioning. To begin, DSM-I (American Psychiatric Association, 1952) provided four categories of psychiatric disorder: (1) disturbances of pattern; (2) disturbances of traits; (3) disturbances of drive, control, and relationships; and (4) sociopathic disturbances. These and subsequent categories of personality disorder in DSM-II (American Psychiatric

Association, 1968) were used only when the patient did not fit comfortably in other categories. The personality disorders defined on a separate axis, whether or not a symptomatic disorder was present, first appeared in DSM-III in 1980. The interested reader is referred to Millon (1995) for one of the best historical reviews of both the process of DSM-III's construction and its formulation of personality disorders as well as a more general prior history of personality disorders.

The advent of DSM-III and its successors (DSM-III-R, DSM-IV, DSM-IV-TR), which use a multiaxial diagnostic system that makes a distinction between clinical syndromes (Axis I) and personality disorders (Axis II), both brought into sharp focus and encapsulated the controversy concerning the nature and role of personalty/personality pathology in the history of psychiatry and the history of modern personality research. The introduction of a distinction between clinical syndromes and personality disorders as well as explicit description of personality pathology within DSM-III by no means brought about unanimity and intellectual peace. In many ways, the introduction of the formal Axis II classification scheme in 1980 ushered in what would begin an exceedingly active initial phase of personality disorder research—namely, clarification and validation of the personality disorder constructs and beginning efforts at illumination of the relations between personality and personality disorder (see section "Normal Personality and Personality Disorder").

Numerous examples can be cited of active productive discussion resulting from the introduction of DSM-III and subsequent DSM nomenclatures. Some workers have argued from accumulated clinical experience that the particular disorders defined in Axis II do not adequately match clinical reality. For example, distinctions between hysterical and histrionic personality disorders have been neglected in Axis II (see Kernberg & Caligor, Chapter 3, this volume); or the very existence of pathological masochism has been only variably recognized and fraught with debate; or clinically rich concepts related to the classic psychopathy notion have been given diminished attention in favor of a behaviorally defined antisocial personality disorder concept. Others have argued at a more basic level that DSM Axis II criteria do not meet scientific standards (Clark, 1992). For example, Clark (1992) suggested that the Axis II personality criteria were not optimally grouped into "disorders" and do not accurately reflect trait dimensions.

These issues highlight some of the difficulties that coexist with the alleged benefits of an "atheoretical" approach proclaimed by the architects of DSM-III and its successors. The development of DSM-III, really the culminating event of the so-called neo-Kraepelinian revolution in psychiatry (see Blashfield, 1984), justifiably sought a diagnostic system that would provide explicit, usually behavioral, criteria that could be reliably assessed.

Such a methodological approach to the definition and operationalization of constructs was long known in psychology (see Cronbach & Meehl, 1955) and its utility was established. Therefore, many psychiatric and clinical psychology researchers welcomed the overhaul of the diagnostic system with open arms. Unfortunately, however, it is our sense that during the rush for diagnostic reliability in the 1970s, the value placed on reliability (something all could agree on) became conflated with or necessarily implied the need for an "atheoretical" approach to diagnosis. The reasons for adopting an atheoretical approach in the contemporary DSM systems were surely complex and were likely a necessity in order to have the diagnostic systems adopted despite parochial interests of the various schools of psychotherapy and clinical practice. In other words, such an atheoretical approach was necessary given that the product (i.e., the DSM) was a quasi-political one, albeit one with important scientific impact. Our point should be obvious; we firmly endorse a methodological approach to diagnosis that is rigorous and displays adequate reliability and validity; however, such an approach need not necessarily be "atheoretical." In 1996 when we initially presented the first edition of this volume it stood in sharp relief to the atheoretical approach of the DSM system. Since that time there has been an increase in research interest in model-guided research in personality disorders, which, to our minds, represents some of the most exciting work in this area. Nonetheless, we still see the need for a compilation of current substantive models of personality disorder as the official nomenclature (DSM-IV) as well as planned revisions (DSM-V) are likely to continue with the atheoretical perspective on personality disorders. We present the second edition of this volume precisely because the theories and models herein will not only guide empirical measurement of personality pathology but also provide a continuing context in which empirical results can be examined and understood; new hypotheses may be generated; and, ideally, etiology, pathogenesis, and development of personality disorders shall be illuminated.

ISSUES OF CONCERN FOR SCIENTIFIC THEORIES OF PERSONALITY DISORDER

As we noted earlier, the advent of Axis II in the multiaxial system introduced by DSM-III and the explicit definition of personality disorders has stimulated scientific and clinical interest in personality pathology. DSM-III's effect on both research and practice was unambiguous and rather dramatic, primarily leading to an increase in the rate at which Axis II diagnoses were made in clinical settings (e.g., Loranger, 1990) but also a marked increase in the number of research studies directed at personality pathology. A review of articles in the prominent scientific psychopathology journals (e.g., *Archives of General Psychiatry* and *Journal of Abnormal Psychology*) since 1980 will reveal a noteworthy increase in the number of research reports on Axis-II-related topics. This era of scientific growth was rapid and substantial enough, in fact, to warrant development and publication of the specialty journal *Journal of Personality Disorders* as well as the formation of the International Society for the Study of Personality Disorders. The *Journal of Personality Disorders* continues to thrive and more and more reports on personality disorders have appeared in the general psychopathology and psychiatry journals (*Archives of General Psychiatry, American Journal of Psychiatry, Journal of Abnormal Psychology*). There is evidence as well that research funding has begun to increase in the area of personality disorders. By almost any objective index, the rate of scholarly inquiry into personality pathology has seen dramatic growth in the 25 years since the advent of DSM-III and the decades to come are almost certain to see sustained interest in the personality disorders.

The contributors to this volume once again have articulated their respective views on the nature and organization of personality pathology, with numerous updates and revisions to their 1996 positions. In contrast to the "atheoretical" position of DSM-IV, each of our contributors has taken a stand with respect to the fundamental nature of personality disorder, transcending an approach (i.e., DSM-IV) that explicitly describes, but, unfortunately, eschews, explanation. Consistent with the contents of this volume, our hope is that future scientific work in personality disorders will continue to become increasingly theory-guided. The benefit of such a development in the scientific approach to personality pathology lies in the power achieved through formulating testable and falsifiable models that are not merely descriptive but, rather, emphasize etiology, mechanism, and lifespan developmental sequelae of personality pathology. An additional benefit of theory-guided and empirically based models of personality pathology, of course, would be the further development and refinement of rational treatments for personality disorders that are more closely tailored to the specific deficits and dysfunctional attributes presented by individual personality pathologies, an aim embodied in the clinical approach known as "differential therapeutics" or "systematic treatment selection" (Beutler & Clarkin, 1990). Those involved in interventions research have pointed out that the field has focused on a few questions, such as the impact of a few described treatments as compared to no treatment or treatment as usual, and the generalization of treatments across problem areas and settings (National Institute of Mental Health, 2002). Other questions, most relevant to practical clinical work, such as how and why specific psychotherapeutic interventions work, have been ignored. From a technical point of view, this concern about how treatments work involves the search for moderators and mediators of change, necessitating hypothesis-generating analyses. This effort to examine the mediators and moderators of change in psychotherapy will necessitate clear articulation of the theory of personality disorders and their key elements (Clarkin & Levy, in press). Finally, with increased knowledge of etiology and mechanism, one could ultimately consider issues related to the prevention of personality disorders, though clearly a Herculean task that challenges the imagination at present. The importance of theory-guided approaches to personality pathology is only amplified when one considers the pervasiveness of personality disorders in general clinical practice, clinic populations, and the population at large. High-quality epidemiologically derived estimates of the prevalence of Axis II disorders are now available (see below) and they suggest a prevalence between 9 and 13% in the community (Lenzenweger, Loranger, Korfine, & Neff, 1997; Torgersen, Kringlen, & Cramer, 2001; Samuels et al., 2002). These figures accord well with the initial "guesstimates" of between 10 and 15% (Weissman, 1993). Clearly, assuming 1 in 10 persons is affected by personality pathology, it is safe to assert that personality pathology is ubiquitous and we are, therefore, challenged to understand the "hows" and "whys" of personality disorder development as well as to discern the most efficient and valid classification approach for such disorders. On a related note, these prevalence estimates suggest personality disorders do represent a public health concern, and funding for research on the personality disorders is deserving of a nontrivial enhancement.

We are committed to and advocate a scientific approach to the study of psychopathology and the study of personality disorders is no exception. In this framework the necessity of reliable assessments, measures, and procedures that possess suitable validity is axiomatic; however, despite good instrumentation, we anticipate future personality disorder theories and research will be characterized by "false starts," forays down "blind alleys," and the customary slow progress of "normal science" punctuated by periodic substantive advances and moments of genuine clarity. This section of our introductory chapter is intended to highlight issues that any scientific theory of personality disorder must consider. We intend to raise more questions than provide answers. As most research in personality disorders is probably best considered as occurring within the "context of discovery" (Reichenbach, 1938), it seems prudent to us to draw attention to a variety of substantive and methodological issues that should guide research in this rapidly developing area in psychopathology research. We highlighted these issues in the first edition of this volume and most, if not all, of them remain unresolved and in need of continued examination. Personality disorders research, we suggest, is particularly interesting as it will need draw on the lessons we have learned, methodological and otherwise, from the study of other forms of severe psychopathology (e.g., schizophrenia and affective illness). However, it is particularly ripe with challenges that are relatively unique to this domain of pathology. For example, Where are the boundaries between "normal" personality and personality disorder? Can one define a "case" of personality disorder in the absence of marked impairment or distress? Furthermore, one could argue that some of the specific research challenges that personality disorder psychopathology affords may not be readily illuminated by the clues we have gleaned from other areas of study and reliance on previous insights may be less useful than having the wrong map for a territory. In short, in the study of personality pathology we rely on the efforts and insights many psychopathologists—including those contributing to this volume—to chart these new territories.

In citing several methodological and/or substantive issues below, it is not our intention to suggest previous personality disorders research that has addressed these issues, directly or in part, has been somehow lax (though some clearly has been!). We are mindful that personality disorders research has only just "taken off" in the last 25 years and many would regard model-guided work in this area as just beginning to emerge (much effort in the 1980s concerned development of assessment technologies). We seek, therefore, to encourage more extensive and ambitious model-guided work in this area. We remain convinced that it continues to be sensible to highlight themes that remain troubling, challenging, and unresolved in personality disorders research. Finally, as in the first edition, we would like to stress the fact that the literature we cite later is necessarily highly selected due to space constraints and our review is not intended to be exhaustive. Our examples, as one might anticipate, will hail primarily from recent research in personality disorders and will, therefore, be heavily influenced by the prevailing DSM nomenclature. Although many of the issues we shall raise derive from studies that focus on DSM defined personality pathology, our comments are not intimately linked to that taxonomy. We continue to view the following issues, not ordered in terms of importance, as largely unresolved and in need of further work as well as worthy of considerable attention by any comprehensive theory of personality disorder, including those contained in this volume.

Normal Personality and Personality Disorder: Questions of Continuity and Structure?

With the advent of specific diagnostic criteria and a polythetic approach to classification, Axis II of DSM-III represented an opportunity for rich theoretical discussion of and empirical research on the relations between personality disorders as conceptualized by psychopathologists and normal personality as studied by academic personality psychologists. Theoretical discussion to date has focused on three key conceptual issues, namely, (1) the dimensional versus categorical nature of personality disorders (Costa &

Widiger, 2002); (2) the distinction between normal and pathological personality features (e.g., social isolation as possibly representing low sociability vs. suicidal attempts as unrepresented on any "normal" dimension of personality; e.g., Wiggins, 1982); and (3) the nature of the basic processes and structure underlying both personality disorders and normal personality (cf. Cloninger, Svrakic, & Przybeck, 1993; Depue & Lenzenweger, 2001, Chapter 8, this volume; Rutter, 1987; Livesley, Jang, & Vernon, 1998). In short, the "normal" personality correlates, if any, of specific personality disorders remain but tentatively specified. Most important, it remains unclear to what extent personality disorder symptoms are *continuous*, albeit exaggerated, extensions of normal traits. For example, although there are now 15 studies of the associations between the "five-factor model" and personality disorder dimensions (Saulsman & Page, 2004), these studies *cannot* address the issue of continuity between personality and personality disorder domains due to their fundamental design (i.e., cross-sectional correlations). Furthermore, research to date has not effectively addressed, using techniques such as confirmatory factor analysis, the comparability or goodness of fit between the overall DSM personality disorder taxonomy *and* the empirically based dimensional structures observed in contemporary personality research such as the interpersonal circumplex (Leary, 1957; Wiggins, 1982) and established multidimensional/factorial models (e.g., the "big five" model; see Digman, 1990, or John & Srivastava, 1999, for excellent reviews, and Block, 1995, 2001; Westen, 1996; and Shedler & Westen, in press; for strident criticism; the "three superfactor" model of Tellegen, 1985, and the three-factor temperament model, e.g., Buss & Plomin, 1984). That is, it is not clear how comparably organized personality pathology is at the latent level *vis-à-vis* normal personality—stated differently, do three, four, or five major dimensions also *continuously* underlie personality disorders? Although normal personality research now suggests that somewhere between three and five factors adequately capture the variation in the primary descriptors of personality, the same cannot be said readily for personality pathology. Moreover, the correspondence between the primary factors of personality and personality disorder remains to be explored in a fine-grained manner beyond simple correlational analyses (e.g., Saulsman & Page, 2004). This is a critical issue as it is not an uncommon experience to see reviewer comments on manuscripts or hear comments at conferences and National Institute of Mental Health (NIMH) study sections suggestive of the (mis)impression that the five-factor approach is an adequate conceptualization of normal personality and the personality disorders (see Depue & Lenzenweger, Chapter 8, this volume).

Most efforts at searching for the personality correlates of personality disorder focus principally on any obtained correlations; however, the meaning of such discovered associations looms large. A large number of studies have focused on the relations between normal personality and personality disorder in recent years, and many more will do so in the future. However, it is worth noting that it is likely that most of these studies will *not* address directly the issue of whether or not personality disorder symptoms are continuously versus discontinuously distributed in the population if they rely primarily on demonstrating correlations among these variables (i.e., Are personality disorder symptoms exaggerations of normal traits?). An implicit assumption of the work generating associations between normative and personality pathology measures has been that an association between such variables suggests a *continuity* between the phenomena (e.g., Costa & McCrae, 1990; Costa & Widiger, 2002). This implicit assumption is fraught with substantive and statistical pitfalls. It could quite conceivably be that in some instances no genuine (i.e., real and natural) connection between a dimension of personality and a personality disorder variable exists even though a statistically significant correlation may exist between them. To begin to address this issue an exceptionally large randomly ascertained general population sample of individuals would need to be assessed for personality disorder symptoms and the distributions of these symptoms should be examined for the existence of qualitative discontinuities as evidenced, possibly, by "bimodality" (see Grayson, 1987, for a provocative review of this concept) *and* through application of complex statistical procedures such as such as admixture analysis (e.g., Lenzenweger & Moldin, 1990), finite mixture modeling (Titterington, Smith, & Makov, 1985; McLachlan & Peel, 2000), or taxometric analysis (Meehl, 1992, 1995; cf. Korfine & Lenzenweger, 1995, Lenzenweger & Korfine, 1992; Waller & Meehl, 1998). Comparable work will, of course, need to be done on normative "dimensions" of personality as well before proceeding to inferences concerning the continuous relations between personality and personality disorder (Endler & Kocovski, 2002).

A question concerning the very existence of "dimensional" continuities and "categorical" (or "typological") discontinuities in either the personality or personality disorder realms itself remains controversial (see Meehl, 1992). In short, regardless of the application of appropriate statistical procedures to such problems, there remain quasi-ideological preferences for either dimensional or categorical conceptualizations of personality-related phenomena. The "dimensional versus categorical" issue was been discussed extensively in relation to personality pathology through the 1980s, with some psychologists advocating a dimensional approach (Widiger, 1992), whereas the psychiatric community remained essentially wed to a categorical framework (American Psychiatric Association, 1994). The "dimensions versus categories" discussion with respect to personality disorders continues to this day. The reasons for such preferences are not always immediately discernible, though psychiatry has long preferred a typological approach to psychopathology (consistent with traditional medicine) and this approach is therefore familiar, facilitates communication, and is consistent with clinical decision making (American Psychiatric Association, 1994; Widiger, 1992). Although much of the "categories" versus "dimensions" debate concerns professional diagnostic or assessment-style preferences, there is a deeper level of analysis to this problem that has garnered the attention of a number of psychopathologists with interest in the structure of nature in psychopathology. Normal personality research has long preferred a dimensional or continuum view of personality and other behavioral phenomena (Meehl, 1992, 1995), due perhaps in part to reliance on parametric statistics and a focus on the study of normative aspects of psychological functioning. Interestingly, as a "dimensional" approach to personality pathology has become increasingly of interest to psychiatry (cf. American Psychiatric Association, 1994), psychological research has seen a resurgence of interest in the detection of discontinuities, "types," or "taxa" in a variety of psychological and psychopathologic realms (see Meehl, 1992, 1995; cf. Lenzenweger & Korfine, 1992). For example, taxometric data generated using the MAXCOV technique developed by Meehl suggests that schizotypy (Lenzenweger & Korfine, 1992; Korfine & Lenzenweger, 1995) and psychopathy (Harris, Rice, & Quinsey, 1994) are taxonic at the latent level; the published taxometric data for borderline personality disorder (Trull, Widiger, & Guthrie, 1990; Haslam, 2003) are also consistent with a taxonic model[1] (but see also Rothschild, Cleland, Haslam, & Zimmerman, 2003). The proper application of taxometric techniques to the study of psychopathology requires great care and guidelines have recently been proposed for future studies to avoid some of the difficulties that appeared in some earlier efforts (Lenzenweger, 2004).

Other than the need for an appropriate methodological approach in the determination of continuity versus discontinuity between personality and personality disorder constructs, theoretical conjectures concerning the relationships between personality disorders (and personality disorder symptoms) and normal personality must take into account the divergent behavioral, affective, attitudinal, and cognitive domains covered by these two broad areas of scientific inquiry. Are there normative counterparts of accepted personality disorder symptoms? Clearly, some personality disorder symptoms will not be expected to have normative personality counterparts (e.g., suicidal behaviors and self-mutilation). The normative construct sociability, on the other hand, clearly ranges from "high" to "low" and, perhaps, an individual with schizoid personality disorder shares much in common with a person described as displaying low sociability. All things considered, though, it is somewhat unrealistic to conceive of precise *one-to-one* correspondences between personality disorder symptoms and normative personality traits. We readily predict that noteworthy correspondences will be observed between several of the major dimensions underlying normal personality (or temperament) and personality disorder symptomatology; however, the meaning and interpretation of such correspondences should prove a challenge to personality disorder theorists. At a minimum, we suggest that models seeking to relate personality systems with personality disorder features do so in a manner that works rationally from the underlying personality systems to possible personality disorder configurations.

Finally, although DSM-IV has presented us with a "structure" for organizing personality pathology, namely, the disorders of Axis II, any meaningful consideration of the relations between personality pathology and normal personality must be cognizant of the possibility that the Axis II arrangement may have little genuine correspondence to the true (or, natural) latent organization of personality disorder symptomatology. By this we mean, in short, that DSM-IV presents us with 10 disorders grouped into three so-called clusters, the odd–eccentric, the impulsive–erratic, and the anxious–avoidant clusters. However, there are no published data derived from a large sample ($N > 1,300$, assuming 10 subjects per Axis II diagnostic criterion) of carefully clinically assessed cases in which analyses, conducted at the level of *individual items* (i.e., criterion level), confirm the DSM-IV cluster structure, or even the disorder structures themselves. Some factor-analytic studies have obtained three-factor solutions, corresponding broadly to the three "clusters" of the DSM-III-R/DSM-IV Axis II taxonomy. However, these studies analyzed data at the level of disorders and they seemed unaware of the fact that the data that were analyzed had been structured *a priori* by being organized into 10 or 11 predefined disorders.

Given the relatively high degree of overlap that can be found among the currently defined Axis II personality disorders, in the form of both correlations among symptom dimensions and/or rates of co-occurrence of categorical diagnoses (Korfine & Lenzenweger, 1991; Widiger et al., 1991), it seems quite reasonable to hypothesize that item-level multivariate analyses of the domain of symptoms found on Axis II will reveal perhaps but a handful of meaningful (i.e., interpretable) factors. While the preliminary work on this problem would by definition need to be more exploratory in nature, a confirmatory approach could be adopted for assessing the fit between an emergent structure or model and new sets of data. An illustration of such an approach can be found in the schizophrenia literature wherein the latent structure of positive and negative symptoms was resolved through application of confirmatory factor analysis and the systematic comparison of multiple competing models of latent structure (Lenzenweger & Dworkin, 1996). Efforts to discern the latent structure of personality disorder symptomatology, whether specified by DSM or an alternative model such as one of those in this volume, must bear in mind the effect of the use of cases selected solely from clinical settings on obtained results. In short, those individuals who come to hospitals and clinics for treatment tend to be more severely affected in general and this fact alone will likely increase the degree of overlap (or correlation) seen across forms of personality pathology. Moreover, the more ill a sample is on the whole, the less likely will be subthreshold cases, which are important of "filling in" the range of personality pathology as it occurs naturally. Thus the impact of sampling on efforts to illuminate the latent structure of personality pathology must be considered.

The State–Trait Issue in Relation to the Definition and Diagnosis of Personality Disorders

Implied in the DSM definition of personality disorders is the assumption that state factors such as anxiety and depression should not substantively affect the assessment of personality pathology. DSM-IV clearly acknowledges that personality disorder symptoms may be manifested during periods of acute illness (e.g., major depression); however, it is equally clear that personality disorder symptomatology should be typical of a person's long-term functioning and shall not be limited only to periods of acute illness (American Psychiatric Association, 1994, p. 629). Although some data do suggest that certain normative personality features, assessed via self-report instruments (not necessarily personality disorder symptoms), among clinically depressed patients do vary over time as a function of changing levels of depression (Hirschfeld et al., 1983), at present neither the relationship between personality disorder symptoms and state disturbance within the context of the cross-sectional diagnostic process nor the relationship between longitudinal symptom stability and state variability is resolved unambiguously for DSM personality disorders. A well-known study that employed structured interviews administered by experienced clinicians (Loranger et al., 1991) found that changes in clinical state (i.e., anxiety and depression) did *not* correspond significantly with changes in the number of DSM-III-R personality disorder criteria met at two points in time; this finding has subsequently been replicated by Loranger and Lenzenweger (1995; cf. Zimmerman, 1994). Trull and Goodwin (1993) reported that changes in mental state were not associated with either self-reported or interview-assessed personality pathology, although the levels of depression and anxiety characterizing the patients in his study are unusually low (perhaps not clinically significant in intensity). Current normal personality research also acknowledges the importance of determining the influence of state factors on trait assessment (Tellegen, 1985) and normative trait-oriented lifespan research methodologists have long advocated the inclusion of state factors as important causal factors in longitudinal developmental models and research (Nesselroade, 1988). Therefore, a major focus of future research in personality pathology should be further clarification of the effect of anxiety and depression on both cross-sectional personality disorders symptom and personality trait assessment as well as the effect of such state factors on the longitudinal stability and change of personality disorders symptoms and traits. Any major theory of personality disorder must incorporate and address the role of state disturbances in the development and manifestation of personality pathology.

On a broadly related theme, the relatively robust association between personality pathology and affective disturbance also raises an important issue specifically concerning less severe affective pathology that is frequently accompanied by personality pathology (Loranger et al., 1991; Klein, Riso, & Anderson, 1993; Klein & Shih, 1998). For example, focusing on but one possible issue, we suggest that future research on personality-disordered populations as well as theories of personality disorder needs to address more directly the precise relationship between dysthymia and personality disorder. Klein et al. (1993, p. 234) in a careful examination of the dysthymia construct outlines *four* plausible, though competing, conceptualizations of dysthymia in relation to personality disorder:

1. Dysthymia is a "characterological depression," essentially an attenuated form of major affective disorder, and this depression has an adverse impact on normative developmental processes, giving rise to the frequently co-occurring features of borderline, dependent, avoidant, and other personality disorder features;
2. Dysthymia is an "extreme" form of normally occurring depressive personality traits, a view deriving largely from psychodynamic theorists;
3. Dysthymia is the result or consequence of life stressors, notably those elicited by personality pathology; and
4. Dysthymia is a "character spectrum disorder" in which the low-grade dysphoria of the illness is a complication of a primary personality disorder traits.

Simply stated, any theory of personality disorder must not only take into account the role of dysphoric emotional states in the assessment and definition of personality pathology but also make explicit its assumptions about the relations hypothesized to exist between personality pathology, affect/emotion, and affective disorder (see Klein & Shih, 1998, for an excellent discussion).

Study Populations and the Epidemiology of Personality Disorders

An essential issue of concern in both future personality disorder research and theory is the representativeness of findings from studies and substantive conceptualizations based on hospitalized and/or clinic patient populations (*vis-à-vis* the general population at large) for furthering our understanding of the nature, course, and development of personality disorders (cf. Drake, Adler, & Vaillant, 1988; Kohlberg, LaCrosse, & Rickey, 1972). There can be little doubt that additional studies using inpatient and/or outpatient samples represent a necessity in future personality disorder research. However, we suggest it is critical to recognize that many individuals with personality disorders exist in the community at large and these people may never present themselves for psychiatric treatment (Dohrenwend & Dohrenwend, 1982) even though they may be quite impaired (Drake & Vaillant, 1985; Drake et al., 1988). This may be especially true for certain personality disorder diagnoses. For example, two studies that used clinically experienced raters found very low rates of schizoid and paranoid personality disorder in patient samples (Loranger, 1990; Pfohl, Coryell, Zimmerman, & Stengl, 1986), although population prevalence estimates for such pathology suggest that many more people are affected by these conditions than those who seek treatment (see Lenzenweger et al., 1997; Torgersen et al., 2001; Samuels et al., 2002). Furthermore, given the polythetic nature of DSM-IV, individuals with personality disorders who are hospitalized may be defined by substantively different configurations of symptoms than those who are not hospitalized. For example, hospitalized borderline patients with personality disorders might display more life-threatening and self-mutilating phenomenology than individuals who are also diagnosed borderline but who have not been hospitalized, although both would be validly diagnosed (the reader can surmise there are many "ways" to be diagnosed with borderline personality disorder according to DSM-IV). Moreover, as was established long ago in epidemiology, those individuals who present for hospital care for one condition are frequently afflicted with other conditions as well as driven by other factors to seek such care, and, consequently, generalizations based on the study of such patient populations must always be made cautiously (i.e., "Berkson's bias"; Berkson, 1946). Therefore, we argue that a future studies of personality disorders that employ subjects drawn from nonclinical (i.e., community) sources will likely represent useful adjuncts to the more traditional study of hospitalized patients and, moreover, may lead to insights that reflect noteworthy differences between personality pathology that is observed in clinical versus nonclinical settings (see Korfine & Hooley, 2001).

Since 1996, significant strides forward have been made in our understanding of the epidemiology of the personality disorders through the use of well-characterized community samples. In 1993 Myrna Weissman hypothesized that the base rate of personality disorder in the community would be approximately 10–13% (Weissman, 1993). Since that time, three high-quality epidemiological studies of personality disorders in nonclinical community samples have been completed. Lenzenweger et al. (1997) applied two-stage procedure for case identification (Shrout & Newman, 1989) to a large nonclinical sample and estimated the point prevalence of DSM-III-R personality pathology to be approximately 11%. The results of this study were subsequently replicated by Torgersen et al. (2001), who found a prevalence of 13% in a Norwegian community sample, and Samuels et al. (2002), who found a prevalence of 9% in an urban community sample (Baltimore, MD). Also currently under way is the National Comorbidity Study—Replication (NCS-R), which is under the direction of R. Kessler. The NCS-R seeks to estimate the prevalence of specified personality disorders in the U.S. population using a rigorous sampling strategy and two-stage procedure for case identification (following Lenzenweger et al., 1997). The effective use of the two-stage procedure for case identification has helped to allay some of the concerns expressed earlier regarding the feasibility and cost of undertaking epidemiological work on the personality disorders (see Loranger, 1992). The appearance of empirically grounded prevalence rates for specific personality disorders will not only advance knowledge but also facilitate public health planning. For example, we now know that the community prevalence of borderline personality disorder is not 2% as suggested by DSM-IV, but is in the range of .3% (Lenzenweger et al., 1997) to .7% (Torgersen et al., 2001), and this information should prove useful to many parties.

Longitudinal Course/Lifespan Perspectives on Natural History of Personality Disorders

One of the cardinal assumptions, and perhaps most important from a theoretical perspective, concerning the nature of personality disorders is that they represent *enduring* conditions that are trait-like and, therefore, relatively stable over time (American Psychiatric Association, 1980, 1987, 1994). In fact, DSM-IV states, "The features of Personality Disorders usually become recognizable during adolescence or early adult life. . . . Some types of Personality Disorder . . . tend to become less evident or remit with age" (American Psychiatric Association, 1994, p. 632). However, with the possible exception of antisocial personality disorder (Glueck & Glueck, 1968; Robins, 1966, 1978), it remains safe to say, as we did in 1996, that very little is known about the long-term longitudinal course, development, or natural history of personality disorders. Although there had been a variety of studies that have used the basic test–retest study design in the examination of personality disorder stability and change over time (see Perry, 1993, for review), it is essential to note that as Rogosa (Rogosa, Brandt, & Zimowski, 1982), the lifespan research methodologist, remarks pointedly, "Two waves of data are better than one, but maybe not much better" (p. 744). Due to regression toward the mean effects (Nesselroade, Stigler, & Baltes, 1980) and other difficulties (e.g., inability to estimate individual growth curves; inadequacy for study of individual differences in change; Rogosa, 1988) fundamentally inherent in simple test–retest design studies, these test–retest studies did not address the fundamental issues concerning stability and change in personality disorders.

In contrast to the situation with personality disorders, as of the mid-1990s, there were abundant data in support of the general longitudinal stability of *normal* personality traits and features in a variety of age groups, including college students and young adults, (Block, 1971; Costa & McCrae, 1986, 1988; Finn, 1986; Haan & Day, 1974; Helson & Moane, 1987; McCrae & Costa, 1984; Mortimer, Finch, & Kumka, 1982; Nesselroade & Baltes, 1974; Vaillant, 1977; Roberts & DelVecchio, 2000; Srivastava, John, Gosling, & Potter, 2003). In this context, it should be noted that although the impression for normal personality is one of stability, the issue is far from closed and active discussion remains on this general issue (see Caspi & Roberts, 1999; Roberts & DelVecchio, 2000; Srivastava et al., 2003). Moreover, lifespan methodologists had already articulated the preferable way to conduct such research, namely the use of *multiwave* panel design studies (Baltes, Reese, & Nesselroade, 1977; Kessler & Greenberg, 1981; Nesselroade et al., 1980) with multiple indicators for all of the disorders (constructs) of interest. What this literature implied in practical terms would be studies in which a large number of cases are examined at least three, and preferably more, times for personality pathology across meaningfully lengthy time intervals, with all cases being examined using the same measures (procedures) at each assessment point. The scientific utility of a multiwave design lies in the fact that it provides an opportunity for the most informative statistical analysis of empirical relationships among constructs over time (Baltes & Nesselroade, 1973; Collins & Horn, 1991; Collins & Sayer, 2001; Nesselroade & Baltes, 1979, 1984; Rogosa, 1979, 1988; Singer & Willett, 2003), a fact that has been well established in the lifespan developmental research realm for many years.

As suggested in 1996, we continue to urge the reader to bear in mind that stability, however, is not necessarily as easy to investigate as one might initially think because changes over time in personality pathology could be the result of aging, period, treatment, and/or retest effects, although retest effects appear less relevant to personality assessments (Costa & McCrae,

1988). Longitudinal stability (and, by definition, change) of personality disorder features can be evaluated from at least four different perspectives (following Kagan, 1980; Mortimer et al., 1982; Lenzenweger, 1999; cf. Collins & Horn, 1991; Collins & Sayer, 2001), namely, structural invariance, rank-order stability, level stability, and ipsative (or intraindividual) stability. Structural invariance, or the maintenance of a temporally consistent factor structure and configuration of factor loadings, can be assessed using both confirmatory factor analysis (CFA) and causal modeling techniques (Bentler, 1984; Joreskog, 1979; Nesselroade & Baltes, 1984; Rogosa, 1979). These statistical techniques are ideally suited for use in longitudinal research as they allow the investigator to use all available panel data simultaneously (Kessler & Greenberg, 1981; Rogosa, 1979) and they allow for direct comparison of alternative structural models of stability (Bentler, 1984; Nesselroade & Baltes, 1984). Rank order, or "normative stability," concerns the extent to which individuals maintain their relative position within a group ranking on a variable of interest from time 1 to time 2. Level stability concerns the extent to which group means remain invariant over time on a variable (or disorder) of interest. Finally ipsative stability concerns *intra*individual consistency in the organization of personality disorder features or personality traits over time (cf. Mortimer et al., 1982). Finally, growth and change in a psychological attribute or behavior can be studied in a fine-grained manner using the powerful methods of individual growth curve analysis (Rogsoa & Willett, 1985; Singer & Willett, 2003), which allows one to illuminate important parameters of change such as level and slope within a statistical context that can be either descriptive or explanatory.

Given the body of evidence supporting the stability of normal personality, it is not unreasonable to expect that at least some personality disorder features would display significant *long-term* temporal stability, on the assumption they are reflective of normal personality variation in some manner—particularly, for example, features such as schizoid social withdrawal, compulsive rigidity, and the "extraverted" or outwardly directed interpersonal style of the psychopath. Although several early studies supported the temporal stability of personality disorder features and diagnoses over relatively short time spans (e.g., 1 year or less) (Perry, 1993), evidence concerning long-term or lifespan stability of operationally defined personality disorders was conspicuously lacking in the published empirical research literature (Drake & Vaillant, 1988; Drake et al., 1988) through the 1980s and well into the 1990s. By the late 1980s, it was recognized that long-term longitudinal work was sorely needed in the area of personality disorders, but no studies were under way.

This situation changed in 1990 due to the initiation of a large-scale prospective multiwave longitudinal study of personality disorders. The

Longitudinal Study of Personality Disorders (LSPD), under the direction of M. F. Lenzenweger, was begun in 1990 as the first NIMH-funded longitudinal study of personality disorders of any type. The LSPD concerns the stability and change of personality disorders, personality, temperament and many other aspects of psychological functioning over time. An initial report from the LSPD (Lenzenweger 1999), using three waves of data, described impressive evidence of rank-order stability in personality features over time as well as some nontrivial evidence of change in the level of personality disorder features over time. Thus, stability emerged as a complex issue for the personality disorders in these data—individuals retained their position in an ordinal sense; however, there was clear evidence that change was happening. Further analysis of the LSPD data set using state of the art individual growth curve methodology (Lenzenweger, Johnson, & Willett, in press) suggests a considerable amount of change occurring in personality disorder features over time, change that was not clearly detectable using more traditional analytic techniques. Such findings raise profound and fundamental questions regarding the very basic nature of personality disorders as defined in the DSM systems.

A second longitudinal study of personality disorders was begun in 1996, also with the support of the NIMH, known as the Collaborative Longitudinal Personality Disorders Study (CLPS) under the direction of a team of investigators at several sites (Gunderson et al., 2000; Shea et al., 2002). The CLPS focuses on four personality disorders: schizotypal, borderline, avoidant, and obsessive–compulsive personality disorders. Early reports from the CLPS suggest some degree of rank-order stability over time, with evidence of relatively substantial symptom declines with time (Shea et al., 2002). Specifically, Shea et al. (2002) found that 66% of their CLPS patients dropped below diagnostic thresholds in 1 year with highly significant declines (revealing substantial effects) for continuously measured personality disorder symptoms. These CLPS findings replicate those reported earlier from the LSPD (Lenzenweger, 1999); however, the CLPS data have not been analyzed yet with more advanced techniques. Unfortunately, complicating factors in the CLPS methodology such as the absence of blinded assessors in their personality disorder assessment protocol and the fact that all study subjects have been in treatment during the study cannot be ignored. These factors make the extraction of meaning and direction from the CLPS study less than straightforward. Finally, two other studies have taken a focus on DSM personality pathology, the Johnson et al. (2000) study that focuses on a retrospective assessment of personality disorder phenomenology from case records, which include various clinical data, for a cohort of adolescents, and the study by Zanarini, Frankenburg, Hennen, and Silk (2003) of borderline personality disorder. What is remarkable about both of these latter studies is that, despite methodological limitations, they suggest evidence of considerable *change* in the level of personality disorder features over time, consistent with LSPD (Lenzenweger, 1999; Lenzenweger et al., in press). For example, Zanarini et al. (2003) found massive declines in symptoms such that 73.5% of previously diagnosed borderline personality disorder subjects were "remitted" at 6-year follow-up, suggesting nontrivial mean level changes in borderline personality disorder symptoms. Johnson et al. (2000) found 28–48% reductions in personality disorder symptoms (continuous format) with time.

What is particularly fascinating about the emerging corpus of data from the longitudinal study of personality disorders is that the picture appears to be one of *change*. This is especially interesting as DSM-IV maintains its view that the personality disorders are stable and trait-like over time and it is not uncommon to see reviewer comments on manuscripts, NIMH study section "pink sheet" comments, or psychology textbooks reflecting the assumption that personality disorders are stable, enduring, and "set like plaster." In short, the assumption regarding the stability of personality disorders may be just that, an assumption that will erode in time with the accrual of empirical data that actually specify the true developmental and longitudinal nature of personality disorders over time. We continue to advocate the need for additional longitudinal studies of personality disorder, from both community and clinical settings. However, in advocating the careful study of the longitudinal stability of personality disorders, we do not intend to suggest that inquiry into stability represents an end in itself, one that is but merely descriptive and statistical. Rather such study it should be viewed as a necessary step in the ongoing exploration of the lifespan developmental course of personality pathology. Once established, we foresee studies moving away from simple demonstrations of stability (or lack thereof) but toward a lifespan view with an emphasis on discerning those biobehavioral and psychosocial processes and mechanisms that underlie the etiology and development of personality pathology (i.e., moving from description toward an explanatory framework) (see Lenzenweger et al., in press).

Genetic and Biological Underpinnings of Personality Pathology

The role of genetic influences in the development and stability of normal personality as well as individual differences in personality is now well established and beyond dispute (Plomin & Caspi, 1999; Plomin, DeFries, McClearn, & McGuffin, 2000; Plomin, DeFries, Craig, & McGuggin, 2003; McGue, Bacon, & Lykken, 1993), contrarian views being most likely expressed by those with sociopolitical agendas rather than rigorous scientific interests. Though the heritability estimates for features or dimensions of personality tend to be lower than those observed for intelligence or other cognitive abilities, it can be safely said that genetic factors play an influential role in determining personality—they have the status of "fact" at this point (see DiLalla, 2004; Plomin & Caspi, 1999; Plomin et al., 2000; Plomin et al., 2003). The situation for personality disorders, however, remains considerably less clear with respect to the role of genetic factors in the etiology of personality pathology. This is *not* to say that genetic factors do not play a role in determining these disorders but, rather, that the studies bearing on the determination of both familiality and heritability of personality disorders are only just beginning to appear; twin and adoption studies remain a rarity and familial aggregation work is accumulating slowly (see Livesley et al., 1998). To date, the greatest amount of genetically relevant data can be found for schizotypal personality disorder, which by most accounts appears related genetically to schizophrenia as well as to borderline, antisocial, and obsessive–compulsive personality disorders. However, the genetic picture for even these disorders is unclear due in large part to an absence of data for the disorders themselves or putatively correlated dimensions (e.g., sociability in schizoid personality disorder) (Lang & Vernon, 2001; Nigg & Goldsmith,1994). Finally, quite apart from research on genetic factors, it is necessary to point out that the psychobiological underpinnings of personality pathology in terms of prominent central nervous system neurotransmitters and meaningful neurobehavioral circuitry remain in infancy (see Cloninger et al., 1993; Coccaro, 1993; Coccaro et al., 1989; Coccaro, 2001; Depue & Lenzenweger, 2001, Chapter 8, this volume; Siever, Kalus, & Keefe, 1993).

The Axis I and Axis II Interface: Comorbidity, Causality, or Confusion?

As we noted in 1996, the nature of observed comorbidity among the personality disorders was both ubiquitous and poorly understood, a view echoed by others (Pfohl, 1999), and it remains an area of active discussion. In fact, an online search using PsycINFO that tracked the joint appearance of the keywords "comorbidity" and "personality disorder" yielded nearly 800 citations, many reports appearing in the 1990s.

All models of personality disorder are, by necessity, required to deal with the relationship between personality pathology and other major forms of psychopathology, such as affective illness, anxiety disorders, and even schizophrenia. Both clinical practice and available research data suggest strongly that an individual can suffer from both a major Axis I condition as well as a personality disorder simultaneously—a clinical reality typically discussed under the rubric of "comorbidity" (Widiger & Shea, 1991). The comorbidity issue is laden with a number of complex questions that speak not only to description, diagnosis, and classification but also to etiology. For example, at the level of diagnosis, is it the case that comorbidity arises out of the fact that our current multiaxial system encourages multiple diagnoses (is it an artifact of the system) or is it the case that people can actually suffer from two or more disorders simultaneously? Clearly, one could have both pneumonia and heart disease simultaneously; can one have both depression and schizotypal personality disorder at the same time? Can one have a personality disorder even in the face of a psychotic illness—if so, what limitations or qualifications must attend the diagnosis of a personality disorder in such circumstances?

Future research needs to focus on the careful dissection of putatively highly comorbid conditions such as major depression and borderline personality disorder (e.g., Loranger, 1991b) along a variety of meaningful dimensions such as phenomenology, familiality, medication response, psychobiology, and pathogenesis (see Gunderson & Phillips, 1991, for an excellent demonstration). Such careful dissection of comorbid conditions will likely enhance our understanding not only of the boundaries existing between personality pathology and other major syndromes but also of our notions regarding the development and etiology of personality disorders. What possible roles could a major Axis I disorder play in relation to personality pathology? For example, could the presence of a major psychiatric syndrome be shown to "causally" facilitate the development of a personality disorder or merely increase the statistical risk for the development of a personality disorder? Can an Axis I syndrome represent the more severe version of a broad class of psychopathology of which the related personality disorder is but a spectrum variant (cf. schizophrenia and schizotypal personality disorder)? Could it also not be that there is no etiologically relevant connection whatsoever between a major syndrome and a comorbid personality disorder?

For research into the comorbidity issue(s) to be maximally beneficial to the field, two fundamental methodological issues should be kept in mind. First, comorbidity work is badly in need of large n studies. If the natural association between conditions (e.g., borderline personality disorder and depression) is to emerge from data, then the most stable estimate of this association will come from data drawn from large samples. Second, future comorbidity research should be done on either a consecutive admissions basis at a clinical setting or in the general population from an epidemiological perspective (cf. National Comorbidity Survey [NCS]; Kessler et al., 1994). The NCS-R, under the direction of Ronald Kessler, which includes a personality disorders component as noted earlier, should provide useful information on the personality disorders and Axis I disorder comorbidity patterns. Future reports on the comorbid diagnoses of those patients who happen to be in one's personality disorder protocol are not likely to be informative as any inherent sampling bias will misrepresent the natural rate of comorbidity. An excellent example of the application of multivariate statistical technique in the dissection of a large data, the original NCS data, in an effort to address comorbidity can be found in Krueger (1999). Krueger's (1999; Krueger & Tackett, 2003) speculations regarding potentially core common processes in general psychopathology should serve to inspire comparable work on the personality disorders at the item-level of analysis in an effort to resolve comorbidity issues (see above).

Validity of Personality Pathology

Last, but by no means least, is the issue of validity in relation to personality disorder constructs. Despite the 25 years since the publication of DSM-III, the validity of specific DSM personality disorder diagnoses remains a relatively open issue in psychopathology research; however, the base of validity information is growing for most disorders, particularly schizotypal, borderline, and antisocial personality disorders. We take this opportunity to remind our reader that although reliable ratings of personality disorder symptoms are now possible, this does not necessarily ensure that the validity of the diagnoses has been established (Carey & Gottesman, 1978). This statement holds true for the DSM taxonomy as well as all those models described in this volume. Furthermore, no clear and compelling criteria of validity (Cronbach & Meehl, 1955) currently exist against which personality disorder diagnoses can be compared to assess their validity—not unlike other areas of psychopathology, there is no "gold standard" for validity in the personality disorder realm. Although Spitzer (1983) has proposed that the validity of personality disorder diagnoses might ultimately best be established by longitudinal studies of personality disorders that employ well-known expert raters as well as all available data useful for psychiatric diagnosis (the so-called LEAD standard), such a definitive study conducted on a large scale has yet to be undertaken due to the logistical difficulties and formidable expense most likely involved in such a project (cf. Pilkonis, Heape, Ruddy, & Serrao, 1991; see also Zimmerman, 1994). However, we do not wish to suggest that advances have not been made in aggregating data that can ultimately ensure the validity of personality disorder diagnoses. Many have sought to use informants to help validate clinician assigned diagnoses from the reports taken from individuals; however, the use of informant reports to validate the reports of individuals assessed for personality disorders remains a highly problematic and unclear area open to alternative interpretation (Klonsky, Oltmanns, & Turkheimer, 2003). There have been advances in other approaches to assessment that have implications for construct validity. Creative new approaches to the assessment of personality disorders, motivated in part by an interest in increasing validity, can be found, for example, in the novel prototype matching/Q-sort approach developed by Westen and colleagues (Westen & Shedler, 1999, 2000; cf. Westen & Muderrisoglu, 2003) and in the work of Turkheimer, Oltmanns, and colleagues on peer nomination (Oltmanns, Turkheimer, & Straus, 1998; Oltmanns, Melley, & Turkheimer, 2002). Finally, we should like to suggest that the methods of the experimental psychopathology laboratory (Bornstein, 2003; Lenzenweger & Hooley, 2003) hold considerable promise for the elucidation of fundamental processes that may be impaired in personality pathology and illumination of such processes may move personality disorder research away from nearly complete reliance on clinical features (see Korfine & Hooley, 2000, for an excellent example). Not only would such laboratory work speak to construct validity, but it might also discern reliable and valid endophenotypes for personality disorders (Gottesman & Gould, 2003).

LANDMARKS, CRITICAL JUNCTURES, AND FRONTIERS: A GUIDE TO EXPLORING THE MAJOR THEORIES OF PERSONALITY DISORDER

In closing this introductory chapter, as we did in 1996, we look back and see that we have raised a number of specific issues that we believe can be counted among the most challenging and important in the area of personality disorders research. For this area of psychopathology research to move forward, greater clarity must be sought along each of the dimensions noted previously. Our contributors, one and all, speak to various aspects of the foregoing issues we have raised and they can be fit into broader theoretical and scientific contexts as well. At the same time we encourage, our readers, to find how the theoreticians and researchers contributing to this volume deal with the specific substantive issues noted herein, we should also like to encourage each of them to examine the following chapters using a common set of broader guidelines. By evaluating each of the following chapters along the general dimensions specified next, we believe consistencies and inconsistencies across the models as well as possibilities for new theory, research, and treatment will emerge. Readers should consider the following dimensions with respect to each of the following theoretical models of personality disorder.

What Are the Substantive Foundations of the Model?

Can the roots of the model be traced to major historical or research traditions in psychology and/or psychiatry (e.g., psychoanalysis and behaviorism)? Does the author identify the level from which the data are derived that constitute the basis for classification, measurement, and treatment (e.g., intrapsychic, interpersonal, and cognitive)? What is the primary focus of the model (e.g., etiologically oriented or therapeutically oriented)?

What Is the Formal Structure of the Model?

Have the core assumptions of the model been formally stated and are the major explanatory principles clearly articulated? While models in psychopathology, unlike comprehensive theories, can be somewhat incomplete in their effort to explain a form of psychopathology (cf. Matthysse, 1993; see also Webb, 2001), has the model nonetheless been formulated in a manner that allows for its testability and falsifiability (and, therefore, possible refutation) (cf. Meehl, 1978, 1993)?

What Taxonomy Derives from the Model?

What is the nature of the taxonomy that derives from the model? For example, does the model admit of a structure that is hierarchical, based on a circumplex or some alternative form of a multiaxial approach? Is the classification approach based on a prototypal, categorical, or dimensional methodology? Is variation personality pathology discussed in terms of degree (quantitative) or kind (qualitative)? How independent are the personality disorder syndromes in terms of etiological origins and does this independence affect the taxonomy in any fashion? How does the model relate to DSM-III-R and the more recent DSM-IV?

If the model does not subscribe to the DSM (i.e., DSM-IV) approach to personality disorders, what is the nature of the taxonomy that derives from the model? For example, does the model admit of a structure that is hierarchical, based on a circumplex or some alternative form of a multiaxial approach? Is the classification approach based on a prototypal, categorical, or dimensional methodology? Is variation personality pathology discussed in terms of degree (quantitative) or kind (qualitative)? How independent are the personality disorder syndromes in terms of etiological origins and does this independence affect the taxonomy in any fashion?

Etiological and Developmental Considerations?

Does the model transcend a purely descriptive stance and speak to issues of "mechanisms" and "processes" that determine the development of a personality disorder? In short, does the model attempt to answer the question "how" with respect to the emergence of personality pathology? What are the principal components of the processes and mechanisms theorized to be etiologically relevant (e.g., genetic influences, neurobehavioral factors, and temperamental dispositions; cognitive deficits; learned characteristics; and other sources of disorder such as familial conflict and trauma or abuse)?

In the theories presented in this volume one trend is quite clear—all our contributors have clearly eschewed a merely descriptive approach in favor of an explanatory effort with clear up implications for etiology. Furthermore, all our contributors have proposed theoretical models that presume interaction across multiple levels of the individual, emphasizing not only behavioral and personality characteristics and factors but also neurobiological and environmental components as well. For example, although Otto Kernberg and Eve Caligor (Chapter 3) see character pathology largely in terms of a developmental pathology of aggression, their theory incorporates temperament, affect, and trauma components in interaction. Depue and Lenzenweger (Chapter 8) present a fundamental model of personality as defined by interacting dimensions known to be rooted in neurobiological functions and, according to neurobehavioral model personality pathology, which can also be viewed as the interactive result of these dimensions. For Theodore Millon and Seth Grossman (Chapter 7), personality pathology emerges from a complex interaction of three fundamental polarities, self versus other, pleasure versus pain, and activity versus passivity. James Pretzer and Aaron Beck (Chapter 2) see personality pathology largely emerging from and being maintained by systematic biases in information processing and memory of events eliciting pathological cognitive, emotional, and behavioral responses. Meyer and Pilkonis (Chapter 5), Pincus (Chapter 6), and Benjamin (Chapter 4) all stress the role of interpersonal experiences in the emergence of personality disorders.

How Are Assessment and Diagnosis Accounted for in the Model?

Does the model have an associated assessment and diagnostic approach? If so, what are the sources of the empirical data that are used for diagnosis according to the model? Does the assessment approach rely on therapeutic contexts, self-report inventories, or structured interviews? Has the author presented adequate information concerning the reliability and validity of the assessment and diagnostic procedures associated with the model?

Millon and Grossman (Chapter 7), Pincus (Chapter 6), Benjamin (Chapter 4), Meyer and Pilkonis (Chapter 5), and, to a lesser extent, Pretzer and Beck (Chapter 2) have exerted a great deal of effort in operationalizing their personality pathology conducts in the form of assessment instruments covering the taxonomy of the personality disorders. Millon and Grossman are guided by the DSM taxonomy to a great extent, whereas Benjamin, Pincus, and Meyer and Pilkonis have shown the *consistency* of their approaches with the DSM system but do not attempt to map their positions with the DSM landmarks.

Does the Model Articulate Therapeutic Procedures or, at Least, Highlight Implications for Treatment?

According to the model, how does one go about treating personality pathology and what are the treatment goals (e.g., symptom relief vs. reconstructive work)? In what tradition is the therapeutic work carried out (e.g., insight oriented vs. cognitive vs. biological therapy)? Are the principles of change/improvement clearly articulated by the model? What are the limits of the therapeutic approach (i.e., Are there personality disorders for which the therapy would not be appropriate)?

While Benjamin (Chapter 4), Kernberg and Caligor (Chapter 3), and Pretzer and Beck (Chapter 2) all relate their personality pathology constructs and theories to interventions, it is Kernberg and Beck who have articulated treatment manuals for these disorders. This translation of theories of personality disorder to treatment interventions is a necessary step to the current important focus of psychotherapy research on the mechanisms of change (National Institute of Mental Health, 2002). From this prospective, Kernberg and colleagues emphasize the importance of change in identity diffusion (conception of self and others), and Beck points out the importance of faulty cognitions, especially those relating to the self. When one overlooks the somewhat esoteric jargon of each of these orientations, there is an interesting similarity in the focus on the patients' guiding conceptions of self and interactions with others.

Prospects for the Future: Integration of Mind, Brain, and Behavior

To our minds, the task of future theorizing and empirical research in personality disorders is the effective integration of mind, brain, and behavior. Any comprehensive model of complex human behavior, particularly forms of psychopathology, will require a clear and genuine integration of ideas and research findings that cut across the levels of analysis linking mind, brain, and behavior. One thing is quite clear to us, as well as to the contributors of this volume, monolithic theories existing at but one level of analysis are sure to fail in their explanation of complex human behavior. For example, for years normative developmental psychologists have viewed personality and emotional development almost exclusively in terms of psychosocial influences, much to the exclusion of genetic and biological factors. Indeed, David Rowe (1994), the late developmental behavioral geneticist, has termed this view of personality and psychological development "socialization science," and he has offered a pungent criticism of such a monolithic model, demonstrating effectively the relative importance of genetic factors vis-a-vis psychosocial influences for personality development. We maintain a similar position with respect to personality disorders—for example, personality disorders are not likely to be understood or explained solely in terms of psychosocial influences. A genuine integration of genetic factors, neurotransmitter models, and other neurobiological processes with psychosocial, cognitive, and environmental factors will be required to advance our knowledge of the personality disorders. The best models in some ultimate sense will be those that integrate across these levels (e.g., Meehl, 1990; see also Meehl, 1972). The importance of genetic factors in both normative and pathological development is indisputable (DiLalla, 2004; Plomin et al., 2000; Plomin et al., 2003; Rowe, 1994; Rutter, 1991; Rutter & Silberg, 2002) and the essential role of neurobiological factors in temperament (e.g., Kagan, 1994), emotion (Ekman & Davidson, 1994), personality development (e.g., Depue & Lenzenweger, 2001, Chapter 8, this volume), and the emergence of psychopathology (e.g., Breslin & Weinberger, 1990; Cocarro & Murphy, 1990; Davidson, Pizzagalli, Nitschke, & Putnam, 2002; Grace, 1991) is axiomatic, some would even say confirmed. The meaningful integration of brain, emotion, behavior, and environmental influences currently represents an exceptionally active research area in various areas of psychological science, especially cognition and personality—our belief is that personality disorders research will necessarily have to strive for similar integrative work for genuine advances to occur. Our contributors are clearly leading the way in this connection. For example, Depue and Lenzenweger (Chapter 8) seek to integrate personality, behavior, and neurobiology in their model, Kernberg and Caligor (Chapter 3) propose complex interactions among temperament, trauma, and early experience, and Pretzer and Beck (Chapter 2) suggest that biased cognition must be understood within a matrix that incorporates affect and emotion as well as interpersonal factors. Indeed, interesting differences have emerged among our theorists, for example, Kernberg and Caligor (Chapter 3) argue that neurobiological factors, operating through temperament, have more of a *mediating* role in the determination of personality pathology, whereas Depue and Lenzenweger (Chapter 8) cast neurobiological processes, especially the role of serotonin, in *modulating* framework. This is precisely the type of debate and discussion that will not only provide useful heuristics for future research directed at integrating mind, brain, and behavior but will ultimately allow us to better understand and care for our patients.

At this point we should like to end our discussion of points of introduction and orientation and invite readers to sample from what we believe are the leading theories of personality disorder. We encourage readers to view each of these chapters as an independent position statement by their authors as well as the building blocks for what may ideally become a more comprehensive theory of personality pathology.

ACKNOWLEDGMENTS

We thank Richard Depue, Otto F. Kernberg, Lauren Korfine, Kenneth Levy, Armand W. Loranger, and many others for useful discussions concerning critical substantive issues in personality disorders research. Initial development and preparation of this chapter was supported in part by Grant No. MH-45448 from the National Institute of Mental Health to Mark F. Lenzenweger.

NOTE

1. The MAXCOV data reported in Trull et al. (1990) for borderline personality disorder reveal the characteristic right-end peak suggestive of a low base-rate latent taxon (see Meehl, 1992, 1995, or Korfine & Lenzenweger, 1995) for conceptual and mathematical rationale. The data reported in the Rothschild, Cleland, Haslam, and Zimmerman (2003) report are somewhat ambiguous; however, they reveal considerable evidence of taxonicity although the authors have chosen to view the data as supporting a dimensional model (see Haslam, 2003, for a taxonic interpretation of these same data).

REFERENCES

Alexander, F. (1930). The neurotic character. *International Journal of Psycho-Analysis, 11*, 292–311.

Allport, G. W. (1937). *Personality: A psychological interpretation.* New York: Henry Holt.

American Psychiatric Association. *Diagnostic and statistical manual of mental disorders.* Washington, DC: Author.

American Psychiatric Association. (1968). *Diagnostic and statistical manual of mental disorders* (2nd ed.). Washington, DC: Author.

American Psychiatric Association. (1980). *Diagnostic and statistical manual of mental disorders* (3rd ed.). Washington, DC: Author.

American Psychiatric Association. (1987). *Diagnostic and statistical manual of mental disorders* (3rd ed., rev.). Washington, DC: Author.

American Psychiatric Association. (1994). *Diagnostic and statistical manual of mental disorders* (4th ed.). Washington, DC: Author.

American Psychiatric Association. (2000). *Diagnostic and statistical manual of mental disorders* (4th ed., text rev.). Washington, DC: Author.

Baltes, P., & Nesselroade, J. (1973). The developmental analysis of individual differences on multiple measures. In J. Nesselroade & H. Reese (Eds.), *Life-span developmental psychology: Methodological issues.* (pp. 219–251). New York: Academic Press.

Baltes, P., Reese, H., & Nesselroade, J. (1977). *Life-span developmental psychology: Introduction to research methods.* Monterey, CA: Brooks/Cole.

Bentler, P. (1984). Structural equation models in longitudinal research. In S.

Mednick, M. Harway, & K. M. Finelo (Eds.), *Handbook of longitudinal research* (pp. 88–105). New York: Praeger.

Berkson, J. (1946). Limitations of the application of fourfold table analysis to hospital data. *Biometrics, 2,* 339–343.

Beutler, L., & Clarkin, J. F. (1990). *Systematic treatment selection: Toward targeted therapeutic interventions.* New York: Brunner/Mazel.

Blashfield, R. K. (1984). *The classification of psychopathology: Neo-Kraepelinian and quantitative approaches.* New York: Plenum Press.

Block, J. (1971). *Lives through time.* Berkeley, CA: Bancroft Books.

Block, J. (1995). A contrarian view of the five-factor approach to personality description. *Psychological Bulletin, 117,* 187–215.

Block, J. (2001). Millennial contrarianism: The five-factor approach to personality description 5 years later. *Journal of Research in Personality, 35,* 98–107.

Bornstein, R. F. (2003). Behaviorally referenced experimentation and symptom validation: A paradigm for 21st-century personality disorder research. *Journal of Personality Disorders, 17,* 1–18.

Breslin, N. A., & Weinberger, D. R. (1990). Schizophrenia and the normal functional development of the prefrontal cortex. *Development and Psychopathology, 2,* 409–424.

Buss, A., & Plomin, R. (1984). *Temperament: Early developing personality traits.* Hillsdale, NJ: Erlbaum.

Carey, G., & Gottesman, I. (1978). Reliability and validity in binary ratings: Areas of common misunderstanding in diagnosis and symptom ratings. *Archives of General Psychiatry, 35,* 1454–1459.

Caspi, A., & Roberts, B. W. (1999). Personality continuity and change across the life course. In L. A. Pervin & O. P. John (Eds.), *Handbook of personality: Theory and research* (2nd ed., pp. 300–326). New York: Guilford Press.

Clark, L. A. (1993). *Manual for the schedule for nonadaptive and adaptive personality (SNAP).* Minneapolis: University of Minnesota Press.

Clark, L. A. (1992). Resolving taxonomic issues in personality disorders: The value of large-scale analyses of symptom data. *Journal of Personality Disorders, 6,* 360–376.

Clarkin, J. F., & Levy, K. F. (in press). The mechanisms of change in the treatment of borderline personality disorder. Special Issue, *Journal of Clinical Psychology.*

Cloninger, C., Svrakic, D., & Przybeck, T. (1993). A psychobiological model of temperament and character. *Archives of General Psychiatry, 50,* 975–990.

Coccaro, E. (1993, Spring). Psychopharmacologic studies in patients with personality disorders: Review and perspective. *Journal of Personality Disorders,* 7(Suppl.), 181–192.

Coccaro, E. (2001). Biological treatments and correlates. In W. J. Livesley (Ed.), *Handbook of personality disorders* (pp.124–135). New York: Guilford Press.

Coccaro, E., Siever, L., Klar, H., Maurer, G., Cochrane, K., Cooper, T., Mohs, R., & Davis, K. (1989). Serotonergic studies in patients with affective and borderline personality disorders: Correlates with suicidal and impulsive aggressive behavior. *Archives of General Psychiatry, 46,* 587–599.

Coccarro, E. F., & Murphy, D. L. (Eds.). (1990). *Serotonin in major psychiatric disorders.* Washington, DC: American Psychiatric Press.

Collins, L., & Horn, J. (Eds.). (1991). *Best methods for the analysis of change: Recent advances, unanswered questions, future directions.* Washington, DC: American Psychological Association.

Collins, L., & Sayer, A. G. (2001). *New methods for the analysis of change.* Washington, DC: American Psychological Association.

Costa, P., & McCrae, R. (1986). Personality stability and its implications for clinical psychology. *Clinical Psychology Review, 6,* 407–423.

Costa, P., & McCrae, R. (1988). Personality in adulthood: A six-year longitudinal study of self-reports and spouse ratings on the NEO personality inventory. *Journal of Personality and Social Psychology, 54,* 853–863.

Costa, P., & McCrae, R. (1990). Personality disorders and the five-factor model of personality. *Journal of Personality Disorders, 4,* 362–371.

Costa, P. T., & Widiger, T. A. (2002). *Personality disorders and the five-factor model of personality* (2nd ed). Washington, DC: American Psychological Association.

Cronbach, L., & Meehl, P. (1955). Construct validity in psychological tests. *Psychological Bulletin, 52,* 281–302.

Davidson, R. J., Pizzagalli, D., Nitschke, J. B., & Putnam, K. (2002). Depression: Perspectives from affective neuroscience. *Annual Review of Psychology, 53,* 545–574.

Depue, R. A., & Collins, P. (1999). Neurobiology of the structure of personality: Dopamine, facilitation of incentive motivation, and extraversion. *Behavioral and Brain Sciences, 22,* 491–569.

Depue, R. A., & Lenzenweger, M. F. (2001). A neurobehavioral dimensional model of personality disorders. In W. J. Livesley (Ed.), *Handbook of personality disorders* (pp. 136–176). New York: Guilford Press.

Digman, J. (1990). Personality structure: Emergence of the five-factor model. *Annual Review of Psychology, 41,* 417–440.

Dilalla, L. F. (2004). *Behavior genetics principles: Perspectives in development, personality, and psychopathology.* Washington, DC: American Psychological Association.

Dohrenwend, B., & Dohrenwend, B. (1982). Perspectives on the past and future of psychiatric epidemiology. *American Journal of Public Health, 72,* 1271–1279.

Drake, R., Adler, D. A., & Vaillant, G. E. (1988). Antecedents of personality disorders in a community sample of men. *Journal of Personality Disorders, 2,* 60–68.

Drake, R., & Vaillant, G. (1985). A validity study of Axis II. *American Journal of Psychiatry, 142,* 553–558.

Drake, R., & Vaillant, G. (1988). Introduction: Longitudinal views of personality disorder. *Journal of Personality Disorders, 2,* 44–48.

Ekman, P., & Davidson, R. J. (1994). *The nature of emotion: Fundamental questions.* New York: Oxford University Press.

Endler, N. S., & Kocovski, N. (2002). Personality disorder at the crossroads. *Journal of Personality Disorders, 16,* 487–502.

Finn, S. (1986). Stability of personality self-ratings over 30 years: Evidence for an age/cohort interaction. *Journal of Personality and Social Psychology*, *50*, 813–818.

First, M. B., Spitzer, R. L., Gibbon, M., & Williams, J. B. W. (1997). *User's guide for the Structured Clinical Interview for DSM-IV Axis II Disorders*. Washington, DC: American Psychiatric Press.

Frances, A. (1980). The DSM-III personality disorders section: A commentary. *American Journal of Psychiatry*, *137*, 1050–1054.

Freud, S. (1959). Character and anal erotism. In J. Strachey (Ed. and Trans.), *The standard edition of the complete psychological works of Sigmund Freud* (vol. 9, pp. 167–175). London: Hogarth Press. (Original work published 1908)

Funder, D. C. (2001). Personality. *Annual Review of Psychology*, *52*, 197–221.

Glueck, S., & Glueck, E. (1968). *Delinquents and non-delinquents in perspective*. Cambridge, MA: Harvard.

Gottesman, I. I., & Gould, T. D. (2003). The endophenotype concept in psychiatry: Etymology and strategic intentions. *American Journal of Psychiatry*, *160*, 636–645.

Grace, A. A. (1991). Phasic versus tonic dopamine release and the modulation of dopamine system responsivity: A hypothesis for the etiology of schizophrenia. *Neuroscience*, *41*, 1–24.

Grayson, D. (1987). Can categorical and dimensional views of psychiatric illness be distinguished? *British Journal of Psychiatry*, *151*, 355–361.

Gunderson, J., & Phillips, K. (1991). A current view of the interface between borderline personality disorder and depression. *American Journal of Psychiatry*, *148*, 967–975.

Gunderson, J. G., Shea, M. T., Skodol, A. E., McGlashan, T. H., Morey, L. C., Stout, R. L., Zanarini, M. C., Grilo, C. M., Oldham, J. M., & Keller, M. B. (2000). The Collaborative Longitudinal Personality Disorders Study: Development, aims, design, and sample characteristics. *Journal of Personality Disorders*, *14*, 300–315.

Haan, N., & Day, D. (1974). A longitudinal study of change and sameness in personality development: Adolescence to early adulthood. *International Journal of Aging and Human Development*, *5*, 11–39.

Harris, G. T., Rice, M. E., & Quinsey, V. L. (1994). Psychopathy as a taxon: Evidence that psychopatho are a discrete class. *Journal of Consulting and Clinical Psychology*, *62*, 387–397.

Haslam, N. (2003). The dimensional view of personality disorders: A review of the taxometric evidence. *Clinical Psychology Review*, *23*, 75–93.

Hathaway, S. R., & McKinley, J. R. (1983). *The Minnesota Multiphasic Personality Inventory manual*. New York: Psychological Corporation. (Original work published 1943)

Helson, R., & Moane, G. (1987). Personality change in women from college to midlife. *Journal of Personality and Social Psychology*, *53*, 176–186.

Hirschfeld, R., M. A., Klerman, G. L., Clayton, P. J., Keller, M. B., MacDonald-Scott, P., & Larkin, B. H. (1983). Assessing personality: Effects of the depressive state on trait measurement. *American Journal of Psychiatry*, *140*, 695–699.

Hogan, R., Johnson, J., & Briggs, S. (Eds). (1997). *Handbook of personality psychology.* San Diego, CA: Academic Press

Jacob, F. (1982). *The logic of life: A history of heredity.* New York: Pantheon Books.

John, O. (1990). The "big five" factor taxonomy: Dimensions of personality in the natural language and in questionnaires. In L. Pervin (Ed.), *Handbook of personality: Theory and research* (pp. 66–100). New York: Guilford Press.

John, O. P., & Srivastava, S. (1999). The big five trait taxonomy: history, measurement, and theoretical perspectives. In L. A. Pervin & O. P. John (Eds.), *Handbook of personality: theory and research* (2nd ed., pp. 102–138). New York: Guilford Press.

Johnson, J. G., Cohen, P., Kasen, S., Skodol, A. E., Hamagami, F. , & Brook, J. S. (2000). Age-related change in personality disorder trait-levels between early adolescence and adulthood: A community-based longitudinal investigation. *Acta Psychiatrica Scandinavica, 102,* 265–275.

Joreskog, K. G. (1979). Statistical estimation of structural equations in longitudinal-developmental investigations. In J. Nesselroade & P. Baltes (Eds.), *Longitudinal research in the study of behavior and development.* New York: Academic Press.

Kagan, J. (1980). Perspectives on continuity. In O. Brim & J. Kagan (Eds.), *Constancy and change in human development.* Cambridge, MA: Harvard.

Kagan, J. (1994). *Galen's prophecy: Temperament in human nature.* New York: Basic Books.

Kessler, R., & Greenberg, D. (1981). *Linear panel analysis: Models of quantitative change.* New York: Academic Press.

Kessler, R., McGonagle, K., Zhao, S., Nelson, C., Hughes, M. Eshleman, S., Wittchen, H-U., & Kendler, K. (1994). Lifetime and 12-month prevalence of DSM-III-R psychiatric disorders in the United States: Results from the National Comorbidity Survey. *Archives of General Psychiatry, 51,* 8–19.

Klein, D., Riso, L., & Anderson, R. (1993). DSM-III-R dysthymia: Antecedents and underlying assumptions. In L. Chapman, J. Chapman, & D. Fowles (Eds.), *Progress in experimental personality and psychopathology research* (Vol. 16, pp. 222–253). New York: Springer.

Klein, D., & Shih, J. H. (1998). Depressive personality: Associations with DSM-III-R mood and personality disorders and negative and positive affectivity, 30-month stability, and prediction of course of Axis I depressive disorders. *Journal of Abnormal Psychology, 107,* 319–327.

Klonsky, E., Oltmanns, T. F., & Turkheimer, E. F. (2003). Informant reports of personality disorder: Relation to self-reports and future research directions. *Clinical Psychology: Science and Practice, 9,* 300–311.

Kohlberg, L., LaCrosse, J., & Ricks, D. (1972). The predictability of adult mental health from childhood behavior. In B. Wolman (Ed.), *Manual of child psychopathology* (pp. 1217–1284). New York: McGraw-Hill.

Korfine, L., & Hooley, J. M. (2000). Directed forgetting of emotional stimuli in borderline personality disorder. *Journal of Abnormal Psychology, 109,* 214–221.

Korfine, L., & Hooley, J. M. (2001). *Detecting individuals with borderline person-*

ality disorder in the community: An ascertainment strategy and comparison with a hospital sample. Unpublished manuscript, Harvard University, Cambridge, MA.

Korfine, L., & Lenzenweger M. F. (1991, December). *The classification of DSM-III-R Axis II personality disorders: A meta-analysis.* Paper presented at the 6th annual meeting of the Society for Research in Psychopathology, Harvard University, Cambridge, MA.

Korfine, L., & Lenzenweger, M. F. (1995). The taxonicity of schizotypy: A replication. *Journal of Abnormal Psychology, 104,* 26–31.

Kraepelin, E. (1907). *Clinical psychiatry.* London: Macmillan.

Krueger, R. F. (1999). The structure of common mental disorders. *Archives of General Psychiatry, 56,* 921–926.

Krueger, R. F., & Tackett, J. L. (2003). Personality and psychopathology: Working toward the bigger picture. *Journal of Personality Disorders, 17,* 109–128.

Lang, K. L., & Vernon, P. A. (2001). Genetics. In W. J. Livesley (Ed.), *Handbook of personality disorders* (pp. 177–195). New York: Guilford Press.

Leary, T. (1957). *Interpersonal diagnosis of personality.* New York: Ronald.

Lenzenweger, M. F. (1999). Stability and change in personality disorder features: The Longitudinal Study of Personality Disorders. *Archives of General Psychiatry, 56,* 1009–1015.

Lenzenweger, M. F. (2004). Consideration of the challenges, complications, and pitfalls of taxometric analysis. *Journal of Abnormal Psychology, 113,* 10–23.

Lenzenweger, M. F., & Dworkin, R. H. (1996). The dimensions of schizophrenia phenomenology? Not one or not two, at least three, perhaps four. *British Journal of Psychiatry, 168,* 432–440.

Lenzenweger, M. F., & Hooley, J. M. (Eds.). (2003). *Principles of experimental psychopathology: Essays in honor of Brendan A. Maher.* Washington, DC: American Psychological Association.

Lenzenweger, M. F., Johnson, M. D., & Willett, J. B. (in press). Individual growth curve analysis illuminates stability and change in personality disorder features: The Longitudinal Study of Personality Disorders. *Archives of General Psychiatry.*

Lenzenweger, M. F., & Korfine, L. (1992). Confirming the latent structure and base rate of schizotypy: A taxometric approach. *Journal of Abnormal Psychology, 101,* 576–571.

Lenzenweger, M. F., Loranger, A. W., Korfine, L., & Neff, C. (1997). Detecting personality disorders in a nonclinical population: Application of a two-stage procedure for case identification. *Archives of General Psychiatry, 54,* 345–351.

Lenzenweger, M. F., & Moldin, S. (1990). Discerning the latent structure of hypothetical psychosis proneness through admixture analysis. *Psychiatry Research, 33,* 243–257.

Lilienfeld, S. O., Wood, J. M., & Garb, H. M. (2000). The scientific status of projective techniques. *Psychological Science in the Public Interest, 1*(2), 27–66.

Livesley, W. J. (2003). Diagnostic dilemmas in classifying personality disorder. In K. A. Phillips & M. B. First (Eds.), *Advancing DSM: Dilemmas in psychiatric diagnosis* (pp. 153–189). Washington, DC: American Psychiatric Association.

Livesley, W. J., Jang, K. L., & Vernon, P. A. (1998). Phenotypic and genetic structure of traits delineating personality disorder. *Archives of General Psychiatry*, 55, 941–948.

Loranger, A. (1988). *The Personality Disorder Examination (PDE) manual.* Yonkers, NY: DV Communications.

Loranger, A. (1990). The impact of DSM-III on diagnostic practice in a university hospital: A comparison of DSM-II and DSM-III in 10,914 patients. *Archives of General Psychiatry*, 47, 672–675.

Loranger, A. (1991a). Diagnosis of personality disorders: General considerations. In R. Michels, A. Cooper, S. Guze, L. Judd, G. Klerman, A. Solnit, & A. Stunkard (Eds.), *Psychiatry* (rev. ed., Vol. 1, pp. 1–14). New York: Lippincott.

Loranger, A. W. (1991b, May). *Comorbidity of borderline personality disorder.* Paper presented at the 144th annual meeting of the American Psychiatric Association, New Orleans, LA.

Loranger, A. W. (1992). Are current self-report and interview measures adequate for epidemiological studies of personality disorders? *Journal of Personality Disorders*, 6, 313–325.

Loranger, A. W. (1999). *The International Personality Disorder Examination (IPDE) DSM-IV and ICD-10 Modules.* Odessa, FL: Psychological Assessment Resources.

Loranger, A. W. (2000). Personality disorders: General considerations. In M. G. Gelder, J. J. Lopez-lbor, & N. Andreasen(Eds.), *The New Oxford textbook of psychiatry* (vol. 1, pp.923–926). New York: Oxford University Press

Loranger, A. W. (2002). *OMNI personality inventory and OMNI-IV personality disorder inventory manual.* Odessa, FL: Psychological Assessment Resources.

Loranger, A. W., & Lenzenweger, M. (1995). *Trait–state artifacts and the diagnosis of personality disorders: A replication.* Unpublished data.

Loranger, A., Lenzenweger, M., Gartner, A., Susman, V., Herzig, J., Zammit, G., Gartner, J., Abrams, R., & Young, R. (1991). Trait–state artifacts and the diagnosis of personality disorders. *Archives of General Psychiatry*, 48, 720–728.

Loranger, A. W., Sartorius, N., Andreoli, A., Berger, P., Buchheim, P., Channabasavanna, S. M., Cold, B., Dahl, A., Diekstra, R. F. W., Ferguson, B., Jacobsberg, L. B., Mombour, W., Pull, C., Ono, Y., & Regier, D. A. (1994). The International Personality Disorder Examination: The World Health Organization/Alcohol, Drug Abuse and Mental Health Administration International Pilot Study of Personality Disorders. *Archives of General Psychiatry*, 51, 215–224.

Matthysse, S. (1993). Genetics and the problem of causality in abnormal psychology. In P. Sutker & H. Adams (Eds.), *Comprehensive handbook of psychopathology* (pp. 178–186). New York: Springer-Verlag.

McCrae, R., & Costa, P. (1984). *Emerging lives, enduring dispositions: Personality in adulthood.* Boston: Little, Brown.

McGue, M., Bacon, S., & Lykken, D. (1993). Personality stability and change in early adulthood: A behavioral genetic analysis. *Developmental Psychology*, 29, 96–109.

McLachlan, G., & Peel, D. (2000). *Finite mixture models.* New York: Wiley.

Meehl, P. E. (1972). Specific genetic etiology, psychodynamics, and therapeutic nihilism. *International Journal of Mental Health*, 1, 10–27.

Meehl, P. E. (1978). Theoretical risks and tabular asterisks: Sir Karl, Sir Ronald, and the slow progress of soft psychology. *Journal of Consulting and Clinical Psychology, 46,* 806–834.

Meehl, P. E. (1990). Toward an integrated theory of schizotaxia, schizotypy, and schizophrenia. *Journal of Personality Disorders, 4,* 1–99.

Meehl, P. E. (1992). Factors and taxa, traits and types, differences of degree and differences in kind. *Journal of Personality, 60,* 117–174.

Meehl, P. E. (1993). Philosophy of science: Help or hindrance? *Psychological Reports, 72,* 707–733.

Meehl, P. E. (1995). Bootstraps taxometrics: Solving the classification problem in psychopathology. *American Psychologist, 50,* 266–275.

Millon, T. (Ed.). (1981). *Disorders of personality: DSM-III Axis II.* New York: Wiley.

Millon, T. (1990). The disorders of personality. In L. A. Pervin (Ed.), *Handbook of personality: Theory and research* (pp. 339–370). New York: Guilford Press.

Millon, T. (1995). *Disorders of personality: DSM-IV and beyond* (2nd ed.). New York: Wiley.

Morey, L. C. (1991). *Personality Assessment Inventory professional manual.* Odessa, FL: Psychological Assessment Resources.

Morey, L. C., Gunderson, J. G., Quigley, B. D., & Lyons, M. (2000). Dimensions and categories: The "big five" factors and the DSM personality disorders. *Assessment, 7*(3), 203–216.

Mortimer, J., Finch, M., & Kumka, D. (1982). Persistence and change in development: The multidimensional self-concept. In P. Baltes & O. Brim (Eds.), *Life-span development and behavior* (Vol. 4, pp. 263–313). New York: Academic Press.

Murray, H. A. (1938). *Explorations in personality.* New York: Wiley.

Nesselroade, J. (1988). Some implications of the trait-state distinction for the study of development over the life-span: The case of personality. In P. Baltes, D. L. Featherman, & R. M. Lerner (Eds.), *Life-span development and behavior* (Vol. 8, pp. 163–189). Hillsdale, NJ: Erlbaum.

Nesselroade, J., & Baltes, P. (1974). Adolescent personality development and historical change: 1970–1972. *Monographs of the Society for Research in Child Development, 39*(1, Whole No. 154).

Nesselroade, J., & Baltes, P. (1979). *Longitudinal research in the study of behavior and development.* New York: Academic Press.

Nesselroade, J., & Baltes, P. (1984). From traditional factor analysis to structural causal modeling in developmental research. In V. Sarris & A. Parducci (Eds.), *Perspectives in psychological experimentation: Toward the year 2000.* Hillsdale, NJ: Erlbaum.

Nesselroade, J., Stigler, S., & Baltes, P. (1980). Regression toward the mean and the study of change. *Psychological Bulletin, 88,* 622–637.

Nigg, J., & Goldsmith, H. (1994). Genetics of personality disorders: Perspectives from psychology and psychopathology research. *Psychological Bulletin, 115,* 346–380.

National Institute of Mental Health. (2002). *Psychotherapeutic interventions: How and why they work.* Rockville, MD: Author. Available from: *www.nimh.nih. gov/research/interventions/cfm*

Oltmanns, T. F., Melley, A. H., & Turkheimer, E. (2002). Impaired social functioning and symptoms of personality disorders assessed by peer and self-report in a nonclinical population. *Journal of Personality Disorders, 16,* 437–452.

Oltmanns, T. F., Turkheimer, E., & Strauss, M. E. (1998). Peer assessment of personality traits and pathology in female college students. *Assessment, 5,* 53–65.

Perry, J. (1993, Spring). Longitudinal studies of personality disorders. *Journal of Personality Disorders, 7* (Suppl.), 63–85.

Pervin, L. A. (1990). A brief history of modern personality theory. In L. A. Pervin (Ed.), *Handbook of personality: Theory and research* (pp. 3–18). New York: Guilford Press.

Pervin, L. A., & John, O. P. (Eds.). (1999). *Handbook of personality: Theory and research* (2nd ed). New York: Guilford Press.

Pfohl, B. (1999). Axis I and Axis II: Comorbidity or confusion? In C.R. Cloninger (Ed.), *Personality and psychopathology* (pp. 83–98). Washington, DC: American Psychiatric Association.

Pfohl, B., Blum, N., & Zimmerman, M. (1997). *Structured interview for DSM-IV personality* (SIDP-IV). Washington, DC: American Psychiatric Press.

Pfohl, B., Coryell, W., Zimmerman, M., & Stangl, D. (1986). DSM-III personality disorders: Diagnostic overlap and internal consistency of individual DSM-III criteria. *Comprehensive Psychiatry, 27,* 21–34.

Pilkonis, P., Heape, C., Ruddy, J., & Serrao, P. (1991). Validity in the diagnosis of personality disorders: The use of the LEAD standard. *Psychological Assessment: A Journal of Consulting and Clinical Psychology, 3,* 46–54.

Plomin, R., & Caspi, A. (1999). Behavioral genetics and personality. In L. Pervin & O. P. John (Eds.), *Handbook of personality: Theory and research* (2nd ed., pp. 251–276). New York: Guilford Press.

Plomin, R., DeFries, J. C., Craig, I. W., & McGuggin, R. (Eds.). (2003). *Behavioral genetics in the postgenomic era.* Washington, DC: American Psychological Association.

Plomin, R., DeFries, J. C., McClearn, G. E., & McGuffin, P. (2000). *Behavioral genetics* (4th ed.). New York: Worth.

Rapaport, D., Gill, M. M., & Schafer, R. *Diagnostic psychological testing* (rev. ed., R. R. Holt, ed.). (1968). New York: International Universities Press.

Reich, W. (1945). *Character-analysis: Principles and technique for psychoanalysts in practice and in training.* New York: Orgone Institute Press.

Reichenbach, H. (1938). *Experience and prediction.* Chicago: University of Chicago Press.

Roberts, B. W., & DelVecchio, W. F. (2000). The rank-order consistency of personality traits from childhood to old age: A quantitative review of longitudinal studies. *Psychological Bulletin, 126,* 3–25.

Robins, L. (1966). *Deviant children grown up.* Baltimore: Williams & Wilkins.

Robins, L. (1978). Sturdy childhood predictors of adult anti-social behavior: Replications from longitudinal studies. *Psychological Medicine, 8,* 611–622.

Rogosa, D. (1979). Causal models in longitudinal research: Rationale, formulation, and interpretation. In J. Nesselroade & P. Baltes (Eds.), *Longitudinal research in the study of behavior and development* (pp. 263–302). New York: Academic Press.

Rogosa, D. (1988). Myths about longitudinal research. In K. Shaie, R. Campbell, W. Meredith, & S. Rawlings (Eds.), *Methodological issues in aging research* (pp. 171–209). New York: Springer.

Rogosa, D., Brandt, D., & Zimowski, M. (1982). A growth curve approach to the measurement of change. *Psychological Bulletin, 90,* 726–748.

Rogosa, D. R., & Willett, J. B. (1985). Understanding correlates of change by modeling individual differences in growth. *Psychometrika, 50,* 203–228.

Rotschild, L., Cleland, C., Haslam, N., & Zimmerman, M. (2003). A taxometric study of borderline personality disorder. *Journal of Abnormal Psychology, 112,* 657–666.

Rowe, D. C. (1994). *The limits of family influence: Genes, experience, and behavior.* New York: Guilford Press.

Rutter, M. (1987). Temperament, personality, and personality disorder. *British Journal of Psychiatry, 150,* 443–458.

Rutter, M. (1991). Nature, nurture, and psychopathology: A new look at an old topic. *Development and Psychopathology, 3,* 125–136.

Rutter, M., & Silberg, J. (2002). Gene–environment interplay in relation to emotional and behavioral disturbance. *Annual Review of Psychology, 53,* 463–490.

Samuels, J. E., Eaton, W. W., Bienvenu, O. J., Brown, C., Costa, P. T., & Nestadt, G. (2002). Prevalence and correlates of personality disorders in a community sample. *British Journal of Psychiatry, 180,* 536–542.

Saulsman, L. M., & Page, A. C. (2004). The five-factor model and personality disorder empirical literature: A meta-analytic review. *Clinical Psychology Review, 23,* 1055–1085.

Schroeder, M. L., Wormworth, J. A., & Livesley, W. J. (1994). Dimensions of personality disorder and the five-factor model of personality. In: P. T. Costa & T. A. Widiger (Eds.), *Personality disorders and the five-factor model of personality* (pp. 117–130). Washington, DC: American Psychological Association.

Schroeder, M. L., Wormworth, J. A., & Livesley, W. J. (2002). Dimensions of personality disorder and the five-factor model of personality. In P. T. Costa & T. A. Widiger (Eds.), *Personality disorders and the five-factor model of personality* (2nd ed., pp. 149–160). Washington, DC: American Psychological Association.

Shea, M. T., Stout, R., Gunderson, J. G., Moery, L. C., Grilo, C. M., McGlashan, T. H., Skodol, A. E., Dolan-Sewell, R., Dyck, I., Zanarini, M. C., & Keller, M. B. (2002). Short-term diagnostic stability of schizotypal, borderline, avoidant, and obsessive–compulsive personality disorders. *American Journal of Psychiatry, 159,* 2036–2041.

Shedler, J., & Westen, D. (in press). Dimensions of personality pathology: An alternative to the Five Factor Model. *American Journal of Psychiatry.*

Shrout, P., & Newman, S. C. (1989). Design of two-phase prevalence studies of rare disorders. *Biometrics, 45,* 549–555.

Siever, L., Kalus, O., & Keefe, R. (1993). The boundaries of schizophrenia. *Psychiatric Clinics of North America, 16,* 217–244.

Singer, J. D., & Willett, J. B. (2003). *Applied longitudinal data analysis: Modeling change and event occurrence.* New York. Oxford University Press.

Spitzer, R. (1983). Psychiatric diagnosis: Are clinicians still necessary? *Comprehensive Psychiatry, 24,* 399–411.

Spitzer, R., Williams, J., & Gibbon, M. (1987). *Structured clinical interview for DSM-III-R personality disorders (SCID-II).* New York: New York State Psychiatric Institute.

Srivastava, S., John, O. P., Gosling, S. D., & Potter, J. (2003). Development of personality in early and middle adulthood: Set like plaster or persistent change? *Journal of Personality and Social Psychology, 84,* 1041–1053.

Tellegen, A. (1985). Structure of mood and personality and their relevance for assessing anxiety, with an emphasis on self-report. In A. Tuma & J. Maser (Eds.), *Anxiety and the anxiety disorders* (pp. 681–706). Hillsdale, NJ: Erlbaum.

Titterington, D. M., Smith, A. F. M., & Makov, U. E. (1985). *Statistical analysis of finite mixture distributions.* New York: Wiley.

Torgersen, S., Kringlen, E., & Cramer, V. (2001). The prevalence of personality disorders in a community sample. *Archives of General Psychiatry, 58,* 590–596.

Trull, T., & Goodwin, A. (1993). Relationship between mood changes and the report of personality disorder symptoms. *Journal of Personality Assessment, 61,* 99–111.

Trull, T., Widiger, T., & Guthrie, P. (1990). Categorical versus dimensional status of borderline personality disorder. *Journal of Abnormal Psychology, 99,* 40–48.

Vaillant, G. E., & Perry, J. C. (1985). Personality disorders. In H. I. Kaplan & B. J. Sadock (Eds.), *Comprehensive textbook of psychiatry/IV* (Vol. 1, 4th ed., pp. 958–986). Baltimore: Williams & Wilkins.

Waller, N. G., & Meehl, P. E. (1998). *Multivariate taxometric procedures: Distinguishing types from continua.* Thousand Oaks, CA: Sage.

Webb, B. (2001). Can robots make good models of biological behavior? *Behavioral and Brain Sciences, 24,* 1033–1050.

Weissman, M. (1993, Spring). The epidemiology of personality disorders: A 1990 update. *Journal of Personality Disorders, 7*(Suppl.), 44–62.

Westen, D. (1996). A model and method for uncovering the nomothetic from the idiographic: An alternative to the five factor model? *Journal of Research in Personality, 30,* 400–41.

Westen, D., & Muderrisoglu, S. (2003). Assessing personality disorders using a systematic clinical interview: Evaluation of an alternate to structured interviews. *Journal of Personality Disorders, 17,* 351–369.

Westen, D., & Shedler, J. (1999). Revising and assessing Axis II, Part I: Developing a clinically and empirically valid assessment method. *American Journal of Psychiatry, 156,* 258–272.

Westen, D., & Shedler, J. (2000). A prototype matching approach to diagnosing personality disorders: Toward DSM-V. *Journal of Personality Disorders, 14,* 109–126.

Widiger, T. (1992). Categorical versus dimensional classification. *Journal of Personality Disorders, 6,* 287–300.

Widiger, T., Frances, A., Harris, M., Jacobsberg, L., Fyer, M., & Manning, D. (1991). Comorbidity among Axis II disorders. In J. Oldham (Ed.), *Personality disorders: New perspectives on diagnostic validity* (pp. 163–194). Washington, DC: American Psychiatric Press.

Widiger, T., & Shea, T. (1991). Differentiation of Axis I and Axis II disorders. *Journal of Abnormal Psychology, 100,* 399–406.

Wiggins, J. (1982). Circumplex models of interpersonal behavior in clinical psychology. In P. Kendall & J. Butcher (Eds.), *Handbook of research methods in clinical psychology* (pp. 183–221). New York: Wiley.

Wiggins. J., & Pincus, A. (1989). Conceptions of personality disorders and dimensions of personality. *Psychological Assessment: A Journal of Consulting and Clinical Psychology, 1,* 305–316.

Wiggins, J. S., & Pincus, A. L. (2002). Personality structure and the structure of personality disorders. In P. T. Costa & T. A. Widiger (Eds.), *Personality disorders and the five-factor model of personality* (2nd ed., pp. 103–124). Washington, DC: American Psychological Association.

Zanarini, M. C., Frankenburg, F. R., Hennen, J., & Silk, K. R. (2003). The longitudinal course of borderline psychopathology: 6-year prospective follow-up of the phenomenology of borderline personality disorder. *American Journal of Psychiatry, 160,* 274–283.

Zimmerman, M. (1994). Diagnosing personality disorders: A review of issues and research methods. *Archives of General Psychiatry, 51,* 225–245.

CHAPTER 2

■ ■ ■

A Cognitive Theory
of Personality Disorders

JAMES L. PRETZER
AARON T. BECK

Clients with personality disorders present particularly complex and demanding problems. Personality disorders are encountered frequently in many clinical settings and often co-occur with Axis I disorders (e.g. Black, Yates, Noyes, Pfohl, & Kelley, 1989; Freidman, Shear, & Frances, 1987; Overholser, 1991; Turner, Bidel, Borden, Stanley, & Jacob, 1991). When this is the case, the presence of an Axis II disorder can have a significant effect on the clinical presentation, development, and course of the Axis I disorder. It has even been suggested that clients with personality disorders may account for a substantial proportion of those individuals for whom psychotherapy proves ineffective or deleterious (Mays & Franks, 1985). Clearly, the development of effective approaches to understanding and treating individuals with personality disorders is of great importance. In recent years, major advances have been made in applying the principles of cognitive therapy[1] with this difficult population.

Cognitive therapy is an active, problem-focused approach to psychotherapy based on contemporary understandings of the role of thought, feeling, and action in psychopathology. This approach may have particular potential for overcoming some of the problems encountered in attempting to understand and treat individuals with personality disorders. First, persons with personality disorders are often difficult to conceptualize clearly. Cognitive therapy provides a conceptual framework that is straightforward and easy to grasp and which can make therapy with complex clients less

43

confusing and frustrating. Second, individuals with personality disorders often present a wide range of symptoms which demand immediate attention. Cognitive therapy provides a coherent framework within which a wide range of interventions can be used flexibly and strategically. These interventions include specialized cognitive-behavioral techniques which provide powerful tools for both alleviating current distress and accomplishing the lasting changes needed to head off future difficulties. Finally, many approaches to psychotherapy have only a limited empirical base. Cognitive therapy is supported by a large body of empirical research on both the validity of the theory and the effectiveness of the treatment. While research into cognitive therapy with personality disorders is in its initial stages, there are preliminary indications that it will prove to be an effective treatment for these complex disorders.

Despite these arguments in favor of cognitive therapy as an approach to understanding and treating personality disorders, there is evidence that cognitive-behavioral treatment frequently proves ineffective or counterproductive for individuals with Axis II diagnoses if the treatment approach is not modified to account for the presence of a personality disorder (Fleming & Pretzer, 1990; Pretzer & Fleming, 1990). For example, Turner (1987) found that social phobics without concurrent Axis II diagnoses improved markedly during a 15-week time-limited cognitive-behavioral treatment for social phobia whereas patients who had concomitant Axis II diagnoses failed to respond to this treatment regimen. Similarly, Persons, Burns, and Perloff (1988) found that premature termination of "standard" cognitive therapy and the consequent ineffectiveness of therapy were more likely when depressed patients had concurrent personality disorders.

Personality disorders are among the most difficult and least understood problems faced by therapists regardless of the therapist's orientation. The treatment of clients with these disorders can be just as complex and frustrating for cognitive therapists as it is for other therapists. For example:

> Gary, a young radiologist, contacted a therapist (the first author) seeking treatment for persistent anxiety which aggravated a long-standing problem with irritable bowel syndrome. Initially, the case seemed fairly straightforward and initial interventions directed toward helping him to learn more effective ways of coping with stress and to learn to control his excessive worries proved effective. However, after six sessions of apparently successful treatment, Gary reported that the relaxation techniques which had been quite effective up to that point had now "quit working" and he seemed increasingly unwilling to relax his vigilance and worry. As treatment progressed, his therapist discovered that Gary had a persistent belief that others were hostile and malicious, that he had recurrent encounters with his family of origin and with coworkers which seemed to confirm this negative view of others,

and that he was enmeshed in a complex dysfunctional relationship with his alcoholic girlfriend. It turned out that in addition to the generalized anxiety disorder which initially brought him to treatment, Gary met DSM-IV-R criteria for dysthymic disorder and paranoid personality disorder as well.

"Standard" interventions were proving ineffective with Gary, as they do with many individuals with personality disorders. Is it necessary to abandon cognitive therapy and switch to some other type of therapy? Are major revisions of cognitive therapy called for? Or is it simply a matter of taking Gary's personality disorder into account in planning therapeutic interventions?

For cognitive therapy to live up to its promise as an approach to understanding and treating personality disorders, it is necessary to tailor the approach to the characteristics of individuals with personality disorders rather than simply using "standard" cognitive therapy without modification. Actually, it is not surprising that Gary's treatment reached an impasse because the interventions which were being used were based on a very incomplete understanding of Gary's problems. His paranoia had not been apparent before this impasse in treatment and the treatment plan the therapist had in mind did not take it into account at all. To intervene effectively, Gary's therapist needed to develop a treatment plan based on a clear conceptualization which encompassed Gary's problems with both anxiety and his personality disorder. However, this presents a problem: How is one to understand personality disorders in cognitive-behavioral terms?

PHILOSOPHICAL FOUNDATIONS OF COGNITIVE THERAPY

Cognitive therapy's basic philosophical orientation is phenomenological. It assumes that the individual's perception and interpretation of situations shapes his or her emotional and behavioral responses to the situation. This is hardly a radical view. Thinkers from Buddha and the ancient Stoic philosophers up to the present have emphasized the idea that humans react to their interpretation of events, not to the actual events themselves, and have argued that misperceptions and misinterpretations of events result in much unnecessary distress.

Cognitive therapy is based on the proposition that much psychopathology is the result of systematic errors, biases, and distortions in perceiving and interpreting events. These cognitive factors are seen as resulting in dysfunctional responses to events which, in turn, may have consequences that serve to perpetuate the dysfunctional cognitions. Theoretically, the focus is strongly on the interaction between the individual and his or her environment rather than emphasizing either individual or situational factors in isolation (for a detailed example, see Pretzer, Beck, & Newman, 1990). Individuals' interpretations of events are seen as playing a central role in many forms of psychopathology, and these interpretations are seen as being the product of the interaction between the characteristics of the individual and the nature of the events the individual encounters. However, in discussing treatment, much more emphasis is placed on individual factors (such as dysfunctional beliefs) than on situational factors (such as negative life events) because therapist and client are more able to modify individual factors than situational ones.

Some phenomenological approaches are highly subjective in orientation and assume that objective reality is unknowable. Cognitive therapy, however, has a strongly empirical orientation. Given our assumption that individuals' perceptions are subject to errors, biases, and distortions which can lead to misperceptions, misunderstandings, and dysfunctional responses, we also assume that we need to be aware of the potential for errors, biases, and distortions in our own thinking as therapists. Thus we need to make efforts to both minimize biases and distortions in our observations and to test the validity of our conclusions rather than assuming that clinical observation and logical analysis will lead us to "the truth."

Cognitive therapy has a strong tradition of empirical research, but our empirical orientation goes far beyond conducting outcome research, testing hypotheses based on cognitive models of specific forms of psychopathology, or making use of the available empirical research in developing cognitive conceptualizations of various disorders. The idea of "collaborative empiricism" is central to the practice of cognitive therapy. In the course of therapy, the cognitive therapist works with his or her client to collect detailed information regarding the specific thoughts, feelings, and actions that occur in problem situations. These observations are used as a basis for developing an individualized understanding of the client which provides a basis for strategic intervention. Collaborative empiricism continues to play an important role as the focus of therapy shifts from assessment to intervention. Many of the specific techniques used to modify dysfunctional thoughts, beliefs, and strategies emphasize using firsthand observation and "behavioral experiments" to test the validity of dysfunctional automatic thoughts or dysfunctional beliefs and to develop more adaptive alternatives. Rather than relying on the therapist's expertise, theoretical deductions, or logic, cognitive therapy assumes that empirical observation is the most reliable means for developing valid conceptualizations and effective interventions.

This emphasis on an empirical approach does not mean that we emphasize objective reality over subjective experience but that we try to develop accurate understandings of both. Cognitive theory asserts that it is the subjective experience of events which shapes the individual's emotional and behavioral responses, but it also asserts that the individual's emotional and behavioral responses are likely to prove to be dysfunctional when there is a substantial discrepancy between subjective experience and objective reality. For the cognitive therapist to intervene effectively, he or she must endeavor both to understand the individual's subjective experience and to perceive objective reality accurately. In attempting to do this, it is often necessary to rely on client self-reports because some of the factors of interest to cognitive therapists, such as automatic thoughts and dysfunctional beliefs, are not directly observable and because it is often impractical for the therapist to do extensive *in vivo* observation. We recognize that self-reports may be an imperfect source of data as they are open to a wide range of potential biases and distortions. However, they are often the most practical source of information regarding the client's day-to-day experiences[2].

In considering the role of cognition in psychopathology, cognitive therapy uses the term "cognition" broadly to refer to much more than verbal thought of which the individual is self-consciously aware. "Cognition" is treated as synonymous with information processing and no *a priori* assumption is made that all important aspects of cognition are verbally mediated, are easily accessible to the individual's awareness, or are subject to the individual's volitional control. In fact, much cognition occurs outside awareness simply because the individual is not paying attention to it. Many of the processes involved are automatic and occur without a need for awareness or volitional control. Cognition is not necessarily verbally mediated. It can also be mediated by mental imagery or can involve more abstract modes of information processing.

In discussing cognition and other aspects of individual functioning, cognitive investigators have tried to avoid the tendency to generate specialized technical terms and instead have relied heavily on "natural language" along with terms borrowed from cognitive psychology. The advantages of using a straightforward, easily understood vocabulary greatly outweigh the supposed advantages of a more precise technical vocabulary.

Above all, cognitive therapy is a practical approach which has emphasized effective treatment rather than abstract theory. We emphasize basing interventions on an individualized conceptualization of the client's problems not because of any inherent commitment to theory but because strategic interventions based on a clear conceptualization are more efficient and more effective. Similarly, cognitive therapy's emphasis on the "here-and-now" is a matter of practicality rather than philosophy. We find that time spent investigating the factors that perpetuate the psychopathology in the present is usually more productive than time spent investigating the individual's past. This does not mean that cognitive therapists ignore the individual's past. In fact, it can be quite valuable for therapist and client to revisit previous traumatic experiences at times (e.g., see Bedrosian & Bozicas, 1994; J. Beck, 1995; Padesky, 1994). Cognitive therapists, however, attempt to focus on the past only to the extent that this contributes to understanding and/or modifying the factors that perpetuate the disorder in the present.

To return to the question of how to develop a cognitive conceptualization of a person such as Gary, the young radiologist discussed earlier, cognitive therapy's orientation is toward attempting to develop an accurate understanding of both Gary's subjective experience of events and the objective reality he faces. To minimize the problems that can arise from the therapist's own misperceptions and misunderstandings, an attempt will be made to make use of knowledge acquired through empirical research and direct observation insofar as possible; however, due to practical constraints it will be necessary to rely heavily on Gary's reports both of the situations he encounters and of his cognitive, emotional, and behavioral responses to them. The focus in therapy will be primarily on the here-and-now, on the interaction between Gary and the situations in which he finds himself, and on identifying the factors or processes that perpetuate Gary's problems. It is anticipated that when Gary's perception of a situation differs substantially from the reality of the situation, his responses are likely to prove dysfunctional. However, this general philosophical orientation does not provide a detailed enough conceptual framework to permit us to develop a clear understanding of Gary's problems or to develop a promising approach to intervention. A more detailed theoretical framework is needed.

THEORETICAL FOUNDATIONS OF COGNITIVE THERAPY

Precursors

The evolution of cognitive therapy has been influenced by a wide range of theorists and clinicians and it can be argued that cognitive therapy is a highly integrative approach (Alford & Norcross,1991; Beck, 1991). The three primary theoretical influences on cognitive therapy have been the phenomenological approach to psychology, psychodynamic depth psychology, and cognitive psychology. The clinical practice of cognitive therapy has been strongly influenced by client-centered therapy and by contemporary behavioral and cognitive-behavioral approaches to therapy. Among the influences Beck considers to have been most important are phenomenological perspectives dating back to the Greek Stoic philosophers and presented more recently by Adler, Rank, and Horney; the structural theory and depth psychology of Kant and Freud; the cognitive perspectives of George Kelley, Magda Arnold, and Richard Lazarus; the emphasis on a specific, here-and-now approach to problems taken by Austen Riggs and Albert Ellis; Rogers's client centered therapy; the idea of preconscious cognition from writers such as Leon Saul; and the work of cognitive-behavioral investigators including Albert Bandura, Marvin Goldfried, Michael Mahoney, Donald Meichenbaum, and G. Terrence Wilson (Weishaar, 1993).

The Development of Cognitive Therapy

Aaron Beck's initial training and therapeutic orientation were psychodynamic. He accepted the psychodynamic view of the day that depression, anxiety disorders, and other disorders were only the surface manifestation of an underlying personality defect or disorder. Cognitive therapy developed out of his attempts to substantiate Freud's theory that the core of depression was "anger turned on the self." Beck initially set out to examine the thoughts and dreams of depressed individuals expecting to discover indications of hostility turned inward and thus provide empirical support for psychoanalytic theory. However, he consistently noted themes of defeat, deprivation, and despair rather than the hostility turned inward which Freud postulated. Further empirical research and clinical observation led him to the realization that an understanding of the content of depressed individuals' appraisals of the situations and events they encountered did much to explain their mood and behavior and revealed a consistent negative bias in information processing. Beck initially developed a cognitive model of emotional disorders to explain the biases and distortions in information processing which he observed in depressed individuals.

This cognitive understanding of psychopathology led naturally to attempts to modify the cognitive processes that appeared to play a major role in psychopathology. It was soon discovered that when the therapist engaged in an active dialogue with depressed clients and focused on the clients' thoughts and beliefs, it was possible to help them to consciously correct the biases and distortions in their information processing and consequently to alleviate their depression. Albert Ellis's (1962) initial work on rational-emotive therapy was concurrent with Beck's research and shared a focus on the client's thoughts and beliefs and an active, problem-focused approach to therapy. Despite important conceptual and stylistic differences, the two approaches have developed concurrently and have influenced each other in many ways.

The "cognitive revolution" in behavior therapy occurred at the same time as cognitive therapy was evolving and had important influences on both the theory and the clinical practice of cognitive therapy. Bandura's social learning theory (Bandura, 1977) emphasized the interaction between the individual and the environment, modeling, vicarious learning, and concepts of expectancy of reinforcement and self- and outcome-efficacies. Similarly, Mahoney's (1974) emphasis on the cognitive mediation of human learning was an important theoretical influence. Behavior therapy also had important influences on cognitive therapy's developing approach to clinical intervention with its emphasis on detailed, objective clinical observation, its problem-focused approach to intervention, its emphasis on empirical evaluation of interventions, and its wide range of specific intervention techniques.

The investigators who have collaborated with Beck in the development of cognitive therapy have come from a variety of backgrounds but have not clung to their preconceptions or theoretical assumptions. The emphasis within cognitive therapy has been on treating theoretical concepts, whatever their origin, as hypotheses to be tested empirically and clinically with the goal of developing a coherent, empirically validated understanding of psychopathology and an effective approach to psychotherapeutic intervention. The result has been a truly integrative approach (Alford & Beck, 1997; Alford & Norcross, 1991; Beck, 1991) which emphasizes the importance of understanding individuals' subjective experience, of accurately observing the objective situation and the individual's response to it, and of addressing the discrepancies between subjective experience and objective reality. While the individual's cognitive processes have been an important focus of cognitive therapy, affect and interpersonal behavior have always played an important role as well and they have received increasing attention in recent years.

COGNITION AND PSYCHOPATHOLOGY

Core Assumptions

The cognitive view of psychopathology is essentially an information-processing model. It assumes that to function in the wide range of life situations which they encounter, humans are constantly perceiving, recalling, interpreting, and storing data from the environment and that these continuous, automatic processes elicit the individual's cognitive, emotional, and behavioral responses to events. It also assumes that biases, distortions, or defects in perception and interpretation of experiences can result in maladaptive responses and that persistent, systematic errors in information processing play an important role in many forms of psychopathology. Thus an individual who accurately perceives a particular situation as benign is likely to respond adaptively. In contrast, an individual who erroneously perceives a single benign situation as dangerous will experience a "false alarm" and will respond as though the situation is dangerous. This reaction, by itself, is not likely to result in a significant problem; however, the individual who consistently misperceives benign situations as dangerous is likely to manifest problematic levels of anxiety and avoidance behavior.

This view might seem to presume that individuals normally respond to events in a logical, rational, computer-like manner and that psychopathology is the result of irrational or illogical responses, but this is not our assumption at all. We argue that much information processing occurs automatically and outside awareness. Furthermore, the processes involved are not necessarily logical, rational, or veridical. The processes through which humans interact with their environment evolved to serve the basic requirements of the organism in an environment that was substantially different from the environments in which humans find themselves today. Some biases in information processing may have had important advantages for the organism. For example, an optimistic bias in mate selection may have promoted bonding and reproductive success while a tendency to exaggerate the degree of danger presented by risk situations may have maximized the likelihood of avoiding real danger and have promoted survival (Beck, 1992). On the one hand, humans may have biases in information processing which prove to be more adaptive than purely objective information processing would be. On the other hand, as human social change has outstripped physiological evolution, we may well have also retained some biases in information processing which now tend to be maladaptive.

The cognitive view of human functioning (Figure 2.1) emphasizes three aspects of cognition. First, an individual's "automatic thoughts," his or her immediate, spontaneous appraisal of the situation, are seen as playing a central role in eliciting and shaping an individual's emotional and behavioral response to a situation. For example, when Gary (the young radiologist described earlier) and his therapist examined one of the situations in which the progressive relaxation exercises "didn't work," Gary reported remembering[3] that his immediate reaction as a colleague approached was, "He'll catch up with me and see what I'm doing. I don't want him stealing my idea." Given that he perceived the situation as one in which he needed to be vigilant in order to prevent a rival at work from "stealing" his ideas, it is not surprising that he was unable to relax. Unfortunately for Gary, he was prone to conclude that he had to be vigilant and on guard in a wide range of situations in which vigilance was actually unnecessary and in which the resulting tension and anxiety was seriously maladaptive.

How could an intelligent, perceptive person like Gary consistently misperceive mundane situations? Certainly one possibility is that the type of evolutionarily based biases in information processing discussed previously could contribute to a tendency to misperceive certain types of situations. However, our view is that many misperceptions and misinterpreta-

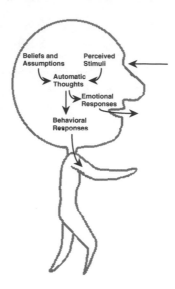

FIGURE 2.1. The basic cognitive model.

tions result from the effects of schemas, cognitive structures containing the individual's basic beliefs and assumptions, which shape the individuals' perceptions of events and their responses to them. Humans do not "start from scratch" in perceiving and interpreting each event or situation they encounter. For example, when an individual encounters a large quadruped covered with shaggy hair, he or she can easily classify it as a dog and interpret its wagging tail as indicative of benign intentions even if he or she has not previously encountered a Briard (a French breed of sheep dog) and has never seen a dog that looks quite like this one. This is because the individual has retained a set of related concepts regarding the characteristics which characterize dogs, important aspects of canine behavior, and human–canine interaction. These concepts are automatically used in interpreting a relevant stimulus. This set of related concepts, termed a "schema," is based on the individual's previous experience with dogs, his or her observations of other persons' experience with dogs, verbal and non-verbal communications from others regarding dogs, and so on.

A given individual will have an assortment of schemas which are relevant to hairy quadrupeds, but these are not simply applied randomly in perceiving our Briard. The context automatically influences the selection of schemas so that those that seem most likely to be relevant to the situation are tried first and a series of schemas are tried until a "good fit" is achieved. Thus, if the Briard is encountered at a dog show, the individual's "dog schema" is likely to be applied first and the Briard is likely to be perceived correctly at once. If the Briard is encountered in a cage at the zoo, more exotic schemas are likely to be applied first and it is likely to take longer for the individual to correctly perceive it as a dog. If the Briard is encountered among a collection of rare breeds of sheep and goats, its size, shaggy coat, and so on may well result in its being misperceived as an unusual type of goat until it emits some behavior, such as barking, which is incompatible with the individual's "goat schema." As soon as the animal is correctly identified as an unfamiliar breed of dog, the individual automatically uses an assortment of generalizations about canine behavior to interpret the dog's current behavior and to anticipate what the dog is likely to do in the future.

Normally, schemas greatly facilitate our responses to the situations we encounter. Life would be impossibly cumbersome if we had to start *de novo* in interpreting each organism and object we encountered. However, they can also play an important role in maladaptive responses to stimuli. For example, an individual with a dog phobia is likely to have a schema regarding dogs which differs from the average individual's "dog schema" by emphasizing potentially dangerous aspects of dogs and canine behavior. As a result, the dog phobic correctly identifies the Briard as a dog but is likely to automatically classify it as dangerous and to respond with a range of physiological reactions, a subjective surge of anxiety, and an abrupt departure.

Gary, had operated on a long-standing conviction that other persons were malicious, deceptive, and hostile and would take advantage of him or attack him if given a chance (see Figure 2.2). These assumptions had important effects on the way in which Gary interpreted experiences. First, because he anticipated that others would be malicious and deceptive, he was alert for signs of deceit, deception, and malicious intentions. This selective attention resulted in his being quick to recognize those occasions when others were being dishonest or untrustworthy. In addition, many interpersonal interactions are ambiguous enough to be open to a variety of interpretations. Given his hypervigilance, Gary was quick to respond to ambiguous situations on the assumption that others had malicious intentions without pausing to consider other possibilities. Thus, his world view resulted in his being vigilant for signs of maliciousness and deception in a way that tended to result in his perceiving many of his experiences in a way which was congruent with his world view. Furthermore, when he did have an experience of someone's proving trustworthy or benevolent, his assumption that others are deceptive led to his concluding that the other person was trying to "set him up" rather than his concluding that the person was genuinely being trustworthy. In short, Gary's vigilance for experiences which appeared to confirm his preconceptions and his tendency to discount

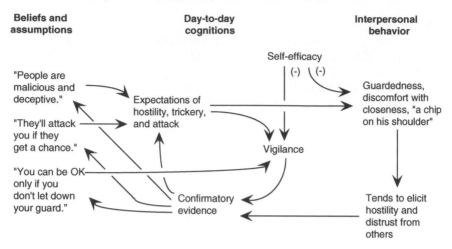

FIGURE 2.2. Cognitive conceptualization of paranoid personality disorder.

experiences which appeared to be inconsistent with his world view tended to confirm and perpetuate his assumptions about others.

In addition to their beliefs and assumptions about "the way things are," individuals also hold beliefs and assumptions about what one should do about this which can be termed "interpersonal strategies." For example, in addition to his assuming that others were malicious and deceptive, Gary believed that the way to be safe was to be vigilant, on guard, and quick to react to any offense. This reaction had a major impact on his interpersonal relationships. He tended to be quite guarded and defensive in interpersonal interactions, to avoid closeness, and to react quickly and strongly to any perceived mistreatment. He also assumed that assertion would prove ineffective or counterproductive, so instead of speaking up for himself when he felt mistreated, he often overreacted dramatically.

A third aspect of cognition which can contribute to persistent misperceptions of situations are systematic errors in reasoning, termed "cognitive distortions." Humans are prone to a variety of errors in logic which can contribute to misinterpretations of events and which can amplify the impact of schemas (see Table 2.1). Gary viewed trustworthiness in a dichotomous manner (see "dichotomous thinking" in Table 2.1). As he saw it, one is either trustworthy or untrustworthy, with no gradation in between. As he approached interpersonal interactions he was vigilant for signs of deceit, deception, or malicious intentions, and once he observed any indication that the individual was not perfectly trustworthy, Gary automatically classified the other person as untrustworthy. Because of

TABLE 2.1. Common Cognitive Distortions

Dichotomous thinking. Viewing experiences in terms of two mutually exclusive categories with no "shades of gray" in between. For example, believing that one is *either* a success *or* a failure and that anything short of a perfect performance is a total failure.

Overgeneralization. Perceiving a particular event as being characteristic of life in general rather than as being one event among many. For example, concluding that an inconsiderate response from one's spouse shows that she doesn't care despite her having showed consideration on other occasions.

Selective abstraction. Focusing on one aspect of a complex situation to the exclusion of other relevant aspects of the situation. For example, focusing on the one negative comment in a performance evaluation received at work and overlooking the positive comments contained in the evaluation.

Disqualifying the positive. Discounting positive experiences which would conflict with the individual's negative views. For example, rejecting positive feedback from friends and colleagues on the grounds that "they're only saying that to be nice" rather than considering whether the feedback could be valid.

Mind reading. Assuming that one knows what others are thinking or how others are reacting despite having little or no evidence. For example, thinking "I just know he thought I was an idiot!" despite the other person's having given no apparent indications of his reactions.

Fortune telling. Reacting as though expectations about future events are established facts rather than recognizing them as fears, hopes, or predictions. For example, thinking "He's leaving me, I just know it!" and acting as though this is definitely true.

Catastrophizing. Treating actual or anticipated negative events as intolerable catastrophes rather than seeing them in perspective. For example, thinking "Oh my God, what if I faint!" without considering that while fainting may be unpleasant or embarrassing, it is not terribly dangerous.

Maximization/minimization. Treating some aspects of the situation, personal characteristics, or experiences as trivial and others as very important independent of their actual significance. For example, thinking "Sure, I'm good at my job, but so what, my parents don't respect me."

Emotional reasoning. Assuming that one's emotional reactions necessarily reflect the true situation. For example, concluding that since one feels hopeless, the situation must really be hopeless.

"Should" statements. The use of "should" and "have to" statements which are not actually true to provide motivation or control over one's behavior. For example, thinking "I shouldn't feel aggravated. She's my mother, I have to listen to her."

Labeling. Attaching a global label to oneself rather than referring to specific events or actions. For example, thinking "I'm a failure!" rather than "Boy, I blew that one!"

Personalization. Assuming that one is the cause of a particular external event when, in fact, other factors are responsible. For example, thinking "She wasn't very friendly today, she must be mad at me." without considering that factors other than one's own behavior may be affect the other individual's mood.

Gary's dichotomous view, intermediate categories such as "not very trust-worthy" or "usually reliable" were not considered. Individuals were seen as trustworthy only if they had proven to be completely trustworthy and were considered to be untrustworthy as soon as a single apparent lapse in trust-worthiness was observed. This, of course, contributed to Gary's view that people in general were untrustworthy as very few of the people he knew managed to prove perfectly trustworthy for long.

Ideally, an individual perceives situations accurately, interprets them correctly, and consequently manifests cognitive, emotional, and behavioral responses which are appropriate to the situation and which prove to be adaptive. According to the cognitive model, on those occasions when the individual's perception of the situation is biased or on which the perceived situation is interpreted incorrectly, the cognitive, emotional, and/or behav-ioral responses will be inappropriate to the situation or maladaptive to some extent. However, in most situations the individual's perception and interpretation of subsequent events should provide feedback that reveals the extent to which the responses were inaccurate or maladaptive. Once this feedback is perceived and interpreted, it not only corrects the specific misperceptions and misinterpretations which occurred but also is stored in memory to aid in accurately perceiving and interpreting future events.

Thus, the cognitive view is that given the complexity of daily life and the ambiguity of many interpersonal interactions, occasional mispercep-tions and misinterpretations of events are inevitable. However, isolated misperceptions and misinterpretations give rise to isolated maladaptive responses which are easily corrected by subsequent experiences. For seri-ously maladaptive responses to develop, a systematic bias in perception, recall, or interpretation would be required. This would result in more per-sistent maladaptive responses than would result from "normal" mis-perceptions and misinterpretations. If it also distorted the feedback process either by strongly biasing the interpretation of events or by influencing the responses of others, it could result in very persistent maladaptive responses.

Because the individual's schemas, beliefs, and assumptions have a major impact on the perception, recall, and interpretation of events, they are one possible source of such a systematic bias. However, they are not the only possible source of a systematic bias in the perception, recall, and inter-pretation of events. Despite cognitive therapy's name, the model in not exclusively cognitive. Rather, the cognitive model focuses on the interplay between cognition, affect, and behavior in psychopathology (see Figure 2.3). The effect of Gary's beliefs and assumptions on his perception of events and on his interpersonal behavior was discussed previously, but the cycle does not end with the effects of cognition on behavior. A person's interpersonal behavior influences the responses of others and their re-sponses can, in turn, result in experiences that can influence the first indi-

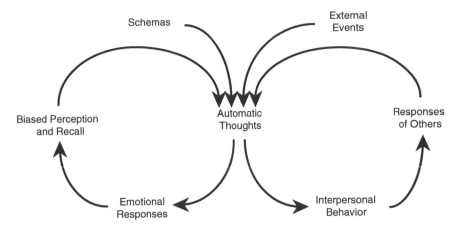

FIGURE 2.3. The role of cognition in psychopathology.

vidual's beliefs and assumptions. For example, Gary's guardedness, defensiveness, and reluctance to be assertive did not endear him to others. Instead, his interpersonal behavior seemed to provoke hostility and bad treatment from others and these responses from others provided additional experiences which seemed to confirm his negative world view.

Also, while the cognitive model assumes that the individual's interpretation of events shapes his or her emotional response to the situation, we also argue that the individual's emotional state has important effects on cognition. A large body of research has demonstrated that affect tends to influence both cognition and behavior in mood-congruent ways (Isen, 1984). A number of studies have demonstrated that even a mild, experimentally induced depressed mood biases perception and recall in a depression-congruent way (see Watkins, Mathews, Williamson, & Fuller, 1992). This means that a depressed mood increases the likelihood that the individual will focus on negative aspects of the situation and preferentially recall negative experiences which occurred in the past. While this phenomenon has not been investigated extensively for most other moods, it appears that many moods tend to bias perception and recall in a mood-congruent way. Thus, as an individual's level of anxiety increases, attentional processes appear to be biased in favor of signs of threat (Watkins et al., 1992). This phenomenon lays the foundation for a potentially self-perpetuating cycle where the individual's automatic thoughts elicit a particular mood, the mood biases perception and recall in a mood-congruent way, which increases the likelihood of additional mood-eliciting automatic thoughts, which elicit more of the mood in question, which further biases perception and recall, and so on, until something happens to disrupt the cycle.

For example, Gary's assumptions led him to interpret mundane interpersonal interactions as presenting a risk of malicious treatment and to interpret unremarkable interpersonal interactions as thinly disguised abuse. As a result, he experienced recurrent feelings of anxiety and resentment. On those occasions when he happened to be feeling relatively calm and peaceful, Gary showed only mild vigilance for interpersonal threats and only mild hypersensitivity to mistreatment. However, as soon as some event or spontaneous thought elicited feelings of anxiety and resentment, his vigilance for interpersonal danger and his sensitivity to mistreatment immediately increased substantially. This increased the likelihood of his interpreting subsequent events in a way which that elicit additional anxiety and resentment and thus his moods tended to "snowball" quite quickly. Once Gary's anxiety and resentment built to clinical levels, they tended to be persistent.

Affect can play an important role in an individual's functioning in another way as well. As Taylor and Rachman (1991, 1992) have noted, individuals may fear certain emotions and may strive to avoid the emotion itself; may seek to escape from experiencing the emotion as quickly as possible; or may attempt to avoid thoughts, memories, or situations they expect to elicit the emotion. Gary was unwilling to tolerate a number of emotions he perceived as "weak," including feelings of sadness, loneliness, and vulnerability. Consequently he avoided situations he perceived as likely to elicit these feelings, was quick to intentionally focus his attention on perceived mistreatment by others in order to feel angry rather than sad, and refused to acknowledge or express these "weak" feelings. This further complicated commonplace interpersonal situations such as coping with periods of estrangement from his girlfriend.

It is important to notice that the cognitive model does *not* assert that cognition causes psychopathology. We view cognition as an important part of the cycle through which humans perceive and respond to events and thus as having an important role in pathological responses to events. However, we view it as a part of a cycle and as a promising point for intervention, not as the cause.

Cognitive Therapy and the Personality Disorders

Beck's initial training was predominantly psychoanalytic, and he believed, in line with the psychodynamic view of the day, that depression, phobias, and other problems which we would now classify as Axis I disorders were only the surface manifestation of underlying personality problems. This view held that the hypothesized personality problems were the "cause" of depression, anxiety, and so on and that, therefore, if the personality problems were cured, the neurosis would be cured as well. However, when

Beck's early research into the psychoanalytic theory of depression produced results that were not compatible with the psychoanalytic views of that day, he began to reevaluate these assumptions. As cognitive therapy of depression evolved, Beck's thinking was influenced by the behavior therapy movement, and he accepted the view that the behavioral (and cognitive and emotional) manifestations of depression *were* the problem and that there was no deeper underlying cause that had to be treated. This formulation fit well with clinical experience and empirical research into cognitive therapy of depression which was available at that time. For example, when patients recovered from depression, their problematic "personality" characteristics such as overdependency, demandingness, and negativism often were no longer apparent. Apparently, curing the "symptoms" made the supposed personality defects go away.

At the same time that cognitive therapy was evolving, behavior therapy first incorporated cognitive perspectives and then began to consider personality disorders. Behaviorists had traditionally rejected the idea that personality traits could be important determinants of behavior and emphasized the situational determinants of behavior. Behavior therapy's rejection of the concept of personality was based in part on the assumption that only variables that can be observed directly can be studied scientifically and in part on a large body of research which appeared to demonstrate that personality variables accounted for little of the variance in human behavior while situational variables accounted for a much larger portion of the variance. Because the term "personality disorder" was regarded as implying that individuals with Axis II diagnoses suffered from a disordered personality, behaviorists' initial reaction was to reject the concept of personality disorder. However, as it became clear that individuals diagnosed as having personality disorders were relatively common in clinical practice and were as difficult for behaviorists to treat as they were for other clinicians, behaviorists began to reconsider these individuals.

Over the interval during which most behaviorally oriented authors had ignored personality disorders, much had changed. First, many behaviorists had accepted the idea of considering cognition and emotion as important aspects of human behavior even though they are not directly observable. Second, more sophisticated research into personality had shown that personality variables can account for a substantial amount of variance in behavior under at least some conditions (Epstein, 1979). Finally, DSM-III redefined personality disorders as "enduring patterns of perceiving, relating to, and thinking about the environment and oneself" which "are exhibited in a wide range of important social and personal contexts" and which "are inflexible and maladaptive and cause either significant functional impairment or subjective distress" (American Psychiatric Association, 1987, p. 335). Some behaviorists began to realize that, given this definition of "personality disorder," one need not presume that such patterns of cognition and behavior are the product of a disordered personality (Turner & Hersen, 1981).

Since the early 1980s behaviorists have seriously considered the topic of personality disorders, and behavioral perspectives on the personality disorders have evolved from simply treating personality disorders as a collection of isolated symptoms which could each be treated separately (Stephens & Parks, 1981) to viewing them as disorders of interpersonal behavior (Turner & Hersen, 1981), then to seeing them as the product of dysfunctional schemas (Beck, 1964, 1967; Young, 1990), and most recently to conceptualizing personality disorders in terms of self-perpetuating cognitive–interpersonal cycles (Beck, Freeman, Davis, & Associates, 2003).

Cognitive therapy itself evolved along with a range of other cognitive-behavioral approaches. It was developed initially as a short-term treatment for depression, and after an extensive focus on understanding and treating depression, it was applied to a wider range of psychopathology. It was not until the early 1980s that the first systematic efforts to apply the cognitive approach with personality disorders began (Fleming, 1983; Pretzer, 1983; Simon, 1983; Young, 1983). In the two decades since then, a clinically based approach has been used by cognitive investigators in developing detailed conceptualizations and treatment strategies for each of the personality disorders (Beck, Freeman, & Associates, 1990; Fleming, 1983, 1985, 1988; Freeman et al., 1990; Pretzer, 1983, 1985, 1988; Simon, 1983, 1985). These authors began with a detailed evaluation of specific clients, developed individualized conceptualization of the client's problems, and generated treatment plans based on the conceptualizations. The conceptualizations were then tested through clinical observation and through noting the results of therapeutic interventions. This approach has led to the development of generalized conceptualizations and treatment strategies for each of the major personality disorders which are based on the commonalties observed among individuals manifesting the same disorder.

Cognitive therapy's general view of psychopathology applies directly to conceptualizing personality disorders. Returning to the case of "Gary," it is important to note that Gary's beliefs and assumptions, his interpretation of events, his affect, his interpersonal behavior, and the reactions he evoked from others interacted in ways that were strongly self-perpetuating. First, his vigilance for signs of untrustworthiness and maliciousness in others resulted in observations that seemed to confirm his preconceptions about others. Second, his guardedness and defensiveness tended to elicit bad treatment from many to his acquaintances and coworkers which again seemed to confirm his preconceptions. Finally, because his experience seemed to demonstrate that his vigilance and guardedness were necessary, he was unwilling either to relax his vigilance or to risk interacting with others less defensively.

This type of self-perpetuating cognitive–interpersonal cycle can be quite persistent and resistant to change. Once such a pattern is established, the individual's schemas tend to bias his or her perception of events in such a way that experiences that otherwise would contradict his or her assumptions are overlooked, discounted, or misinterpreted while, at the same time, his or her interpretation of events and his or her interpersonal behavior result in experiences that seem to confirm his or her dysfunctional schemas. We would argue that the cognitive and interpersonal processes that occur in individuals who qualify for Axis II diagnoses are the same as occur in any other nonpsychotic, neurologically intact individual except that in individuals with Axis II diagnoses, strongly self-perpetuating, dysfunctional cognitive–interpersonal cycles have evolved. The cognitive view of "personality disorder" is that this is simply the term used to refer to individuals with *pervasive, self-perpetuating cognitive–interpersonal cycles* which are dysfunctional enough to come to the attention of mental health professionals.

It is important to note that the conceptualization summarized in Figure 2.2 is specific to Gary and that the details of the cognitive conceptualization of an individual with a personality disorder would be similar to this only for other individuals with paranoid personality disorder. For other personality disorders, there would be major differences in the particular schemas, beliefs, and assumptions that would be emphasized; in the interplay between cognitions and interpersonal behavior that would be anticipated; and in the types of interventions that would be proposed. For comparison, a recent cognitive conceptualization of borderline personality disorder (from Freeman, Pretzer, Fleming & Simon, 2004) is shown in Figure 2.4. It is immediately obvious that there are major differences between this model and the model of paranoid personality disorder shown in Figure 2.2. While individuals with borderline personality disorder are seen as sharing the paranoid's view of the world of the world as a dangerous place where one is open to attack from others, they are not seen as sharing the paranoids' belief that one can stay safe by relying on one's own capabilities. Instead they are seen as believing that they are relatively weak and vulnerable and also as holding a conviction that they are flawed in some way that inherently will lead to rejection. These differences in basic assumptions lead to very different patterns of interpersonal interaction, elicit different responses from others, and establish a cognitive–interpersonal cycle which is strongly self-perpetuating but which is quite different from that manifested in paranoid personality disorder. A discussion of the cognitive conceptualization of each of the personality disorders is beyond the scope of

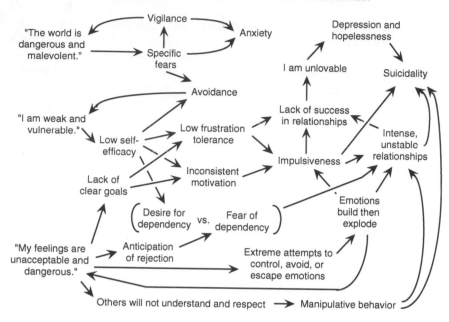

FIGURE 2.4. Cognitive conceptualization of borderline personality disorder.

this chapter. Interested readers can find detailed discussions of cognitive conceptualizations of each of the DSM-IV-TR personality disorders in the second edition of *Cognitive Therapy of Personality Disorders* (Beck et al., 2004) or of *Clinical Applications of Cognitive Therapy* (Freeman et al., 2004).

Some cognitively oriented authors have argued that in order to adequately account for the characteristics of individuals with personality disorders, cognitive therapy needs significant revision and have proposed their own modifications of cognitive therapy (Liotti, 1992; Lockwood, 1992; Lockwood & Young, 1992; Rothstein & Vallis, 1991; Safran & McMain, 1992; Young, 1990; Young & Lindemann, 1992; Young, Klosko, & Weishaar, 2003). These approaches, variously termed "structural," "constructivist," or "post-rationalist" by their advocates, propose adding new concepts or concepts borrowed from other theoretical systems to existing cognitive-behavioral approaches. For example, Young (1990; Young & Lindemann, 1992; Young & Swift, 1988; Young et al., 2003) has advocated adding a "fourth level of cognition" which he terms "early maladaptive schemas" (EMS) to cognitive therapy, Lockwood (1992) advocates integrating concepts from object-relations theory, and Liotti (1992) emphasizes the role of egocentrism in the personality disorders.

These various modifications of theory and therapeutic approach have not been greeted with universal enthusiasm. For example, Padesky (1986, 1988) has argued that there is no need to hypothesize that EMS are qualitatively different from other schemas in order to account for the persistence of dysfunctional cognitive and interpersonal patterns observed in clients with personality disorders. She points out that the tendency of schemas, beliefs, and behavior patterns to persist even after they have become seriously dysfunctional can easily be understood in terms of the effect they have on the perception and processing of new experiences.

It is interesting to note that many of the authors who argued that cognitive therapy needs substantial revision in order to deal adequately with personality disorders made no reference to the extensive work which had been done on conceptualizing and treating personality disorders within the existing cognitive framework (i.e., Beck et al., 1990; Fleming, 1983, 1985, 1988; Freeman et al., 1990; Padesky, 1986, 1988; Pretzer, 1983, 1985, 1988; Simon, 1983, 1985). Many of the points the constructivists emphasize, such as the strongly self-perpetuating nature of personality disorders, the role of family relationships in the etiology of personality disorders, and the importance of the therapist–client relationship in treating these disorders, have been emphasized for some time by the authors who are working within the existing cognitive model. As those who advocate revising cognitive therapy have yet to present detailed conceptualizations of specific personality disorders or to propose treatment strategies that are tailored to the characteristics of specific personality disorders, it is too early to determine whether their proposals contain important new contributions or not.

Propositional Testability

The cognitive theory of personality disorders is empirically testable, at least in principle, in that it generates specific, testable propositions. However, this does not mean that it is testable in its current form. For cognitive conceptualizations of the personality disorders to be truly testable, the general principles embodied in cognitive conceptualizations of the personality disorders will need to be elaborated into unambiguous propositions, more valid methods for quantifying cognitive and interpersonal variables will need to be developed, and experimental designs which overcome the practical problems encountered in attempting to assemble a large sample of subjects with a given personality disorder will need to be developed. There is potential for achieving each of these objectives, and possible methods for doing so are discussed later in this chapter, but much remains to be done to make the cognitive model of personality disorders truly testable.

TOWARD A COGNITIVE TAXONOMY
OF PERSONALITY DISORDERS

Because cognitive therapy's initial emphasis in conceptualizing personality disorders was on clinical practice, the focus has been on developing functional analyses of the various personality disorders to serve as a basis for strategic intervention. Work on developing comprehensive models of personality disorders or on analyzing the similarities and differences between the various personality disorders is of a more recent vintage (e.g. Beck et al., 1990, Chap. 3). The DSM classification system has been used in cognitive discussions of personality disorders for purely practical reasons and cognitive authors generally have not focused on the question of whether there are better ways to classify personality disorders. While there has been no explicit discussion of the merits of the various approaches to classifying personality disorders (categorical vs. dimensional vs. prototypal), a prototypal view is implicit in much that has been written about cognitive therapy with personality disorders. The typical approach used by cognitive authors has been to present conceptualizations and treatment recommendations based on experience with individuals who seem typical of persons with a particular personality disorder. The assumption has been that when an individual presents features of a second personality disorder or meets criteria for two personality disorder diagnoses, the clinician can interpolate between the two conceptualizations and treatment approaches.

While the basic idea that personality disorders are manifestations of self-perpetuating cognitive–nterpersonal cycles, which was discussed earlier applies to all the personality disorders, cognitive therapy's functional approach to conceptualizing personality disorders has resulted in the development of distinct conceptualizations for each of the personality disorders. For example, current cognitive views suggest that while individuals who view the world as a hostile demanding place where one can be safe only by being alert, vigilant, and defensive are seen as being likely to manifest paranoid personality disorder (Beck et al., 2004 ; Freeman et al., 1990, Chap. 7; Pretzer, 1988), individuals who see the world as being a dangerous place but who do not believe that they have the skills and capabilities needed to fend for themselves must find another solution. One obvious alternative is for them to endeavor to find someone strong and capable who can take care of them. Individuals who believe that "the way to be taken care of is to make your helplessness and neediness obvious to others and to passively subordinate your wants and preferences to those who are willing to take care of you" are likely to develop dependent personality disorder (Beck et al., 2004; Fleming, 1985; Freeman et al., 1990, Chap. 12). Individuals who share the same view of the demands of daily life and of their capabilities for coping successfully on their own but who believe that the way to be taken care of is to actively work to attract and hold the other person's attention through being dramatic, seductive, and so on, are seen as being likely to manifest very different interpersonal behavior, elicit very different responses from others, and develop histrionic personality disorder (Beck et al., 2004; Fleming, 1983, 1988; Freeman et al., 1990, Chap. 9).

We would argue that there are commonalties and differences in the underlying assumptions and interpersonal strategies held by individuals which result in systematic differences in momentary cognitions, in interpersonal behavior, and in the responses elicited from others which in turn play important roles in the development of personality disorders. This view suggests that it should be possible to develop a cognitive typology of personality disorders based on the similarities and differences among the underlying assumptions and interpersonal strategies characteristic of different personality disorders. Such a typology might well highlight important commonalties in etiological influences or aid in the selection of appropriate approaches to intervention. A number of authors have begun to work toward such a typology by attempting to list and categorize the cognitive and behavioral characteristics of the various personality disorders (Beck et al., 1990, Chap. 3 and App. A; Beck et al., 2004, Chap. 2; Young, 1990). The most advanced work in this direction is Beck's recent summarization of the cognitive characteristics of nine of the personality disorders which is seen in Table 2.2. However, more work remains to be done in order to develop a comprehensive cognitive typology of the personality disorders.

THE DEVELOPMENTAL ORIGINS
OF PERSONALITY DISORDERS

Inherited Predispositions

A number of heritable characteristics are relevant to understanding the development of personality disorders. First, it can be argued that, over the course of evolution, natural selection molded durable predispositions into humans which served the basic evolutionary goals of survival and reproduction. As our social milieu has changed from small groups subsisting in the wild to an advanced technological society, evolution may well have not kept pace with social change and thus there may well be areas of "poor fit" between our inherited predispositions and the demands of modern society which tend to cause problems for humans in general. If individuals differ in the strength or nature of these inherited predispositions, this could predispose certain individuals toward the development of particular problems. Beck (1992) has hypothesized that inherited predispositions toward certain "primeval strategies" (see Table 2.3) may contribute to the development of certain personality traits.

TABLE 2.2 Profile of Characteristics of Personality Disorders

Personality disorder	View of self	View of others	Main beliefs	Main Strategy
Avoidant	Vulnerable to depreciation, rejection Socially inept Incompetent	Critical Demeaning Superior	It's terrible to be rejected, put down If people know the real me they will reject me. Can't tolerate unpleasant feelings	Avoid evaluative situations Avoid unpleasant feelings or thoughts
Dependent	Weak Needs Helpless Incompetent	(Idealized) Nurturant Supportive Competent	Need people to survive, be happy Need for steady flow of support, encouragement	Cultivate dependent relationships
Passive–aggressive	Self-sufficient Vulnerable to control, interference	Intrusive Demanding Interfering Controlling Dominating	Others interfere with my freedom of action Control by others is intolerable Have to do things my own way	Passive resistance Surface submissiveness Evade, circumvent rules
Obsessive–compulsive	Responsible Accountable Fastidious Competent	Irresponsible Casual Incompetent Self-indulgent	I know what's best Details are crucial People *should* do better, try harder	Apply rules Perfectionism Evaluate, control "Shoulds," criticize, punish

Paranoid	Righteous Innocent, noble Vulnerable	Interfering Malicious Discriminatory Abusive motives	Motives are suspect Be on guard Don't trust	Wary Look for hidden motives Accuse Counterattack
Antisocial	A loner Autonomous Strong	Vulnerable Exploitive	Entitled to *break* rules Others are patsies, wimps Others are exploitative	Attack, rob Deceive, manipulate
Narcissistic	Special, unique Deserve special rules; superior Above the rules	Inferior Admirers	Because I'm special, I *deserve* special rules I'm above the rules I'm better than the others	Use others Transcend rules Manipulative Competitive
Histrionic	Glamorous Impressive	Seducible Receptive Admirers	People are there to serve or admire me They have no right to deny me my just deserts I can go by my feeling	Use dramatics, charm; temper tantrums, crying, suicide gestures
Schizoid	Self-sufficient Loner	Intrusive	Others are unrewarding Relationships are messy, undesirable	Stay away

TABLE 2.3. Primeval Strategies and Their Representation in Personality Disorders

"Strategy"	Personality disorder
Predatory	Antisocial
Help-eliciting	Dependent
Competitive	Narcissistic
Exhibitionistic	Histrionic
Autonomous	Schizoid
Defensive	Paranoid
Withdrawal	Avoidant
Ritualistic	Compulsive

Several cognitive-behavioral authors have hypothesized that inborn defects or deficits play an important role in the development of personality disorders. For example, Linehan (1993) has hypothesized that individuals with borderline personality disorder have an inherent defect in the regulation of emotion. She argues that this inborn defect interacts with a learning history which did not support the adaptive expression of emotion to result in intense, poorly controlled emotional responses. Similarly, Turner (1986) argues that those with borderline personality disorders have a biological predisposition toward low stress tolerance which interacts with maladaptive schemas to distort information processing. However, recent cognitive conceptualizations of borderline personality disorder (Beck et al., 1990, Chap. 9; Freeman et al., 1990, Chap. 8; Pretzer, 1983) have argued that these phenomena can be understood in terms of the effects of dysfunctional beliefs, cognitive distortions, and learning history without any need to postulate any inborn differences between individuals who develop borderline personality disorder and those who do not. Certainly, if inborn defects in information processing, regulation of affect, or interpersonal behavior occur with sufficient frequency, this would be relevant for understanding the development of personality disorders. However, it is not yet clear if such defects actually play a significant role in the development of personality disorders.

A potentially heritable aspect of individual development relevant to understanding the development of personality disorders is the infant's temperament. If one infant inherits a tendency to be extroverted and confident while another inherits a tendency to be shy and retiring, we would expect the shy, retiring infant to be more likely to eventually develop avoidant personality disorder. However, the development of schemas and interpersonal strategies are both strongly influenced by life experience. An inherently shy and retiring child who experiences day-to-day life as calm and secure might gradually risk being a bit more adventuresome. If his or her initial attempts at being somewhat bolder seem to work out well, he or she might conclude that risk taking is a good idea and gradually become less shy and retiring or might develop adaptive ways of coping with his or her shyness. However, a child who experiences daily life as frightening might avoid risk taking as much as possible and therefore not have the experiences that would lead him or her to conclude that risk taking is a good idea. Similarly, a child who experiments with being a bit more adventuresome and perceives his or her boldness to have bad consequences is not likely to persist with risk taking. Either of these children might well persist in being shy and retiring, fall behind his or her peers in developing social skills, and become more and more socially isolated.

However, the role of these possible inherited predispositions toward certain personality disorders is not a simple, straightforward one. First, the interaction between the child's predispositions, his or her family environment, and significant life events would shape development rather than inherited predispositions alone shaping development. Second, it is important to note that it is not objective events but the child's *perception* of events that influences the development of schemas and interpersonal strategies. Because cognitive development occurs in a series of stages over the course of childhood and adolescence, children are at a substantial disadvantage in attempting to understand the complexities of daily life. Misunderstandings and misinterpretations can easily occur because of the child's limited life experience and limitations imposed by the stage of cognitive development which he or she has attained.

Learned Characteristics

The many processes involved in social learning are also likely to play major roles in the development of personality disorders. Parents and significant others influence the developing child through verbal communication and explicit teaching, through their modeling of behaviors, through the contingencies they impose on the child, and through the cultural influences they transmit. A shy, retiring child might be explicitly or implicitly taught by his or her parents that one should avoid uncomfortable situations or might be taught that one should face one's fears. This would have obvious influences on the child's development. However, the parents might well give conflicting messages because the two parents disagree with each other, because one or both of the parents is ambivalent about the wisdom of facing one's fears, or because the parents' words are not consistent with their actions. As the child implicitly experiments with ways of understanding and responding to a particular type of recurrent situation and finds an approach which seems to work, the child may well "specialize" in a particular approach because it is strongly reinforced by the responses of others, because the situation seems risky enough to discourage further experimentation, or simply because it is the best approach the child has been able to discover.

The Developmental Impact of Traumatic Experiences

The long-term effects of traumatic events have been emphasized in many traditional perspectives on personality development. According to cognitive theory, the underlying assumptions and interpersonal strategies that are emphasized in the cognitive model of personality disorders are based on the individual's previous experience, and this certainly would include any traumatic events that have occurred. The extreme experiences some children encounter (see Bowlby, 1985, for striking examples) certainly can have important and lasting impacts on an individual's development. It may be possible for a single, dramatic experience to have lasting effects, but we would expect experiences which are recurrent, which are part of a consistent pattern of events, or which strengthen existing preconceptions to be particularly likely to have lasting effects.

An individual's early experiences play an important role in the development of personality disorders and other psychopathology for several reasons. Childhood experiences occur during the period in which initial schemas are being established, the child is exposed to the family environment daily over a period of years, parents are emotionally important to the growing child, and parents have control over powerful reinforcers and punishers. Childhood experiences are particularly important because once a child's initial schemas and interpersonal strategies are established, they shape the perception and interpretation of subsequent experiences in a way that tends to produce a "confirmatory bias" or "feedforward mechanism" (Mahoney, 1974). Individuals tend to selectively attend to experiences consistent with their preconceptions and to be biased toward interpreting their experiences as confirming these preconceptions in such a way that once schemas are established, they tend to function as self-fulfilling prophecies. Therefore, these cognitive structures tend to persist once they are established.

To return to our case example, Gary believed that people in general were malicious and deceptive, that they would attack him if they got a chance, and that the way to be safe was to be vigilant, on guard, and ready to defend himself. How did he come to hold these views? Gary reported growing up in a family where a suspicious, vigilant approach to the outside world was explicitly taught by his parents both through their words and through their example. In addition, he said that family members had been physically and verbally abusive of him and each other throughout his child-hood and had frequently taken advantage of him from childhood through the present. In short, he reported growing up in a family environment in which his world view and interpersonal strategies were explicitly taught and strongly reinforced by repeated experiences. Of course, we cannot be certain regarding the accuracy of Gary's perception and recall of interactions in his family of origin. However, it was his subjective experience rather than objective reality which, over time, gave rise to generalized beliefs about his world and his role in it. To a certain extent, the objective reality is unimportant because it is the individual's interpretation of experience that gives rise to both immediate responses and more persistent memories, beliefs, and assumptions.

The question of the extent to which there are inherent differences between individuals with personality disorders and individuals who do not have personality disorders is likely to remain a matter of theoretical debate until there are long-term longitudinal studies that examine the extent to which differences observed in infancy predict the subsequent development of personality disorders. When differences between individuals with a given personality disorder and "normal" individuals are identified in cross-sectional research, it can be difficult to determine to what extent an observed difference between groups is an inherent difference which contributed to the development of the disorder, to what extent the difference reflects characteristics acquired in the course of development, and to what extent the difference is a product of the individual's disorder. However, this question is of limited relevance for clinical practice. It is much more important clinically to identify methods for accomplishing therapeutic changes than to identify inherent differences.

ASSESSMENT INSTRUMENTATION

Because many of the concepts central to the cognitive view of psychopathology in general and personality disorders in particular are not directly observable, the development of effective assessment procedures has been an ongoing concern of cognitive therapists. While much progress has been made since the days when behaviorists rejected cognition as being inaccessible to scientific investigation, cognitive therapy's emphasis on variables that cannot be directly observed presents practical problems in both clinical practice and empirical research. The task of identifying individuals' thoughts, feelings, assumptions, interpersonal strategies, and overt behavior is not a simple one. After all, individuals are often oblivious to many of their thoughts, feelings, assumptions, strategies, and even actions. When an individual seems to be able to report this information we are faced by the problem of deciding to what extent their self-reports are inaccurate, biased, or censored.

Many techniques have been developed for assessing cognition (Merluzzi, Glass, & Genest, 1981), emotion (Isen, 1984), and behavior (Cone & Hawkins, 1977). Unfortunately, a great number of these techniques are impractical for regular clinical use due to the time, effort, and expense involved. In practice, cognitive therapists rely heavily on clinical interview, *in vivo* observation and interview, client self-monitoring, and self-report questionnaires. While these methods are not technologically sophisticated, they prove practical and effective in clinical practice (see Freeman et al., 1990, Chap. 2, for a more detailed discussion of clinical assessment in cognitive therapy).

The obvious problems with relying on self-report have received considerable discussion and empirical investigation over the years. It seems clear that the method used in eliciting descriptions of internal processes exercises a strong influence on the validity of the descriptions and that properly obtained reports can be quite useful (Ericsson & Simon, 1980). It is necessary for cognitive therapists to rely on individuals' self reports as an important source of data despite these problems because we have no other way of assessing the content of thoughts, schemas, assumptions, and interpersonal strategies independent of self-report. Freeman et al. (1990, Chap. 2) have summarized a set of guidelines intended to increase the validity of individuals' self-reports (see Table 2.4) and have discussed evaluating the validity of self-reports obtained in clinical practice.

In considering cognitive assessment procedures, it is important to maintain a clear distinction between clinical assessment and assessment procedures to be used in empirical research because these two purposes call for very different approaches to assessment. It can be argued that in clinical practice, the ultimate test of the value of self-reports is their utility in guiding clinical interventions (Kendall & Hollon, 1981). Clinical assessment can be a self-correcting process if therapist and client work together to collect needed information, implement therapeutic interventions based on the resulting conceptualizations, and then use the results of their interventions as a source of corrective feedback. Successful interventions both accomplish desired changes and provide evidence of the clinical utility of the conceptualizations on which the interventions were based. Unsuccessful or partially successful interventions highlight areas in which the current conceptualizations are not adequate. Observations regarding the actual effects of the unsuccessful interventions and the factors that influenced this outcome can serve as a basis for a revised conceptualization which can again be tested in practice. When clinical assessment is integrated with interven-

TABLE 2.4. Guidelines for Increasing the Validity of Self-Reports

1. *Motivate the client to be open and forthright.* Make sure that it is clear that providing full, honest, detailed reports is in the client's interest by (a) providing a clear rationale for seeking the information, (b) demonstrating the relevance of the information being requested to the client's goals, and (c) demonstrating the value of clear, specific information by explicitly making use of the information.

2. *Minimize the delay between event and report.* This will result in more detailed information and will reduce the amount of distortion due to imperfect recall. For events occurring outside the therapist's office, use an *in vivo* interview or self-monitoring techniques when possible.

3. *Provide retrieval cues.* Review the setting and the events leading up to the event of interest either verbally or by using imagery to improve recall.

4. *Avoid possible biases.* Begin with open-ended questions which ask the client to describe his or her experience without suggesting possible answers or requiring inference. Focus on "What happened?" not on "Why?" or "What did it mean?" Do not ask clients to infer experiences they cannot remember. Wait until after the entire experience has been described to test your hypotheses or ask for specific details.

5. *Encourage and reinforce attention to thoughts and feelings.* Clients who initially have difficulty monitoring their own cognitive processes are more likely to gradually develop increased skill if they are reinforced for accomplishments than if they are criticized for failures. Some clients may need explicit training in differentiating between thoughts and emotions, in attending to cognitions, or in reporting observations rather than inferences.

6. *Encourage and reinforce acknowledgment of limitations in recall.* If the therapist accepts only long, detailed reports, this increases the risk of the client's inventing data in order to satisfy the therapist. It is important for the therapist to appreciate the information the client can provide and to encourage the client to acknowledge his or her limits in recalling details, because incomplete but accurate information is much more useful than detailed reports fabricated in order to please the therapist.

7. *Watch for indications of invalidity.* Be alert for inconsistency within the client's report, inconsistency between the verbal report and nonverbal cues, and inconsistency between the report and data obtained previously. If apparent inconsistencies are observed, explore them collaboratively with the client without being accusatory or judgmental.

8. *Watch for factors which may interfere.* Be alert for indications of beliefs, assumptions, expectancies, and misunderstandings which may interfere with the client's providing accurate self-reports. Common problems include (a) the fear that the therapist will be unable to accept the truth and will become angry, shocked, disgusted, or rejecting if the client reports his or her experiences accurately; (b) the belief that the client must do a perfect job of observing and reporting the experiences and that he or she is a failure if the reports are not perfect from the beginning; (c) the fear that the information revealed in therapy may be used against the client or may give the therapist power over him or her; (d) the belief that it is dangerous to closely examine experiences involving strong or "crazy" feelings for fear that the feelings will be intolerable or will "get out of control."

tion in this way, this self-correcting process can make the most of rich data, even if the reliability and validity of a particular observation or self-report are uncertain.

Empirical research, in contrast, generally calls for standardized assessment procedures that produce numerical scores having respectable levels of reliability and validity. A variety of methods ranging from self-report questionnaires to structured self-monitoring to performance on experimental tasks have been used in cognitive-behavioral research with varying degrees of success. Many investigators have relied on minimally validated self-report questionnaires because they are easy to develop and inexpensive to use. While the use of a neatly printed, computer-scored questionnaire gives the appearance that one is proceeding very scientifically, the use of such measures presumes that subjects have sufficient self-knowledge to accurately report the cognitions in question and presumes that the subjects are willing and able to provide unbiased, uncensored reports of their cognitions. While this unsophisticated approach to assessing cognitive variables has produced some useful findings, there is a need for more rigorous approaches to assessment in cognitive-behavioral research.

COGNITIVE THERAPY OF PERSONALITY DISORDERS

Goals of Treatment

In cognitive therapy the goals of treatment are agreed on collaboratively between therapist and client and therefore vary from client to client. The goals typically involve achieving alleviation of the client's distress as efficiently as is feasible and also achieving whatever changes are necessary for the improvement to persist over time and for the client to lead a happy, productive life. When an individual seeks treatment for a specific, focused problem, cognitive therapy may involve very focused interventions which have little impact on the rest of the client's life. However, it is generally true that the greater the extent to which the client's problems have broad effects throughout the client's life, the broader the changes needed to alleviate the client's distress. Because personality disorders, by definition, have pervasive effects throughout the individual's life, cognitive therapy with personality disorders often involves a set of interventions intended to have broad effects throughout the client's life. This does not mean that "personality restructuring" is the goal of cognitive therapy. The primary goals of therapy are generally to alleviate the client's distress, to improve the client's day-to-day functioning, and to accomplish the lasting changes needed for these improvements to persist. Broad personality changes may well be a necessary means toward these ends, but they are not inevitable goals of cognitive therapy. In particular, the practical constraints imposed by limits on health insurance coverage, agency policies, and client motivation mean that the goals of treatment in a given case may be much more limited than this ideal. Cognitive therapy can be used effectively in a very focused, time-limited way to accomplish limited goals or in an open-ended way when the goals are defined much more broadly.

Principles of Cognitive Therapy

The cognitive model of psychopathology emphasizes the effects of dysfunctional automatic thoughts; dysfunctional schemas, beliefs, and assumptions; and dysfunctional interpersonal behavior. Therefore, each of these is an important target for intervention in cognitive therapy. The initial goal of cognitive therapy is to break the cycle or cycles that perpetuate and amplify the client's problems (see Figure 2.3). This could potentially be done by modifying the client's automatic thoughts, by improving the client's mood, by working to counteract the biasing impact of mood on recall and perception, and/or by changing the client's behavior. In theory, these interventions could break the cycle or cycles that perpetuate the problems and thus could alleviate the client's immediate distress. However, if the therapist does only this, the client would be at risk for a relapse whenever he or she experienced events similar to the ones that precipitated the current problems. To achieve lasting results, it would also be important to modify the schemas, beliefs, and assumptions that predispose the client to his or her problems and to help the client plan effective ways to handle situations that might precipitate a relapse.

Our view is that many dysfunctional cognitions persist because (1) many individuals are unaware of the role their thoughts play in their problems, (2) the dysfunctional cognitions often seem so plausible that individuals fail to examine them critically, (3) selective perception and cognitive biases often result in the individual's ignoring or discounting experiences which would otherwise conflict with the dysfunctional cognitions, (4) cognitive distortions often lead to erroneous conclusions, (5) the individual's dysfunctional interpersonal behavior often can produce experiences which seem to confirm dysfunctional cognitions, and (6) individuals who are reluctant to tolerate aversive affect may consciously or nonconsciously avoid memories, perceptions, and/or conclusions that would elicit strong emotional responses.

This view suggests that cognitive interventions should be directed toward identifying the specific dysfunctional beliefs that play a role in the individual's problems and examining them critically while correcting for the effects of selective perception, biased cognition, and cognitive distortions and helping the individual to face and tolerate aversive affect. Logical or intellectual analysis of dysfunctional cognitions is usually not sufficient to accomplish substantive change. Individuals often find that within-session interventions can be intellectually convincing but that to be convinced "on the gut level," and to have the change in cognitions be manifested in their behavior, it is usually necessary to test the new cognitions in real-life situations. These "behavioral experiments" (see Beck, Rush, Shaw, & Emery, 1979, p. 56, or Freeman et al., 1990, pp. 76–77) are often much more convincing than any amount of intellectual insight. When dysfunctional cognitions are strongly supported by interpersonal experience, it may be necessary to accomplish changes in interpersonal behavior and/or in the individual's environment in order to challenge the cognitions effectively.

It is our view that many dysfunctional behaviors persist because (1) they are a product of persistent dysfunctional beliefs, (2) expectations regarding the consequences of possible actions encourage behaviors which actually prove to be dysfunctional and/or discourage behaviors which would prove adaptive, (3) the individual lacks the skills needed to engage in potentially adaptive behavior, or (4) the environment reinforces dysfunctional behavior and/or punishes adaptive behavior. This view suggests that to change dysfunctional behavior it may be necessary to modify long-standing cognitions, to examine the individual's expectations regarding the consequences of his or her actions, to modify the individual's environment, or to help the individual master the cognitive or behavioral skills needed to successfully engage in more adaptive behavior.

It is interesting to note that when dysfunctional behavior is strongly maintained by dysfunctional cognitions, it may be necessary to modify the cognitions first, and that when dysfunctional cognitions are strongly maintained by the effects of dysfunctional behavior, it may be necessary to modify the dysfunctional behavior first. This suggests that if it is true that personality disorders are characterized by self-perpetuating cognitive–interpersonal cycles where dysfunctional cognitions strongly maintain dysfunctional behavior and dysfunctional behavior strongly maintains dysfunctional cognition, it may be difficult to find ways to intervene effectively. We argue that when a self-perpetuating cognitive–interpersonal cycle exists it may not be possible to effectively modify either cognitions or behavior in isolation and that a strategic intervention approach based on a clear conceptualization is likely to be necessary.

The Process of Cognitive Therapy

Obviously, a wide variety of approaches could be used to achieve the changes in cognition and behavior which we see as being necessary to produce lasting improvement. The approach used in cognitive therapy has been described as "collaborative empiricism" (Beck et al., 1979, Chap. 3). The therapist endeavors to work *with* the client to help him or her to recognize the factors that contribute to problems; to test the validity of the thoughts, beliefs, and assumptions that prove important; and to make the necessary changes in cognition and behavior. While it is clear that very different therapeutic approaches ranging from philosophical debate to operant conditioning can be effective with at least some clients, collaborative empiricism has substantial advantages. By actively collaborating with the client, the therapist minimizes the resistance and oppositionality that is often elicited by taking an authoritarian role, yet the therapist is still in a position to structure each session as well as the overall course of therapy to be as efficient and effective as possible (Beck et al., 1979, Chap. 4).

One part of this collaborative approach is an emphasis on a process of "guided discovery." If the therapist guides the client by asking questions, making observations, and asking the client to monitor relevant aspects of the situation, the therapist can help the client develop an understanding of his or her problems, explore possible solutions, develop plans for dealing with the problems, and implement the plans quite effectively. Guided discovery has an advantage over approaches in which the therapist unilaterally develops an understanding of the problems and proposes solutions in that it maximizes client involvement in therapy sessions and minimizes the possibility of the client's feeling that the therapist' ideas are being imposed on the client. In addition, because the client is actively involved in the process of developing an understanding of the problems and coming up with a solution, the client also has an opportunity to learn an effective approach to dealing with problems and should be better able to deal with future problems when they arise.

Conceptualization of the Case

In cognitive therapy, a strategic approach to intervention is emphasized (Persons, 1991). Our view is that therapy is most effective and most efficient when the therapist thinks strategically about intervention and uses a clear conceptualization of the client's problems as a basis for selecting the most productive targets for intervention and the most appropriate intervention techniques. When the therapist intervenes without pausing to develop a conceptualization of the client's problems and without using that conceptualization to select the most appropriate interventions, much time and effort can be expended on interventions that prove ineffective or minimally relevant. This strategic approach is quite unlike therapies in which the therapist uses a standard therapeutic approach with all clients in the hope that by being "therapeutic in general" he or she will eventually address the most important issues. It is also quite different from technique-oriented approaches where intervention A is automatically used with problem A and intervention B is automatically used with problem B.

To take a strategic approach to therapy, the therapist must develop an understanding of the client and his or her problems. Therefore, the first step in cognitive therapy is an initial assessment that provides a foundation for intervention (Beck et al., 1979, Chap. 5). By beginning with a systematic evaluation, the therapist can develop an initial conceptualization quickly rather than waiting for an understanding of the client to develop gradually over the first few months of therapy and thus can be in a position to intervene effectively early in therapy. A clear conceptualization provides a basis for an individualized treatment plan which allows the therapist to be selective and efficient in employing the wide range of interventions and therapeutic techniques that are available.

The Therapeutic Relationship

In cognitive therapy, the initial therapy sessions are also important because they provide an opportunity for the therapist to establish a solid foundation for therapy before plunging into intervention (Beck et al., 1979, Chap. 3; Beck et al., 1990, pp. 64–79). The effectiveness of any psychotherapy depends on a relationship of confidence, openness, caring, and trust established between client and therapist. The cognitive therapist takes an active, directive role in treatment and thus can work actively to develop the therapeutic relationship rather than waiting for it to develop gradually over time. With many clients, this is more easily said than done. The complexities and difficulties encountered in the therapeutic relationship are particularly important in the treatment of clients with personality disorders.

To collaborate effectively, therapist and client must agree on what they are trying to accomplish. Therefore, following the initial evaluation, the therapist works with the client to specify goals for therapy and to prioritize them. These goals include the problems the client wishes to overcome and the positive changes he or she wants to work toward and should be operationalized clearly and specifically enough so that both therapist and client can tell if progress is being made. In considering the sequence in which to work on the goals, a number of factors are considered, including the client's preferences regarding which issues to work on first, the therapist's conceptualization, which problems seem most likely to respond to early interventions, and any practical considerations that are relevant.

There is considerable advantage in working initially toward a goal that appears manageable even if it is not the goal that is most important to the client. If it proves possible to make demonstrable progress toward a valued goal, the client will be encouraged and this will increase his or her motivation for therapy. The process of jointly agreeing on goals and priorities maximizes the likelihood that therapy will accomplish what the client is seeking. At the same time, it establishes the precedent of the therapist's soliciting and respecting the client's input while being open regarding his or her own views. Thus, it lays the foundation for therapist and client to work together collaboratively, and it makes it clear to the client that his or her concerns are understood and respected. The time and effort spent on establishing mutually agreed on goals and priorities is more than compensated for by the resulting increase in client involvement, decrease in resistance, and decrease in time and effort wasted on peripheral topics.

Another issue that is important in a collaborative approach to therapy is to introduce the client to the therapist's understanding of the problems and to his or her approach to therapy. While this could be done as a "mini-lecture" about psychopathology and psychotherapy, it is generally easier and more effective to use a guided discovery approach and to base the explanation on the thoughts and feelings the client reports experiencing on particular occasions when his or her problems were occurring (see Freeman et al., 1990, pp. 94–95).

Intervention Techniques

Cognitive therapy is a "technically eclectic" approach in that a wide range of intervention techniques can be used flexibly within a coherent conceptual framework. As therapist and client endeavor to work together toward their shared goals, the therapist is free to select from the full range of intervention techniques. One of the primary interventions used in cognitive therapy is helping the client to identify the specific automatic thoughts that occur in problem situations, to recognize the effects these thoughts have on his or her emotions and behavior, and to respond effectively to those thoughts that prove problematic (Beck et al., 1979, Chap. 8; Beck et al., 1990, pp. 80–90; Freeman et al., 1990, pp. 49–68). Negative, self-deprecating, or other problematic thoughts typically are a habitual part of the client's life and come "fast and furious" without the client necessarily being aware of their presence or their relationship to his or her distress. By using interview and self-monitoring techniques, the client can learn to recognize dysfunctional thinking, to understand its impact on moods and actions, and to develop increased control over it.

Behavioral interventions are also used frequently in cognitive therapy to alleviate depressed mood, to improve coping skills, to replace dysfunctional interpersonal behavior with more adaptive responses, and to challenge dysfunctional cognitions. However, cognitive therapy is not limited to cognitive and behavioral interventions even though these are the most commonly used interventions. The full range of therapeutic techniques can be used as long as they are appropriate to the goals being pursued at the moment, are compatible with the current conceptualization of the client's problems, and are used collaboratively.

"Homework assignments" are used extensively throughout cognitive therapy (Beck et al., 1979, Chap. 13). Clients who actively engage in some of the work of therapy between sessions accomplish more than those who passively wait for their weekly hour with the therapist (Persons et al., 1988). In addition, clients are in a position to collect data and test the effects of cognitive and behavioral changes in daily life in ways that would be difficult to duplicate within the therapy session. Noncompliance often occurs when homework assignments are used. However, rather than being a problem, noncompliance is often quite useful in identifying problems in the therapist–client relationship and in identifying the factors that block the client from making the desired changes (Beck et al., 1990, pp. 66–77).

The Termination of Therapy

The cognitive model of psychopathology asserts that in addition to modifying dysfunctional automatic thoughts, it is important to address the client's underlying assumptions, and a variety of techniques for doing this have been developed (Beck et al., 1979, Chap. 12; J. Beck, 1995; Padesky, 1994). Otherwise it is possible to resolve the client's current problems but still leave the client prone to relapse. In theory, effectively modifying the client's basic assumptions and any dysfunctional interaction patterns should leave him or her no more prone to future problems than anyone else. However, it is often hard for a therapist to gauge whether interventions have been completely effective. Therefore, cognitive therapy ends by explicitly working to prepare the client to deal with future setbacks (Beck et al., 1979, Chap. 15). This work, based on Marlatt and Gordon's (1985) research on relapse prevention, consists of helping the client to become aware of high-risk situations, to identify early warning signs of impending relapse, and to develop explicit plans for handling high-risk situations and heading off potential relapse.

Preferably, when the client has attained his or her goals for therapy, work on relapse prevention has been completed, and the client's progress has been maintained long enough for him or her to have a reasonable amount of confidence that he or she will be able to cope with problems as they arise, the decision to terminate is made. In the typical case, the therapist and client agree to "taper off" by shifting from weekly sessions to biweekly and, possibly, monthly sessions when the time for termination is near. This not only makes the ending of therapy less abrupt but also provides therapist and client with an opportunity to discover how well the client handles problems without the therapist's help and to discover whether any additional issues need to be addressed. The client is also offered the opportunity to return for "booster sessions" if problems arise, in the hopes that early intervention with future problems may forestall major difficulties.

Cognitive Therapy of Personality Disorders

The basic cognitive therapy approach to treating individuals with personality disorders is the same as cognitive therapy with other clients. However, a number of important modifications are needed to accommodate to the characteristics of individuals with personality disorders and to avoid problems frequently encountered in treating individuals with personality disorders. Pretzer and Fleming have proposed a number of general guidelines for cognitive therapy with clients who have personality disorders (Beck et al., 1990, pp. 351–358; Fleming & Pretzer, 1990; Pretzer & Fleming, 1990):

1. *Interventions are most effective when based on an individualized conceptualization of the client's problems.* Clients with personality disorders are complex, and the therapist is often faced with choosing among many possible targets for intervention and a variety of possible intervention techniques. Not only does this present a situation in which intervention can easily become confused and disorganized if the therapist does not have a clear treatment plan, but the interventions that seem appropriate after a superficial examination of the client can easily prove ineffective or counterproductive. The practice of developing a clear conceptualization of the client's problems on the basis of a detailed evaluation and then revising this conceptualization on the basis of clinical observation and the results of clinical interventions aids in the development of an effective treatment plan and minimizes the risk of the therapist being confused by the sheer complexity of the client's problems.

2. *It is important for therapist and client to work collaboratively toward clearly identified, shared goals.* With clients as complex as those with personality disorders, clear, consistent goals for therapy are necessary to avoid skipping from problem to problem without making any lasting progress. However, it is important for these goals to be mutually agreed on in order to minimize the noncompliance and power struggles that often impede treatment of clients with personality disorders. It can be difficult to develop shared goals for treatment as many of these clients present numerous vague complaints and, at the same time, may be unwilling to modify some of the behaviors the therapist sees as particularly problematic. However, the time and effort spent developing mutually acceptable goals can be a good investment.

3. *It is important to focus more than the usual amount of attention on the therapist–client relationship.* While a good therapeutic relationship is as

necessary for effective intervention in cognitive therapy as in any other approach to therapy, behavioral and cognitive-behavioral therapists are generally accustomed to being able to establish a fairly straightforward therapeutic relationship at the outset of therapy and then proceed without paying much attention to the interpersonal aspects of therapy. However, this is not usually the case when working with clients who have personality disorders. The dysfunctional schemas, beliefs, and assumptions that bias clients perceptions of others are likely to bias their perception of the therapist, and the dysfunctional interpersonal behaviors that clients manifest in relationships outside therapy are likely to manifested in the therapist–client relationship as well. While the interpersonal difficulties that are manifested in the therapist–client relationship can disrupt therapy if they are not addressed effectively, they also provide the therapist with the opportunity to do *in vivo* observation and intervention (Freeman et al., 1990; Mays, 1985; Padesky, 1986) rather than having to rely on the client's report of interpersonal problems occurring between sessions.

One type of problem in the therapist–client relationship which is more common among individuals with personality disorders than among other individuals in cognitive therapy is the phenomenon traditionally termed "transference" when the client manifests an extreme or persistent misperception of the therapist which is based on his or her previous experience in significant relationships rather than on the therapist's behavior. This can be understood in cognitive terms as the individual overgeneralizing beliefs and expectancies acquired in significant relationships. Individuals with personality disorders are typically vigilant for any sign that their fears may be realized, and they are prone to react quite intensely when the therapist's behavior appears to confirm their anticipations. When these strongly emotional reactions occur, it is important for the therapist to recognize what is happening, quickly develop an understanding of what the client is thinking, and directly but sensitively clear up the misconceptions before they disrupt therapy. While these reactions can be quite problematic, it is also true that they provide opportunities to identify the beliefs, expectations, and interpersonal strategies that play an important role in the client's problems and that they provide an opportunity to respond to the client in ways which tend to disconfirm his or her dysfunctional beliefs and expectancies.

4. *Consider beginning with interventions which do not require extensive self-disclosure.* Many clients with personality disorders are quite uncomfortable with self-disclosure due to a lack of trust in the therapist, discomfort with even mild levels of intimacy, fear of rejection, and so on. While it is sometimes necessary to begin treatment with interventions that require extensive discussion of the client's thoughts and feelings, sometimes it can be useful to begin treatment by working on a problem that can be approached through behavioral interventions that do not require extensive

self-disclosure. This allows time for the client to gradually become more comfortable with therapy and for the therapist to gradually address the client's discomfort with self-disclosure (Freeman et al., 1990, Chap. 8).

5. *Interventions that increase the client's sense of self-efficacy[4] often reduce the intensity of the client's symptomatology and facilitate other interventions.* The intensity of the emotional and behavioral responses manifested by individuals with personality disorders is often due in part to the individual's doubting his or her ability to cope effectively with particular problem situations. This doubt regarding one's ability to cope effectively not only intensifies emotional responses to the situation but also predisposes the individual to drastic responses. If it is possible to increase the individual's confidence that he or she will be able to handle these problem situations if they arise, the client's level of anxiety is often lowered, his or her symptomatology is moderated, he or she is able to react more deliberately, and it becomes easier to implement other interventions. The individual's sense of self-efficacy, his or her confidence that he or she can deal effectively with specific situations when they arise, can be increased through interventions that correct any exaggerations of the demands of the situation or minimization of the individual's capabilities, through helping the individual to improve his or her coping skills, or through a combination of the two (Freeman et al., 1990, Chap. 7; Pretzer et al., 1990).

6. *Do not rely primarily on verbal interventions.* The more severe a client's problems are, the more important it is to use behavioral interventions to accomplish cognitive as well as behavioral change (Freeman et al., 1990, Chap. 3). A gradual hierarchy of "behavioral experiments" not only provides an opportunity for desensitization to occur and for the client to master new skills but also can be quite effective in challenging unrealistic beliefs and expectations.

7. *Try to identify and address the client's fears before implementing changes.* Clients with personality disorders often have strong but unexpressed fears about the changes they seek or are asked to make in the course of therapy, and attempts to induce the client to simply go ahead without addressing these fears are often unsuccessful (Mays, 1985). If the therapist makes a practice of discussing the client's expectations and concerns before each change is attempted, it is likely to reduce the client's level of anxiety regarding therapy and improve compliance.

8. *Help the client deal adaptively with aversive emotions.* Clients with personality disorders often experience very intense aversive emotional reactions in specific situations. These intense reactions can be a significant problem in their own right, but in addition, the individual's attempts to avoid experiencing these emotions, his or her attempts to escape the emotions, and his or her cognitive and behavioral response to the emotions often play an important role in the client's problems in living. Often, the

individual's unwillingness to tolerate aversive affect blocks him or her from handling the emotions adaptively and perpetuates fears about the consequences of experiencing the emotions. If the individual is willing to face the emotions long enough to handle them adaptively, he or she may well also need to acquire some of the cognitive and/or behavioral skills needed to handle the emotions effectively (Farrell & Shaw, 1994).

9. *Anticipate problems with compliance.* Many factors contribute to a high rate of noncompliance among clients with personality disorders. In addition to the complexities in the therapist–client relationship and the fears regarding change which were discussed previously, the dysfunctional behaviors of individuals with personality disorders are strongly ingrained and often are reinforced by aspects of the client's environment. However, rather than simply being an impediment to progress, episodes of noncompliance can provide an opportunity for effective intervention. When noncompliance is predictable, addressing the issues beforehand may not only improve compliance with that particular assignment but may also prove helpful with other situations in which similar issues arise. When noncompliance arises unexpectedly, it provides an opportunity to identify issues that are impeding progress in therapy so that they can be addressed.

10. *Do not presume that the client exists in a reasonable environment.* Some behaviors, such as assertion, are so generally adaptive that it is easy to assume that they are always a good idea. However, clients with personality disorders are often the product of seriously atypical families and live in atypical environments. When implementing changes, it is important to assess the likely responses of significant others in the client's environment rather than presuming that they will respond in a reasonable way.

11. *Attend to your own emotional reactions during the course of therapy.* Interactions with clients with personality disorders can elicit emotional reactions from the therapist ranging from empathic feelings of depression to strong anger, discouragement, fear, or sexual attraction. It is important for the therapist to be aware of these responses so that they do not unduly influence or disrupt the therapist's work with the client, and so that they can be used as a source of potentially useful data. Because emotional responses do not occur randomly, an unusually strong emotional response is likely to be a reaction to some aspect of the client's behavior. Because a therapist may respond emotionally to a pattern in the client's behavior long before it has been recognized intellectually, accurate interpretation of one's own responses can speed recognition of these patterns. Careful thought is needed regarding whether to disclose these reactions to the client. On the one hand, clients with personality disorders often react strongly to therapist self-disclosure and may find it very threatening. However, on the other hand, if the therapist does not disclose an emotional reaction which is apparent to the client from nonverbal cues or which the

client anticipates on the basis of experiences in other relationships, it can easily lead to misunderstandings or distrust. Therapists may benefit from using cognitive techniques (such as the Dysfunctional Thought Record; Beck et al., 1979) and/or seeking consultation with an objective colleague.

12. *Be realistic regarding the length of therapy, goals for therapy, and standards for therapist self-evaluation.* Many therapists using behavioral and cognitive-behavioral approaches to therapy are accustomed to accomplishing substantial results relatively quickly. One can easily become frustrated and angry with the "resistant" client when therapy proceeds slowly or become self-critical and discouraged when therapy goes badly. Behavioral and cognitive-behavioral interventions can accomplish substantial, apparently lasting changes in some clients with personality disorders, but more modest results are achieved in other cases, and little is accomplished in others. When therapy proceeds slowly, it is important to neither give up prematurely nor perseverate with an unsuccessful treatment approach. When treatment is unsuccessful, it is important to remember that therapist competence is not the only factor influencing the outcome of therapy.

Just as in cognitive therapy with other problems, the basic strategy in cognitive therapy with personality disorders is to develop an initial conceptualization based on the initial evaluation and then to intervene strategically, focusing both on alleviating the individual's current distress and on accomplishing lasting changes. In the case of Gary, the conceptualization of his problems which was summarized in Figure 2.2 may seem to provide little chance for effective intervention. One goal of therapy would be to modify Gary's basic assumptions as these are the foundation of the disorder. However, how can one hope to challenge Gary's conviction that others are malicious and deceptive effectively while his vigilance and guardedness constantly produce experiences that seem to confirm his assumptions? If it were possible to induce Gary to relax his vigilance and defensiveness, this would simplify the task of modifying his assumptions. But how can we hope to do this as long as Gary is convinced that people have malicious intentions? Fortunately, the client's sense of self-efficacy plays an important role in the model as well and provides a promising point for intervention.

The paranoid individual's intense vigilance and defensiveness is a product of the belief that constant vigilance and defensiveness are necessary in order to stay safe. If it is possible to increase the client's sense of self-efficacy regarding problem situations to the point that he or she is confident of being able to handle problems as they arise, then the intense vigilance and defensiveness seems less necessary and it may be possible for the client to relax both to some extent. This can reduce the intensity of the client's symptomatology substantially, make it much easier to address the client's cognitions through conventional cognitive therapy techniques, and make it more possible to persuade the client to try alternative ways of handling interpersonal conflicts. Therefore, the initial strategy in the cognitive treatment of paranoid personality disorder is to work to increase the client's sense of self-efficacy. This is followed by attempts to modify other aspects of the client's automatic thoughts, interpersonal behavior, and basic assumptions.

Self-efficacy can be increased in two basic ways. Because it is essentially a subjective evaluation of the demands inherent in a situation and the individual's ability to successfully meet those demands, an unrealistically low sense of self-efficacy can result if individuals overestimate the demands of the situation or underestimate their ability to handle the situation. When this is the case, cognitive interventions that result in a more realistic evaluation of the situation can increase self-efficacy. A low sense of self-efficacy can also result when individuals realistically conclude that they do not have the skills or capabilities needed to handle the situation effectively. In that case, self-efficacy can be increased through interventions that increase the client's coping skills. This can be a matter of helping the client master new coping skills, helping the client muster the needed resources, helping the client plan how to best use the skills and resources he or she has, and so on.

Gary's paranoid personality disorder was not recognized until the seventh therapy session, and the stress-management interventions that began therapy had already raised his sense of self-efficacy substantially. However, Gary still felt that vigilance was necessary in many innocuous situations because he doubted his ability to cope if he was not constantly vigilant. This doubt stemmed from his persistently labeling himself as "incompetent" despite Gary's skills and accomplishments. When this was explored in therapy, it became clear that Gary had very strict idiosyncratic standards for competence and viewed competence dichotomously. He believed that one was either fully competent or totally incompetent. Because he manifested a dichotomous view of competence, the "continuum technique," a cognitive technique used specifically to counteract dichotomous thinking, was used:

THERAPIST: It sounds like a lot of your tension and your spending so much time double-checking your work is because you see yourself as basically incompetent and think "I've got to be careful or I'll really screw up."

GARY: Sure. But it's not just screwing up something little, someone's life could depend on what I do.

THERAPIST: Hmm. We've talked your competence in terms of how you were evaluated while you were in training and how well you've done since then without making much headway. It occurs to me that I'm not sure exactly what "competence" means for you. What does it take for somebody to really qualify as competent? For example, if a Martian came down knowing nothing of humans and he wanted to know how to tell who was truly competent, what would you tell him to look for?

GARY: It's someone who does a good job at whatever he's doing.

THERAPIST: Does it matter what the person is doing? If someone does well at something easy, do they qualify as competent in your eyes?

GARY: No, to really be competent they can't be doing something easy.

THERAPIST: So it sounds like they've got to be doing something hard and getting good results to qualify as competent.

GARY: Yeah.

THERAPIST: Is that all there is to it? You've been doing something hard and doing well at it, but you don't feel competent.

GARY: But I'm tense all the time and I worry about work.

THERAPIST: Are you saying that a truly competent person isn't tense and doesn't worry?

GARY: Yeah. They're confident. They relax while they're doing it and they don't worry about it afterward.

THERAPIST: So a competent person is someone who takes on difficult tasks and does them well, is relaxed while he's doing them, and doesn't worry about it afterwards. Does that cover it or is there more to competence?

GARY: Well, he doesn't have to be perfect as long as he catches his mistakes and knows his limits.

THERAPIST: What I've gotten down so far [the therapist has been taking notes] is that a truly competent person is doing hard tasks well and getting good results, he's relaxed while he does this and doesn't worry about it afterward, he catches any mistakes he makes and corrects them, and he knows his limits. Does that capture what you have in mind when you use the word competent?

GARY: Yeah, I guess it does.

THERAPIST: From the way you've talked before, I've gotten the impression that you see competence as pretty black and white, either you're competent or you aren't.

GARY: Of course. That's the way it is.

THERAPIST: What would be a good label for the people who aren't competent? Does incompetent capture it?

GARY: Yeah, that's fine.

THERAPIST: What would characterize incompetent people? What would you look for to spot them?

GARY: They screw everything up. They don't do things right. They don't even care whether it's right or how they look or feel. You can't expect results from them.

THERAPIST: Does that cover it?

GARY: Yeah, I think so.

THERAPIST: Well, let's look at how you measure up to these standards. One characteristic of an incompetent person is that he screws everything up. Do you screw everything up?

GARY: Well, no. Most things I do come out OK but I'm real tense while I do them.

THERAPIST: And you said that an incompetent person doesn't care whether it comes out right or how they look to others, so your being tense and worrying doesn't fit with the idea that you're incompetent. If you don't qualify as incompetent, does that mean that you're completely competent?

GARY: I don't feel competent.

THERAPIST: And by these standards you aren't. You do well with a difficult job and you've been successful at catching the mistakes you do make, but you aren't relaxed and you do worry. By these standards you don't qualify as completely incompetent or totally competent. How does that fit with the idea that a person's either competent or incompetent?

GARY: I guess maybe it's not just one or the other.

THERAPIST: While you were describing how you saw competence and incompetence I wrote the criteria here in my notes. Suppose we draw a scale from 0–10 here where 0 is absolutely, completely incompetent and 10 is completely competent, all the time [see Figure 2.5]. How would you rate your competence in grad school?

GARY: At first I was going to say 3 but, as I think about it, I'd say a 7 or 8 except for my writing, and I've never worked at that until now.

THERAPIST: How would you rate your competence on the job?

GARY: I guess it would be an 8 or 9 in terms of results, but I'm not relaxed, that would be about 3. I do a good job of catching my mistakes as long as I'm not worrying too much, so that would be an 8, and I'd say a 9 or 10 on knowing my limits.

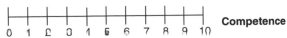

Incompetence	Competence
Screws everything up.	Doing hard tasks well and getting good results.
Doesn't do anything right.	
Doesn't care whether it is right.	Being relaxed while doing tasks.
Doesn't care how he looks to others.	Not worrying re tasks afterwards.
You can't expect results.	Catching and correcting mistakes.
	Knowing his limits.

FIGURE 2.5. "Continuum" of competence.

THERAPIST: How would you rate your skiing?

GARY: That would be a 6 but it doesn't matter, I just do it for fun.

THERAPIST: So I hear several important points. First, when you think it over, competence turns out not to be all or nothing. Someone who's not perfect isn't necessarily incompetent. Second, the characteristics you see as being signs of competence don't necessarily hang together real well. You rate an 8 or 9 in terms of the quality of your work but a 3 in being relaxed and not worrying. Finally, there are times, such as when you're at work, when being competent is very important to you and other times, like skiing, when its not very important.

GARY: Yeah, I guess I don't have to be at my peak all the time.

THERAPIST: What do you think of this idea that if a person's competent they'll be relaxed and if they're tense that means they're not competent?

GARY: I don't know.

THERAPIST: It certainly seems that if a person's sure they can handle the situation they're likely to be less tense about it. But I don't know about the flip side, the idea that if you're tense, that proves you're incompetent. When you're tense and worried does that make it easier for you to do well or harder for you to do well?

GARY: It makes it a lot harder for me to do well. I have trouble concentrating and keep forgetting things.

THERAPIST: So if someone does well despite being tense and worried, they're overcoming an obstacle.

GARY: Yeah, they are.

THERAPIST: Some people would argue that doing well despite having to overcome obstacles shows greater capabilities than doing well when things are easy. What do you think of that idea?

GARY: It makes sense to me.

THERAPIST: Now, you've been doing a good job at work despite being real tense and worried. Up to this point you've been taking your tenseness as proof that you're really incompetent and have just been getting by because you're real careful. This other way of looking at it would say that being able to do well despite being anxious shows that you really are competent, not that you're incompetent. Which do you think is closer to the truth?

GARY: I guess maybe I'm pretty capable after all, but I still hate being so tense.

THERAPIST: Of course, and we'll keep working on that, but the key point is that being tense doesn't necessarily mean you're incompetent. Now, another place where you feel tense and think you're incompetent is in social situations. Let's see if you're as incompetent as you feel there . . .

Once Gary accepted the idea that his ability to handle stressful situations well despite his stress and anxiety was actually a sign of his capabilities rather than being a sign of incompetence, his sense of self-efficacy increased substantially. Following this increase in self-efficacy, he was substantially less defensive and was more willing to disclose his thoughts and feelings in therapy. He also was more willing to look critically at his beliefs and assumptions and to test new approaches to problem situations. This made it possible to use standard cognitive techniques with greater effectiveness.

Another series of interventions used particularly effectively with Gary was using the continuum technique to challenge his dichotomous view of trustworthiness, then introducing the idea that he could learn which persons were likely to prove trustworthy by noticing how well they followed through when trusted on trivial issues. As he reexamined the trustworthiness of the people with whom he interacted, Gary concluded that his family members were truly malicious and deceptive but that they were not typical of people in general. He was able to gradually test his negative view of others' intentions by trusting colleagues and acquaintances in small things and observing their performance. He was pleasantly surprised to discover that the world at large was much less malevolent than he had assumed, that it contained benevolent and indifferent people as well as malevolent ones, and that on those occasions when he was treated badly he could deal with the situation effectively.

Concurrently with these primarily cognitive interventions, it was important to work to modify Gary's dysfunctional interpersonal interactions so that he would be less likely to provoke hostile reactions from others which would support his paranoid views. This required focusing on specific problem situations as they arose and identifying and addressing the cognitions which blocked appropriate assertion. These included, "It won't do any good," "They'll just get mad," and "If they know what I want, they'll use that against me." It was also necessary to work to improve Gary's skills in assertion and clear communication through assertion training. When this resulted in improvements in his relationships with colleagues and in his relationship with his girlfriend, it was fairly easy to use guided discovery to help him recognize the ways in which his previous interaction style had inadvertently provoked hostility from others.

THERAPIST: So it sounds like speaking up for yourself directly has been working out pretty well. How do the other people seem to feel about it?

GARY: Pretty good I guess. Sue and I have been getting along fine and things have been less tense at work.

THERAPIST: That's interesting. I remember that one of your concerns was that people might get mad if you spoke up for yourself. It sounds as though it might be helping things go better instead.

GARY: Well, I've had a few run-ins but they've blown over pretty quickly.

THERAPIST: That's a change from the way things used to be right there. Before, if you had a run-in with somebody it would bug you for a long time. Do you have any idea what's made the difference?

GARY: Not really. It just doesn't seem to stay on my mind as long.

THERAPIST: Could you fill me in on one of the run-ins you had this week?

GARY: (*Discusses a disagreement with his boss in detail.*)

THERAPIST: It sounds like two things were different from the old way of handling this sort of situation, you stuck with the discussion rather than leaving angry and you let him know what was bugging you. Do you think that had anything to do with it blowing over more quickly than usual?

GARY: It might.

THERAPIST: It works that way for a lot of people. If it turns out to work that way for you that would be another payoff to speaking up directly. If they go along with what you want there's no problem and if they don't, at least it blows over more quickly. Do you remember how you used to feel after leaving a disagreement unresolved?.

GARY: I'd think about it for days. I'd be tense and jumpy and little things would bug me a lot.

THERAPIST: How do you think it was for the people at work?

GARY: They'd be pretty tense and jumpy too. Nobody'd want to talk to each other for a while.

THERAPIST: That makes it sound like it would be easy for a little mistake or misunderstanding to set off another disagreement.

GARY: I think you're right.

THERAPIST: You know, it seems pretty reasonable for a person to assume that the way to have as little conflict and tension as possible is to avoid speaking up about things that bug him and to try not to let his aggravation show but it doesn't seem to work that way for you. So far it sounds like when you speak up about things that bug you, there are fewer conflicts and the conflicts that happen blow over more quickly.

GARY: Yeah.

THERAPIST: Do you think that your attempts to keep from aggravating people may have actually made things more tense?

GARY: It sounds like it.

Toward the close of therapy, it was possible to further improve Gary's understanding of others and his interpersonal skills by working to help him to better understand the perspectives of others and to empathize with them. This was done through asking questions which required Gary to anticipate the impact of his actions on others, to consider how he would feel if the roles were reversed, or to infer the thoughts and feelings of the other person from their actions and then to examine the correspondence between his conclusions and the available data. Initially Gary found these types of questions difficult to answer, but as he received feedback both from the therapist and from subsequent interactions with the individuals in question, his ability to grasp the other person's perspective increased steadily. Gary discovered that aggravating actions by others were not necessarily motivated by malicious intentions, that understanding the other person's point of view often made situations less aggravating, and that this increased his ability to deal effectively with interpersonal conflicts.

At the close of therapy, Gary was noticeably more relaxed and was only bothered by symptoms of stress and anxiety at times when it is common to experience mild symptoms, such as immediately before major examinations. He reported being much more comfortable with friends and colleagues, was socializing more actively, and seemed to feel no particular need to be vigilant. When he and his girlfriend began having difficulties, due in part to her discomfort with the increasing closeness in their relationship, he was able to suspend his initial feelings of rejection and his desire to retaliate long enough to consider her point of view. He then was able to take a major role in resolving their difficulties by communicating his understanding of her concerns ("I know that after all you've been through it's pretty scary when we start talking about marriage"), acknowledging his own fears and doubts ("I get pretty nervous about this too"), and expressing his commitment to their relationship ("I don't want this to tear us apart"). Thus this approach to intervention resulted both in substantial improvement in his presenting problems and in substantial changes in the way in which he related to others. He continued to maintain these improvements when he returned to therapy briefly several years later for help in dealing with his girlfriend's excessive drinking and conflicting feelings over a career change.

Differential Treatment for Personality Disorders

It is important to note that the intervention approach used with Gary is specific to paranoid personality disorder. Because cognitive therapy sees each personality disorder as embodying a distinct set of schemas, assumptions, and interpersonal strategies, there are important differences in the intervention approaches used with each. For example, Fleming presents a view of histrionic personality disorder (Beck et al., 1990, Chap. 10; Beck et al., 2004; Fleming, 1983, 1988; Freeman et al., 1990, Chap. 9) which hypothesizes that a history of being rewarded from an early age for enacting certain roles rather than for competence or ability results in the individual learning to focus attention on the playing of roles and "performing" for others rather than on developing his or her own capabilities. As a consequence, the individual comes to assume, "I am inadequate and unable to handle life on my own," and "It is necessary to be loved and approved of by everyone," and to have a very strong fear of rejection.

Fleming argues that histrionic individuals' learning histories result in their adopting interpersonal strategies which account for much of the histrionic's dysfunctional behavior. Because they have been rewarded for the enactment of certain roles rather than for careful observation and planning, they attempt to interact with others on the basis of stereotyped roles rather than systematically planning ways to please or impress their audience. When problems arise, the histrionic's fear of disapproval and rejection leads to indirect manipulation rather than assertive responses. However, because the approval of others is assumed to be a dire necessity, the histrionic is quick to become desperate if these methods seem to be failing and to resort to threats, coercion, and temper tantrums as desperation overcomes fear of rejection. This extreme approach to interpersonal relationships is often effective enough to maintain lasting, if tempestuous, relationships. The histrionic's preoccupation with relationships leads him or her to focus predominantly on interpersonal stimuli while his or her tendency to rely on role enactment and manipulation rather than analysis and planning in dealing with problems results in a characteristic thought style which is global, impressionistic, and vivid but is lacking in detail and focus. Global, impressionistic thoughts about interpersonal interactions lead to dramatic reactions which can be intense, labile, and difficult to control, leaving the person subject to explosive outbursts. The resulting difficulties in coping effectively with problem situations further strengthen the histrionic's belief that he or she is inadequate to cope with life alone and needs to rely on the help of others.

Cognitive therapy with histrionic personality disorder is complicated by the fact that the histrionic patient comes to therapy with an approach to life which is diametrically opposed to the systematic, problem-solving approach typically used by cognitive-behavioral therapists. Fleming argues that with such different basic styles, both the therapist and the patient can find therapy quite difficult and frustrating, but she also argues that, if it is possible to bridge this difference in styles, the skills required simply to take part in therapy can constitute an important and useful part of the treatment. She proposes a treatment approach that involves extensive attention to manifestations of the client's histrionic interpersonal style within the therapist relationship, the gradual shaping of effective problem-solving skills, and the development of a more adaptive approach to interpersonal relationships and emphasizes the interplay between cognitive and interpersonal factors:

> Challenging their immediate thoughts may not be sufficient, however, since histrionic individuals so often use emotional outbursts to as a way to manipulate situations. Thus, if a woman with [histrionic personality disorder] has a tantrum because her husband came home late from work, her immediate thoughts may include, "How can he do this to me? He doesn't love me any more! I'll die if he leaves me!" As a result of her tantrum, however, she may well receive violent protestations of his undying love for her which satisfy her desire for reassurance. Thus, in addition to directly challenging her thoughts when she gets emotionally upset, she also needs to learn to ask herself, "What do I really want now?" and explore alternative options for achieving this.
>
> Once patients can learn to stop reacting and to determine what they want out of the situation (which, with histrionic patients, is often reassurance and

attention), they can apply their problem-solving skills by exploring the various methods for achieving that goal and looking at the advantages and disadvantages of each. Thus, rather than automatically having a temper tantrum, they are confronted with a choice between having a temper tantrum and trying other alternatives. (Beck et al., 1990, p. 228)

Thus, despite a shared theoretical framework and therapeutic approach, cognitive therapy with histrionic personality disorder differs from cognitive therapy with paranoid personality disorder in many ways. Discussion of cognitive therapy's conceptualizations of each of the personality disorders and proposed approaches to intervention with each is beyond the scope of this chapter. The interested reader is referred to Beck et al. (2003) or Freeman et al. (2004) for detailed discussions of cognitive therapy with each of the personality disorders.

EMPIRICAL EVALUATION

In examining the empirical status of the cognitive approach to personality disorders there are two important areas to consider. One is empirical evidence regarding the validity of cognitive conceptualizations of personality disorders and the second is empirical evidence regarding the effectiveness of cognitive therapy as a treatment for individuals with personality disorders. While the ideal would be for a particular approach to any area of psychopathology to provide both a valid conceptualization and an effective approach to treatment, the two do not necessarily go hand in hand.

The Validity of Cognitive Conceptualizations of Personality Disorder

Cognitive conceptualizations of personality disorders are of recent vintage, and, consequently, only limited research into the validity of these conceptualizations has been reported thus far. Two early studies examined the relationship between dysfunctional cognitions and personality disorders. O'Leary et al. (1991) examined the role of dysfunctional beliefs and assumptions in borderline personality disorder. The borderline's scores on a measure of dysfunctional beliefs were significantly higher than those of the normal controls and were among the highest of any diagnostic group reported previously. Furthermore, the borderlines' scores were not related to the presence or absence of a concurrent major depression, to history of a previous major depression, or to clinical status. In another study, Gasperini et al. (1989) investigated the relationship between mood disorders, personality disorders, automatic thoughts, and coping strategies. The relationships among diagnostic status and the measures of automatic thoughts and coping strategies were then explored through factor analyses. These analyses revealed that the first factor which emerged from the factor analysis of Automatic Thoughts Questionnaire (Hollon & Kendall, 1980) and Self-Control Schedule (Rosenbaum, 1980) items reflected the presence of a "Cluster B" personality disorder (narcissistic, histrionic, borderline, and antisocial) while the second factor reflected the presence of a "Cluster C" personality disorder (compulsive, dependent, avoidant, and passive–aggressive). Although "Cluster A" personality disorders (paranoid, schizoid, and schizotypal) were unrelated to any of the factors which emerged from the factor analysis, few subjects received Cluster A diagnoses and the lack of relationship could easily be due to small sample size alone. Both of these studies provide support for the general proposition that dysfunctional cognitions play a role in personality disorders. Unfortunately, they have only a very limited bearing on the theoretical model presented in this chapter which hypothesizes more specific relationships between dysfunctional beliefs and each of the personality disorders.

Recent studies have examined the relationships between the sets of beliefs hypothesized to play a role in each of the personality disorders (Beck et al., 1990; Beck et al., 2003; Freeman et al., 1990) and diagnostic status. These hypotheses have been supported for borderline personality disorder (Arntz, Dietzel, & Dreessen, 1999) and for avoidant, dependent, obsessive–compulsive, narcissistic, and paranoid personality disorders (Beck et al., 2001). The other personality disorders were not studied due to an inadequate number of subjects. These findings support the hypothesis that dysfunctional beliefs are related to personality disorders in ways that are consistent with cognitive theory but do not provide grounds for conclusions about causality or about the effectiveness of cognitive therapy as a treatment for individuals with personality disorders.

The Effectiveness of Cognitive Therapy with Personality Disorders

Cognitive therapy has been found to provide effective treatment for a wide range of Axis I disorders. However, research into the effectiveness of cognitive-behavioral approaches to treating individuals with personality disorders is more limited. Table 2.5 provides an overview of the available evidence regarding the effectiveness of cognitive-behavioral interventions with individuals diagnosed as having personality disorders. It is immediately apparent from this table that there have been many uncontrolled clinical reports which assert that cognitive-behavioral therapy can provide

TABLE 2.5. The Effectiveness of Cognitive-Behavioral Treatment with Personality Disorders

	Uncontrolled clinical reports	Single-case design studies	Effects of personality disorders on treatment outcome	Outcome studies
Antisocial[a]	+	−	+	[a]
Avoidant	+	+	±	±
Borderline	±	−	+	+
Dependent	+	+	+	
Histrionic	+		−	
Narcissistic	+	+		
Obsessive–compulsive	+	−		
Paranoid	+	+		
Passive–aggressive	+		+	
Schizoid	+			
Schizotypal				

Note. + Cognitive-behavioral interventions found to be effective; − cognitive-behavioral interventions found not to be effective; ± mixed findings.
[a] Cognitive-behavioral interventions were effective with antisocial personality disorder subjects only when the individual was depressed at pretest.

effective treatment for personality disorders. However, there are only a limited number of controlled outcome studies to provide support for these assertions. This has led some to be concerned about the risks associated with a rapid expansion of theory and practice which has outstripped the empirical research (Dobson & Pusch, 1993).

Effects of Comorbid Personality Disorders on the Treatment of Axis I Disorders

A number of studies have examined the effectiveness of cognitive-behavioral treatment for Axis I disorders in subjects who are also diagnosed as having personality disorders. A number of studies have found that the presence of an Axis II diagnosis greatly decreases the likelihood of treatment's being effective. For example, Turner (1987) found that socially phobic patients without personality disorders improved markedly after a 15-week group treatment for social phobia and maintained their gains at a 1-year follow-up. However, patients with personality disorder diagnoses in addition to social phobia showed little or no improvement both posttreatment and at the 1-year follow-up. Similarly, Mavissakalian and Hamman (1987) found that 75% of agoraphobic subjects rated as being low in personality disorder characteristics responded well to a time-limited behavioral and pharmacological treatment for agoraphobia, while only 25% of the subjects rated as being high in personality disorder characteristics responded to this treatment. Other studies have found that subjects with personality disorders in addition to their Axis I problems respond to cognitive-behavioral treatment but respond more slowly (Marchand, Goyer, Dupuis, & Mainguy, 1998).

However, the evidence regarding of the impact of comorbid personality disorders on the treatment of Axis I disorders is more complex than this. Some studies have found that the presence of personality disorder diagnoses did not influence outcome (Dreesen, Arntz, Luttels, & Sallaerts, 1994; Mersch, Jansen, & Arntz, 1995) or that subjects with personality disorder diagnoses present with more severe symptomatology but respond equally well to treatment (Mersch et al., 1995). Other studies have found that personality disorder diagnoses influenced outcome only under certain conditions (Fahy, Eisler, & Russell, 1993; Felske, Perry, Chambless, Renneberg, & Goldstein, 1996; Hardy et al., 1995), that clients with personality disorders are likely to terminate treatment prematurely but that those who persist in treatment can be treated effectively (Persons et al., 1988; Sanderson, Beck, & McGinn, 1994), and that some personality disorders predicted poor outcome while others did not (Neziroglu, McKay, Todaro, & Yaryura-Tobias, 1996). Kuyken, Kurzer, DeRubeis, Beck, and Brown (2001) found that it was not the presence of a personality disorder diagnosis per se that predicted outcome but the presence of maladaptive avoidant and paranoid beliefs.

Some studies provide evidence that focused treatment for Axis I disorders can have beneficial effects on comorbid Axis II disorders as well. For example, Mavissakalian and Hamman (1987) found that four of seven subjects who initially met diagnostic criteria for a single personality disorder diagnosis no longer met criteria for a personality disorder diagnosis following treatment for agoraphobia. In contrast, subjects diagnosed as having more than one personality disorder did not show similar improvement. Rathus, Sanderson, Miller, and Wetzler (1995) found that patients with elevated scores on personality disorder subscales of the Millon Clinical Multiaxial Inventory—II responded to treatment as well as patients without such elevations and that all subjects showed lower elevations on these MCMI-II scales following treatment.

One major limitation of the studies that have examined the effectiveness of cognitive-behavioral treatment for Axis I disorders with individuals who also have personality disorders is that the treatment approaches used in these studies typically did not take the presence of personality disorders into account. This leaves unanswered the question whether treatment protocols designed to account for the presence of personality disorders would prove to be more effective.

Studies of Cognitive-Behavioral Treatment of Axis II Disorders

A number of studies have focused specifically on cognitive-behavioral treatment of individuals with personality disorders. Turkat and Maisto (1985) used a series of single-case design studies to investigate the effectiveness of individualized cognitive-behavioral treatment for personality disorders. Their study provides evidence that some clients with personality disorders could be treated effectively, but the investigators were unsuccessful in treating many of the subjects in their study. A recent study has attempted to test the efficacy of the intervention approach advocated by Beck et al. (1990) using a series of single-case studies with repeated measures (Nelson-Gray, Johnson, Foyle, Daniel, & Harmon, 1996). The nine subjects for this study were diagnosed with major depressive disorder and one or more co-occurring personality disorders. Each subject was assessed pretherapy, posttherapy, and at a 3-month follow-up for level of depression and for the number of diagnostic criteria present for their primary personality disorder. After receiving 12 weeks of treatment, six of the eight subjects who completed the 3-month follow-up manifested a significant decrease in level of depression, two subjects manifested a significant decrease on both measures of personality disorder symptomatology, two failed to show improvement on either measure, and four showed mixed results. As the authors note, 12 weeks of treatment is a much shorter course of treatment than Beck et al. (1990) would expect to be required for most clients with personality disorders. Springer, Lohr, Buchtel, and Silk (1995) report that a short-term cognitive-behavioral therapy group produced significant improvement in a sample of hospitalized subjects with various personality disorders and that a secondary analysis of a subset of subjects with borderline personality disorder revealed similar findings. They also report that clients evaluated the group as being useful in their life outside the hospital.

At least three personality disorders have been the subject of controlled outcome studies. In a study of the treatment of opiate addicts in a methadone maintenance program, Woody, McLellan, Luborsky, and O'Brien (1985) found that subjects who met DSM-III diagnostic criteria for both major depression and antisocial personality disorder responded well to both cognitive therapy and a supportive–expressive psychotherapy systematized by Luborsky, McLellan, Woody, O'Brien, and Auerbach (1985). The subjects showed statistically significant improvement on 11 of 22 outcome variables used, including psychiatric symptoms, drug use, employment, and illegal activity. Subjects who met criteria for antisocial personality disorder but not major depression showed little response to treatment, improving on only 3 of 22 variables. This pattern of results was maintained at a 7-month follow-up. While subjects not diagnosed as antisocial personality disorder responded to treatment better than the sociopaths did, sociopaths who were initially depressed did only slightly worse than the nonsociopaths while the nondepressed sociopaths did much worse.

Studies of the treatment of avoidant personality disorder have shown that short-term social skills training and social skills training combined with cognitive interventions have been effective in increasing the frequency of social interaction and decreasing social anxiety (Stravynski, Marks, & Yule, 1982). Stravynski et al. (1982) interpreted this finding as demonstrating the "lack of value" of cognitive interventions. However, it should be noted that the two treatments were equally effective, that all treatments were provided by a single therapist (who was also principal investigator), and that only one of many possible cognitive interventions (disputation of irrational beliefs) was used. In a subsequent study, Greenberg and Stravynski (1985) report that the avoidant client's fear of ridicule appears to contribute to premature termination in many cases, and they suggest that interventions which modify relevant aspects of the clients' cognitions might add substantially to the effectiveness of intervention.

Linehan and her colleagues (Linehan, Armstrong, Suarez, Allmon, & Heard, 1991; Linehan, Heard, & Armstrong, 1993; Linehan, Heard, & Armstrong, 1993) have conducted an outcome study of Linehan's cognitive-behavioral approach, which she terms dialectical behavior therapy (DBT), with a sample of chronically parasuicidal borderline subjects. The patients in the DBT condition had a significantly lower rate of premature termination of therapy, significantly less self-injurious behavior, and a significantly lower rate of hospitalization at the close of 1 year of treatment than did a control group which received "treatment as usual" in the community. The two groups showed equivalent improvement in depression and other symptomatology. While these results are modest, it is important to note that this study was conducted with a sample of subjects who not only met diagnostic criteria for borderline personality disorder but who also were chronically parasuicidal, had histories of multiple psychiatric hospitalizations, and were unable to maintain employment due to their psychiatric symptoms. A subsequent replication by Koons et al. (2001) using a sample with a less extreme history of self-mutilation showed a significantly greater decreases in suicidal ideation, hopelessness, depression, and anger expression than did a "treatment as usual" control condition.

While evidence of the effectiveness of DBT is encouraging, there are important conceptual and procedural differences between the two treatment approaches. A more direct test of the effectiveness of cognitive therapy as a treatment for individuals with borderline personality disorder is provided by Brown, Newman, Charlesworth, Crits-Cristoph, and Beck (2004). In this open clinical trial, 32 patients with borderline personality disorder accompanied by suicidality or self-mutilation received 1 year of weekly cognitive therapy for borderline personality disorder (Layden, Newman, Freeman, & Morse, 1993). The year of treatment resulted in significant decreases in suicidal ideation, reports of self-injury, hopelessness, depression, number of borderline symptoms, and dysfunctional beliefs. These improvements were maintained 6 months following the termination of treatment. Ratings by independent diagnosticians showed that only 48% of the sample (14 of 29) still met DSM-IV criteria for borderline personality disorder when treatment was terminated after 1 year. Only 16% (4 of 24) still met DSM-IV criteria upon follow-up 6 months later. Based on these data it appears that patients are able to integrate their therapeutic experiences over time and continue to progress after the termination of therapy, thus increasing the long-term impact of cognitive therapy. If these results are substantiated by a subsequent randomized, controlled study, they will be quite encouraging.

Comparisons with Other Treatment Approaches

Little research is available which compares cognitive therapy with other approaches to the treatment of individuals with personality disorders. In a study of the treatment of heroin addicts with and without antisocial personality disorder, Woody et al. (1985) found that both cognitive therapy and supportive–expressive psychotherapy were effective for antisocial subjects who were depressed at the beginning of treatment and that neither approach was effective with antisocial subjects who were not depressed. In a large, multisite outcome study, the National Institute of Mental Health Treatment of Depression Collaborative Program found a nonsignificant trend for patients with personality disorders to do slightly better than other patients in cognitive therapy while they did worse than other patients in interpersonal psychotherapy and pharmacotherapy (Shea et al., 1990). Finally, Hardy et al. (1995) found that individuals with Cluster B personality disorders had significantly poorer outcomes in interpersonal psychotherapy than in cognitive therapy (they did not assess Cluster A or Cluster C personality disorders). Clearly, these three studies are encouraging but do not provide adequate grounds for drawing conclusions about how cognitive therapy compares with other treatments for individuals with personality disorders.

The Effect of Personality Disorders
on "Real-Life" Clinical Practice

In clinical practice, most therapists do not apply a standardized treatment protocol with a homogeneous sample of individuals who share a common diagnosis. Instead, clinicians face a variety of clients and take an individualized approach to treatment. A recent study of the effectiveness of cognitive therapy under such "real world" conditions provides important support for the clinical use of cognitive therapy with clients who are diagnosed as having personality disorders. Persons et al. (1988) conducted an interesting empirical study of clients receiving cognitive therapy for depression in private practice settings. The subjects were 70 consecutive individuals seeking treatment from Dr. Burns or Dr. Persons in their own practices. Both therapists are established cognitive therapists who have taught and published extensively and in this study both therapists conducted cognitive therapy as they normally do. This meant that treatment was open-ended, it was individualized rather than standardized, and medication and inpatient treatment were used as needed.

The primary focus of the study was on identifying predictors of dropout and treatment outcome in cognitive therapy for depression. However, it is interesting for our purposes to note that 54.3% of the subjects met DSM-III criteria for a personality disorder diagnosis and that the investigators considered the presence of a personality disorder diagnosis as a potential predictor of both premature termination of therapy and therapy outcome. The investigators found that while patients with personality disorders were significantly more likely to drop out of therapy prematurely than were patients without personality disorders, those patients with personality disorder diagnoses who persisted in therapy through the completion of treatment showed substantial improvement and did not differ significantly in degree of improvement from patients without personality disorders. Similar findings were reported by Sanderson et al. (1994) in a study of cognitive therapy for generalized anxiety disorder. Subjects diagnosed with a comorbid personality disorder were more likely to drop out of treatment, but treatment was effective in reducing both anxiety and depression for those who completed a minimum course of treatment.

Implications for Clinical Practice

The past two decades have seen advances in theory and practice regarding cognitive therapy with personality disorders which outstrip the empirical research (Dobson & Pusch, 1993). While this provides grounds for legitimate concern, it is hardly be feasible to suspend theoretical and clinical work until more empirical research is available. The practicing clinician faces a difficult situation in that one can hardly refuse to provide treatment for a class of disorders which may be present in as many as 50% of clients seen in many outpatient settings. Fortunately, while the available treatment approaches are less fully developed and less well validated than is the case for cognitive therapy with many of the Axis I disorders, there is a growing body of evidence which shows that cognitive-behavioral treatment can be effective for clients with personality disorders.

FUTURE DIRECTIONS

Clearly, cognitive therapy for personality disorders is still under development and is in need of continued theoretical refinement, clinical innovation, and empirical research. With some personality disorders, such as paranoid personality disorder, cognitive conceptualizations have been developed in considerable detail and specific treatment approaches have been proposed. These disorders are ripe for empirical tests of the validity of the conceptualization, of the overall effectiveness of the proposed treatment approach, and of the effects of particular interventions. With other personality disorders, such as schizotypal personality disorder, both the conceptualization and the treatment approach are much less developed and would need further refinement in order to be suitable for empirical testing.

While research to test the effectiveness of cognitive therapy as a treatment for individuals with a number of personality disorders is under way, more than simple outcome studies is needed. Evidence of the effectiveness of a given treatment approach does not necessarily demonstrate the validity of the conceptualization on which the treatment is based or suggest ways in which the treatment approach can be improved. If the cognitive perspective on personality disorders is to advance, it will be important to test specific hypotheses derived from cognitive conceptualizations of each of the personality disorders. It is only through such hypothesis testing that it will be possible to identify the conceptual deficiencies of our current models and refine them into conceptualizations which facilitate more effective intervention.

Empirical tests of the actual effects of the particular intervention approaches have much potential for increasing the effectiveness of cognitive therapy with personality disorders. For example, it has been suggested that the use of the "continuum technique" to counteract dichotomous thinking in clients with borderline personality disorder can decrease the intensity of borderlines' remarkable mood swings and can facilitate other interventions (Beck et al., 1990, pp. 199–201; Freeman et al., 1990,

p. 198). An empirical test of the degree to which this intervention actually produces the desired results and an investigation of conditions which may facilitate or block the technique's effects could be quite useful in refining treatment recommendations. Many other specific cognitive, behavioral, and interpersonal intervention techniques have been recommended in various discussions of cognitive therapy with personality disorders. An empirically based understanding of the effects of various interventions and the factors which influence their effectiveness would be quite useful to the therapist who is faced with the dilemma of choosing between many possible interventions or who must choose the most promising time to attempt a given intervention.

One area that needs theoretical attention and empirical investigation is the question of how to best conceptualize and treat individuals who are diagnosed as having mixed personality disorder or who satisfy diagnostic criteria for more than one personality disorder. This issue has received little explicit attention, and it is not at all clear if one can best conceptualize and treat an individual who meets DSM-IV criteria for both paranoid personality disorder and histrionic personality disorder, for example, simply by combining the conceptualizations and treatment approaches which have been developed for each disorder separately. If it is possible to develop a comprehensive cognitive typology of the personality disorders, it could simplify the task of exploring the similarities and differences among the personality disorders and could make it easier to develop clear conceptualizations of individuals who merit more than one personality disorder diagnosis.

One impediment to empirical research on personality disorders is the difficulty of using traditional research designs which require one to assemble a large, homogeneous sample of subjects. The practical problems encountered in attempting to assemble a group of individuals with a given personality disorder and then to collect detailed data regarding their cognitions and behavior can be substantial. Turkat and his colleagues (see Turkat, 1990; Turkat & Maisto, 1985) have broken important new ground by presenting an innovative single-case experimental design which has proven useful in developing and testing cognitive-behavioral conceptualizations of clients with personality disorders. In their approach, a thorough clinical assessment is used as a basis for developing a detailed formulation of a particular individual's problems. Specific hypotheses based on this conceptualization are then generated and tested using the most appropriate available measures. Positive results from this hypothesis testing are interpreted as validating the conceptualization, while negative results are used to identify portions of the conceptualization which are in need of revision. Finally, a treatment plan is developed on the basis of this case formulation and as treatment is implemented, successful interventions are seen as validating the case formulation while unsuccessful interventions are taken as indicating a need for reevaluation of the case formulation. This experimental method reduces many of the practical problems encountered in trying to assemble a homogeneous sample of individuals with the same personality disorder as well as the logistical problems encountered when attempting to conduct detailed data collection on a large sample of individuals who may well be in need of immediate treatment. At the same time, it avoids many of the biases that can creep into unstructured clinical exploration. While this type of experimental design will not replace traditional nomothetic research, it can provide a practical method for developing and refining conceptualizations of specific personality disorders which can then be tested more conclusively using more traditional experimental designs.

A second impediment to research into the cognitive approach to personality disorders, as well as into other areas, is the tendency of cognitive-behavioral researchers to rely on simple self-report questionnaires as the primary means of assessing cognitive variables. As noted earlier, the use of self-report questionnaires presumes that respondents both are capable of accurately reporting the desired information and are willing to do so. These assumptions may be valid in a one-on-one psychotherapeutic relationship where the client can receive training in monitoring and reporting cognitions, where it is to the client's advantage to provide the therapist with the information needed for effective intervention, and where any inconsistencies within the clients' reports of their cognitions or discrepancies between reports of cognitions and reports of emotions and behavior can be explored. However, self-report measures of cognitions have often been used for research purposes without subjects receiving training in monitoring and reporting cognitions, with responses being based on recollection rather than self-monitoring, without an incentive for subjects to provide uncensored reports of their cognitions, and/or without any attention to inconsistencies within the reports or discrepancies between reports of cognitions and other data. Clearly, more attention to obtaining valid measures of cognitive variables could do much to advance cognitive-behavioral research in many areas.

The wider application of laboratory methods used in basic research into cognitive processes to research on clinically relevant topics has considerable potential for providing more valid and more objective measures of cognitive variables. For example, recent studies have successfully used the Stroop color-naming task to investigate selective processing of threat cues in panic disorder (McNally, Riemann, & Kim, 1990), to examine cognitive aspects of posttraumatic stress disorder (Cassiday, McNally, & Zeitlin, 1992), and to assess the self-schema in an individual diagnosed as having a multiple personality (Scott, 1992). Other examples of promising approaches are the use of measures of eye fixation (Matthews & Antes, 1992) and performance on dichotic listening tasks (Klinger, 1978) to investigate attentional biases and the use of thought-sampling procedures (Hurlburt, Leach, & Saltman, 1984) to obtain more accurate data regarding the content of an individual's thoughts. These sorts of methods for measuring cognition without relying exclusively on self-report questionnaires have much potential for advancing cognitive-behavioral research.

Given the prevalence of personality disorders and the consensus that treatment of clients with personality disorders is difficult and complex no matter what treatment approach is used, it is clearly important that these disorders be a continued focus of empirical research, theoretical innovation, and clinical experimentation. For the time being, treatment recommendations based on clinical observation and a limited empirical base are the best that cognitive therapy can offer to clinicians who must try to work with personality disorder clients today rather than waiting for empirically validated treatment protocols to be developed at some point in the future. Fortunately, the authors' experience has been that when cognitive-behavioral interventions are based on an individualized conceptualization of the client's problems and the interpersonal aspects of therapy receive sufficient attention, many clients with personality disorders can be treated quite effectively.

NOTES

1. A number of different cognitive and cognitive-behavioral approaches to therapy have been developed in recent years. While these various approaches have much in common, there are important conceptual and technical differences among them. To minimize confusion, the specific approach developed by Aaron T. Beck and his colleagues will be referred to as "cognitive therapy," whereas the term "cognitive-behavioral" will be used to refer to the full range of cognitive and cognitive-behavioral approaches.
2. A variety of methods are available for increasing the validity and usefulness of self reports. For an overview, see Freeman, Pretzer, Fleming, and Simon (1990, Chap. 2).
3. It is important to note that individuals are not necessarily aware of automatic thoughts as they occur and that when they do become aware of the automatic thoughts, these thoughts typically are so plausible that the individual does not think of examining them critically.
4. The term "self-efficacy" refers to expectations regarding one's ability to deal effectively with a specific situation (Bandura, 1977). An individual's level of self-efficacy regarding a particular situation is believed to have an important effect both on the individual's anxiety level and his or her coping behavior in that situation.

REFERENCES

Alford, B. A., & Beck, A. T. (1997). *The integrative power of cognitive therapy.* New York: Guilford Press.

Alford, B. A., & Norcross, J. C. (1991). Cognitive therapy as integrative therapy. *Journal of Psychotherapy Integration, 1,* 175–190.

American Psychiatric Association. (1987). *Diagnostic and statistical manual of mental disorders* (3rd ed., rev.). Washington, DC: American Psychiatric Association.

American Psychiatric Association. (2000). *Diagnostic and statistical manual of mental disorders* (4th ed., text rev.). Washington, DC: American Psychiatric Association.

Arntz, A., Dietzel, R., & Dreessen, L. (1999). Assumptions in borderline personality disorder: Specificity, stability and relationship with etiological factors. *Behaviour Research and Therapy, 37,* 545–557.

Bandura, A. (1977). *Social learning theory.* Englewood Cliffs, NJ: Prentice Hall.

Beck, A. T. (1964). Thinking and depression: 2. Theory and therapy. *Archives of General Psychiatry, 10,* 561–571.

Beck, A. T. (1967). *Depression: Clinical, experimental, and theoretical aspects.* New York: Harper & Row. (Reprinted as *Depression: Causes and treatment.* Philadelphia: University of Pennsylvania Press, 1972)

Beck, A. T. (1991). Cognitive therapy as *the* integrative therapy: Comments on Alford and Norcross. *Journal of Psychotherapy Integration, 1,* 191–198.

Beck, A. T. (1992). Personality disorders (and their relationship to syndromal disorders). *Across-Species Comparisons and Psychiatry Newsletter, 5,* 3–13.

Beck, A. T., Butler, A. C., Brown, G. K., Dahlsgaard, K. K., Newman, C. F. & Beck, J. S. (2001). Dysfunctional beliefs discriminate personality disorders. *Behaviour Research and Therapy, 39,* 1213–1225.

Beck, A. T., Freeman, A., & Associates. (1990). *Cognitive therapy of personality disorders.* New York: Guilford Press.

Beck, A. T., Freeman, A., Davis, D. D., & Associates. (2004). *Cognitive therapy of personality disorders* (2nd ed.). New York: Guilford Press.

Beck, A. T., Rush, A. J., Shaw, B. F., & Emery, G. (1979). *Cognitive therapy of depression.* New York: Guilford Press.

Beck, J. S. (1995). *Cognitive therapy: Basics and beyond.* New York: Guilford Press.

Bedrosian, R. C., & Bozicas, G. D. (1994). *Treating family of origin problems: A cognitive approach.* New York: Guilford Press.

Black, D. W., Yates, W. R., Noyes, R., Pfohl, B., & Kelley, M. (1989). DSM-III personality disorder in obsessive compulsive study volunteers: A controlled study. *Journal of Personality Disorders, 3,* 58–62.

Brown, G. K., Newman, C. F., Charlesworth, S. E., Crits-Cristoph, P., & Beck, A. T. (2004). An open clinical trial of cognitive therapy for borderline personality disorder. *Journal of Personality Disorders, 18,* 257–271.

Cassiday, K. L., McNally, R. J., & Zeitlin, S. B. (1992). Cognitive processing of trauma cues in rape victims with post-traumatic stress disorder. *Cognitive Therapy and Research, 16,* 283–295.

108   MAJOR THEORIES OF PERSONALITY DISORDER

Cone, J. D., & Hawkins, R. P. (1977). *Behavioral assessment: New directions in clinical psychology.* New York: Bruner/Mazel.

Dobson, K. S., & Pusch, D. (1993). Toward a definition of the conceptual and empirical boundaries of cognitive therapy. *Australian Psychologist, 28,* 137–144.

Dreesen, L., Arntz, A., Luttels, C., & Sallaerts, S. (1994). Personality disorders do not influence the results of cognitive behavior therapies for anxiety disorders. *Comprehensive Psychiatry, 35,* 265–274.

Ellis, A. (1962). *Reason and emotion in psychotherapy.* New York: Lyle Start.

Ericsson, K. A., & Simon, H. A. (1980). Verbal reports as data. *Psychological Review, 87,* 215–251.

Epstein, S. (1979). The stability of behavior: I. On predicting most of the people much of the time. *Journal of Personality and Social Psychology, 37,* 1097–1126.

Fahy, T. A., Eisler, I., & Russell, G. F. (1993). Personality disorder and treatment response in bulimia nervosa. *British Journal of Psychiatry, 162,* 765–770.

Farrell, J. M., & Shaw, I. A. (1994). Emotion awareness training: A prerequisite to effective cognitive-behavioral treatment of borderline personality disorder. *Cognitive and Behavioral Practice, 1,* 71–91.

Felske, U., Perry, K. J., Chambless, D. L., Renneberg, B., & Goldstein, A. J. (1996). Avoidant personality disorder as a predictor for treatment outcome among generalized social phobics. *Journal of Personality Disorders, 10,* 174–184.

Fleming, B. (1983, August). *Cognitive therapy with histrionic patients: Resolving a conflict in styles.* Paper presented at the meeting of the American Psychological Association, Anaheim, CA.

Fleming, B. (1985). *Dependent personality disorder: Managing the transition from dependence to autonomy.* Paper presented at the meeting of the Association for the Advancement of Behavior Therapy, Houston, TX.

Fleming, B. (1988). CT with histrionic personality disorder: Resolving a conflict of styles. *International Cognitive Therapy Newsletter, 4*(4), 8–9, 12.

Fleming, B., & Pretzer, J. (1990). Cognitive-behavioral approaches to personality disorders. In M. Hersen, R. M. Eisler, & P. M. Miller (Eds.), *Progress in behavior modification* (Vol. 25, pp. 119–151). Newbury Park, CA: Sage.

Freeman, A., Pretzer, J. L., Fleming, B., & Simon, K. M. (1990). *Clinical applications of cognitive therapy.* New York: Plenum Press.

Freeman, A., Pretzer, J. L., Fleming, B., & Simon, K. M. (2004). *Clinical applications of cognitive therapy* (2nd ed.). New York: Plenum Press.

Freidman, C. J., Shear, M. K., & Frances, A. (1987), DSM-III personality disorders in panic patients. *Journal of Personality Disorders, 1,* 132–135.

Gasperini, M., Provenza, M., Ronchi, P., Scherillo, P., Bellodi, L., & Smeraldi, E. (1989). *Cognitive processes and personality disorders in affective patients. Journal of Personality Disorders, 3,* 63–71.

Greenberg, D., & Stravynski, A. (1985). Patients who complain of social dysfunction: I. Clinical and demographic features. *Canadian Journal of Psychiatry, 30,* 206–211.

Hardy, G. E., Barkham, M., Shapiro, D. A., Stiles, W. B., Rees, A., & Reynolds, S. (1995). Impact of Cluster C personality disorders on outcomes of contrasting brief therapies for depression. *Journal of Consulting and Clinical Psychology*, 63, 997–1004.

Hollon, S. D., & Kendall, P. C. (1980). Cognitive self-statement in depression: Development of an automatic thoughts questionnaire. *Cognitive Therapy and Research*, 4, 383–395.

Hurlburt, R. T., Leach, B. C., & Saltman, S. (1984). Random sampling of thought and mood. *Cognitive Therapy and Research*, 8, 263–276.

Isen, A. M. (1984). Toward understanding the role of affect in cognition. In R. S. Wyer & T. K. Skrull (Eds.). *Handbook of social cognition* (pp. 179–236). Hillsdale, NJ: Erlbaum.

Kellner, R. (1986). Personality disorders. *Psychotherapy and Psychosomatics*, 46, 58–66.

Kendall, P.C., & Hollon, S. D. (1981). Assessing self-referent speech: Methods in the measurement of self-statements. In P. C. Kendall & S. D. Hollon (Eds.), *Assessment strategies for cognitive behavioral interventions* (pp. 85–118). New York: Academic Press.

Klinger, E. (1978). Modes of normal conscious flow. In K. S. Pope & J. L. Singer (Eds.), *The stream of consciousness: Scientific investigation into the flow of human experience* (pp. 225–258). New York: Plenum Press.

Koons, C. R., Robins, C. J., Tweed, J. L., Lynch, T. R., Gonzalez, A. M., Morse, J. Q., et al. (2001). Efficacy of dialectical behavior therapy in women with borderline personality disorder. *Behavior Therapy*, 32, 371–390.

Kuyken, W., Kurzer, N., DeRubeis, R. J., Beck, A. T., & Brown, G. K. (2001). Response to cognitive therapy of depression: The role of maladaptive beliefs and personality disorders. *Journal of Consulting and Clinical Psychology*, 69(3), 560–566.

Layden, M. A., Newman, C. F., Freeman, A., & Morse, S. B. (1993). *Cognitive therapy of borderline personality disorder*. Boston: Allyn & Bacon.

Linehan, M. M. (1993). *Cognitive-behavioral treatment of borderline personality disorder*. New York: Guilford Press.

Linehan, M. M., Armstrong, H. E., Suarez, A., Allmon, D. J., & Heard, H. L. (1991). Cognitive-behavioral treatment of chronically suicidal borderline patients. *Archives of General Psychiatry*, 48, 1060–1064.

Linehan, M. M., Heard, H. L., & Armstrong, H. E. (1993). Naturalistic follow-up of a behavioral treatment for chronically parasuicidal borderline patients. *Archives of General Psychiatry*, 50, 971–974.

Linehan, M. M., Tutek, D. A., & Heard, H. L. (1992, November). *Interpersonal and social treatment outcomes in borderline personality disorder*. Paper presented at the 26th annual conference of the Association for the Advancement of Behavior Therapy, Boston.

Liotti, G. (1992). Egocentrism and the cognitive psychotherapy of personality disorders. *Journal of Cognitive Psychotherapy: An International Quarterly*, 6, 43–58.

Lockwood, G. (1992). Psychoanalysis and the cognitive therapy of personality disorders. *Journal of Cognitive Psychotherapy: An International Quarterly*, 6, 25–42.

Lockwood, G., & Young, J. (1992). Introduction: Cognitive therapy for personality disorders. *Journal of Cognitive Psychotherapy: An International Quarterly*, 6, 5–10.

Luborsky, L., McLellan, A. T., Woody, G. E., O'Brien, C. P., & Auerbach, A. (1985). Therapist success and its determinants. *Archives of General Psychiatry*, 42, 602–611.

Mahoney, M. J. (1974). *Cognition and behavior modification*. Cambridge, MA: Ballinger.

Marchand, A., Goyer, L. R., Dupuis, G., & Mainguy, N. (1998). Personality disorders and the outcome of cognitive behavioural treatment of panic disorder with agoraphobia. *Canadian Journal of Behavioural Science*, 30, 14–23.

Marlatt, G. A., & Gordon, J. M. (Eds.). (1985). *Relapse prevention: Maintenance strategies in the treatment of addictive behaviors*. New York: Guilford Press.

Matthews, G. R., & Antes, J. R. (1992). Visual attention and depression: Cognitive biases in the eye fixations of the dysphoric and the nondepressed. *Cognitive Therapy and Research*, 16, 359–371.

Mavissakalian, M., & Hamman, M. S. (1987). DSM-III personality disorder in agoraphobia: II. Changes with treatment. *Comprehensive Psychiatry*, 28, 356–361.

Mays, D. T. (1985). Behavior therapy with borderline personality disorders: One clinician's perspective. In D. T. Mays & C. M. Franks (Eds.), *Negative outcome in psychotherapy and what to do about it* (pp. 301–311). New York: Springer.

McNally, R. J., Reimann, B. C., & Kim, E. (1990). Selective processing of threat cues in panic disorder. *Behaviour Research and Therapy*, 28, 407–412.

Merluzzi, T. V., Glass, C. R., & Genest, M. (1981). *Cognitive assessment*. New York: Guilford Press.

Mersch, P. P. A., Jansen, M. A., & Arntz, A. (1995). Social phobia and personality disorder: Severity of complaint and treatment effectiveness. *Journal of Personality Disorders*, 9, 143–159.

Nelson-Gray, R. O., Johnson, D. Foyle, L. W., Daniel, S. S., & Harmon, R. (1996). The effectiveness of cognitive therapy tailored to depressives with personality disorders. *Journal of Personality Disorders*, 10, 132–152.

Neziroglu, F., McKay , D., Todaro, J., & Yaryura-Tobias, J. A. (1996). Effect of cognitive behavior therapy on persons with body dysmorphic disorder and comorbid axis II diagnosis. *Behavior Therapy*, 27, 67–77.

O'Leary, K. M., Cowdry, R. W., Gardner, D. L., Leibenluft, E., Lucas, P. B., & deJong-Meyer, R. (1991). Dysfunctional attitudes in borderline personality disorder. *Journal of Personality Disorders*, 5, 233–242.

Overholser, J. C. (1991). Categorical assessment of the dependent personality disorder in depressed in-patients. *Journal of Personality Disorders*, 5, 243–255.

Padesky, C. A. (1986, September 18–20). *Personality disorders: Cognitive therapy into the 90's*. Paper presented at the 2nd International Conference on Cognitive Psychotherapy, Umeå, Sweden.

Padesky, C. A. (1988). Schema-focused CT: Comments and questions. *International Cognitive Therapy Newsletter*, 4, 5, 7.

Padesky, C. A. (1994). Schema change processes in cognitive therapy. *Clinical Psychology and Psychotherapy*, 1(5), 267–278.

Persons, J. B. (1991). *Cognitive therapy in practice: A case formulation approach.* New York: Norton.

Persons, J. B., Burns, B. D., & Perloff, J. M. (1988). Predictors of drop-out and outcome in cognitive therapy for depression in a private practice setting. *Cognitive Therapy and Research*, 12, 557–575.

Pretzer, J. L. (1983, August). *Borderline personality disorder: Too complex for cognitive-behavioral approaches?* Paper presented at the meeting of the American Psychological Association, Anaheim, CA. (ERIC Document Reproduction Service No. ED 243 007)

Pretzer, J. L. (1985, November). *Paranoid personality disorder: A cognitive view.* Paper presented at the meeting of the Association for the Advancement of Behavior Therapy, Houston, TX.

Pretzer, J. L. (1988). Paranoid personality disorder: A cognitive view. *International Cognitive Therapy Newsletter*, 4(4), 10–12.

Pretzer, J. L., Beck, A. T., & Newman, C. F. (1990). Stress and stress management: A cognitive view. *Journal of Cognitive Psychotherapy: An International Quarterly*, 3, 163–179.

Pretzer, J. L., & Fleming, B. M. (1990). Cognitive-behavioral treatment of personality disorders. *The Behavior Therapist*, 12, 105–109.

Rathus, J. H., Sanderson, W. C., Miller, A. L., & Wetzler, S. (1995). Impact of personality functioning on cognitive behavioral treatment of panic disorder: A preliminary report. *Journal of Personality Disorders*, 9, 160–168.

Rosenbaum, M. (1980). A schedule for assessing self-control behaviors: Preliminary findings. *Behavior Therapy*, 11, 109–121.

Rothstein, M. M., & Vallis, T. M. (1991). The application of cognitive therapy to patients with personality disorders. In T. M. Vallis, J. L. Howes, & P. C. Miller (Eds.), *The challenge of cognitive therapy: applications to nontraditional populations* (pp. 59–84). New York: Plenum Press.

Safran, J. D., & McMain, S. (1992). A cognitive-interpersonal approach to the treatment of personality disorders. *Journal of Cognitive Psychotherapy: An International Quarterly*, 6, 59–68.

Sanderson, W. C., Beck, A. T., & McGinn, L. K. (1994). Cognitive therapy for generalized anxiety disorder: Significance of co-morbid personality disorders. *Journal of Cognitive Psychotherapy: An International Quarterly*, 8, 13–18.

Scott, W. B. (1992, February). *Self-schema in an individual diagnosed as having multiple personality disorder.* Paper presented at the meeting of the Cleveland Area Behavior Therapy Association, Cleveland, OH.

Shea, M. T., Pilkonis, P. A., Beckham, E., Collins, J. F., Elkins, I., Sotsky, S. M., & Docherty, J. P. (1990). Personality disorders and treatment outcome in the NIMH Treatment of Depression Collaborative Research Program. *American Journal of Psychiatry*, 147, 711–718.

Simon, K. M. (1983, August). *Cognitive therapy with compulsive patients: Re-*

placing rigidity with structure. Paper presented at the annual meeting of the American Psychological Association, Anaheim, CA.

Simon, K. M. (1985, November). *Cognitive therapy of the passive-aggressive personality.* Paper presented at the meeting of the Association for the Advancement of Behavior Therapy, Houston, TX.

Springer, T., Lohr, N. E., Buchtel, H. A., & Silk, K. R. (1995). A preliminary report of short-term cognitive-behavioral group therapy for inpatients with personality disorders. *Journal of Psychotherapy Practice and Research, 5,* 57–71.

Stephens, J. H., & Parks, S. L. (1981). Behavior therapy of personality disorders. In J. R. Lion (Ed.), *Personality disorders: Diagnosis and management* (2nd ed., pp. 456–471). Baltimore: Williams & Wilkins.

Stravynski, A., Marks, I., & Yule, W. (1982). Social skills problems in neurotic outpatients: Social skills training with and without cognitive modification. *Archives of General Psychiatry, 39,* 1378–1385.

Taylor, S., & Rachman, S. J. (1991). Fear of sadness. *Journal of Anxiety Disorders, 5,* 375–381.

Taylor, S., & Rachman, S. J. (1992). Fear and avoidance of aversive affective states: Dimensions and causal relations. *Journal of Anxiety Disorders, 6,* 15–25.

Turkat, I. D. (1990). *The personality disorders: A psychological approach to clinical management.* New York: Pergamon Press.

Turkat, I. D., & Maisto, S. A. (1985) Personality disorders: Application of the experimental method to the formulation and modification of personality disorders. In D. H. Barlow (Ed.), *Clinical handbook of psychological disorders: A step-by-step treatment manual* (pp. 502–570). New York: Guilford Press.

Turner, R. M. (1986, March). *The bio-social-learning approach to the assessment and treatment of borderline personality disorder.* Paper presented at the Carrier Foundation Behavioral Medicine Update Symposium, Belle Meade, NJ.

Turner, R. M. (1987). The effects of personality disorder diagnosis on the outcome of social anxiety symptom reduction. *Journal of Personality Disorders, 1,* 136–143.

Turner, S. M., Bidel, D. C., Borden, J. W., Stanley, M. A., & Jacob, R. G. (1991). Social phobia: Axis I and Axis II correlates. *Journal of Abnormal Psychology, 100,* 102–106.

Turner, S. M., & Hersen, M. (1981). Disorders of social behavior: A behavioral approach to personality disorders. In S.M. Turner, K. S. Calhoun, & H. E. Adams (Eds.), *Handbook of clinical behavior therapy* (pp. 103–124). New York: Wiley.

Watkins, P. C., Mathews, A., Williamson, D. A., & Fuller, R. D. (1992). Mood-congruent memory in depression: Emotional priming or elaboration? *Journal of Abnormal Psychology, 101,* 581–586.

Weishaar, M. E. (1993). *Aaron T. Beck.* Thousand Oaks, CA: Sage.

Woody, G. E., McLellan, A. T., Luborsky, L., & O'Brien, C. P. (1985) Sociopathy and psychotherapy outcome. *Archives of General Psychiatry, 42,* 1081–1086.

Young, J. E. (1983, August). *Borderline personality: Cognitive theory and treatment.* Paper presented at the annual meeting of the American Psychological Association, Anaheim, CA.

Young, J. (1990). *Cognitive therapy for personality disorders: A schema-focused approach*. Sarasota, FL. Professional Resource Exchange.

Young, J. E., & Lindemann, M. D. (1992). An integrative schema-focused model for personality disorders. *Journal of Cognitive Psychotherapy: An International Quarterly*, 6, 11–24.

Young, J., & Swift, W. (1988). Schema-focused cognitive therapy for personality disorders: Part I. *International Cognitive Therapy Newsletter*, 4, 5, 13–14.

Young, J. E., Klosko, J. S., & Weishaar, M. (2003). *Schema therapy: A practitioner's guide*. New York: Guilford Press.

CHAPTER 3

■ ■ ■

A Psychoanalytic Theory
of Personality Disorders

OTTO F. KERNBERG
EVE CALIGOR

The fundamental premise of psychoanalytic theories of personality disorders is that the observable behaviors (personality traits) and subjective disturbances that characterize a particular personality disorder reflect specific pathological features of underlying psychological structures. As a result, treatments that alter psychological structures and mental organization will result in changes in pathological personality traits and subjective disturbances. The psychoanalytic theory of personality disorders that we present is intimately linked with models of treatment. Empirical studies of the treatments derived from our theory of personality pathology (Clarkin et al., 2001; Clarkin, Levy, Lenzenweger, & Kernberg, 2004) enable us to study the utility of the underlying model of mental organization.

In this chapter, we make an effort to formulate an integrated psychoanalytic view of the etiology, structural characteristics, and mutual relations of the personality disorders. Our model is based on advances in the psychoanalytic understanding of particular types of personality disorders and their diagnosis, treatment, and prognosis. The study of patients with personality disorders undergoing psychoanalytic treatment provides a unique opportunity. Specifically, psychoanalytic research allows us to observe the relationships (1) among pathological personality traits, (2) between surface behavior and underlying psychological structures, (3) between various constellations of pathological behavior patterns as they change in the course of treatment, (4) between motivation of behavior and psychological structure, and (5) between changes in behavior and shifts in dominant transference patterns. The model we present in this chapter is to a large degree derived from clinical data acquired from psychoanalytic treatment of patients with personality disorders. We attempt to integrate these data with empirical data from psychoanalytic research and relevant scientific developments in the fields of psychiatry, developmental psychology, cognitive science, neurophysiology, genetics, and infant observation.

The theory we present has led to the development of specific treatments that deal with the clinical features presented by patients with personality disorders (Clarkin, Yeomans, & Kernberg, 1999; Bateman & Fonagy, 2004). Specifically, we have developed a psychotherapeutic treatment for patients with severe personality disorders (Clarkin et al., 1999), a psychotherapeutic treatment for patients with higher-level, or "neurotic," personality disorders (Caligor, Clarkin, & Kernberg, 2004) and a psychotherapeutic approach to treatment of patients with narcissistic personality disorders (Kernberg, 1984, 1992). Ongoing research efforts open the possibility of developing a broad array of treatments, finely tuned to address the clinical demands presented by the different personality disorders. In addition, psychoanalytic approaches to psychopathology facilitate differential diagnosis of subtle aspects of personality disorders, which can be used to establish prognostic indicators and to guide differential treatment planning. In this regard, the differentiation between the narcissistic personality disorder, the malignant narcissism syndrome, and the antisocial personality proper (Bursten, 1989; Hare, 1986; Kernberg, 1989, 1992; Stone, 1990) has been especially influential.

In this chapter, we present a model of mental organization and of mental functioning that accounts for the descriptive features of personality disorders. By "descriptive features" we refer both to the observable behaviors and to the subjective states that characterize a particular personality disorder. After presenting our model of mental organization we look to this model of mind, as it interacts with other factors, to address questions about the etiology of personality disorders, developmental continuities among the personality disorders, and implications for treatment. Our model classifies personality disorders first using a dimensional approach, based on severity of pathology, and makes a second-order diagnosis using a prototypical, or categorical, classification system. We believe that any model of classification that is going to be of use in a clinical setting must combine dimensional and categorical approaches.

PSYCHOANALYTIC OBJECT RELATIONS THEORY AND PSYCHOLOGICAL STRUCTURES

The model we present emerges from contemporary psychoanalytic object relations theory as it has been developed by Otto Kernberg (1975, 1976,

1980, 1984, 1992). This model looks to the organization of psychological structures, derived from the interaction of constitutional and environmental factors early in life, to account for descriptive phenomena. In essence, personality traits and the relationships among pathological personality traits are seen as reflecting specific features of underlying psychological organizations. In this sense, our model is predominantly intrapsychic in its orientation.

The term "structure" as we use it here refers to an organization of related functions or processes that is relatively stable and enduring over time. Structures can be integrated and hierarchically organized to form new structures, organized at increasing levels of complexity. The term "organization" is often used to refer to the structures that are the result of this process. A "psychological structure" is a stable and enduring configuration of mental functions or processes that organize the individual's behavior and subjective experience. In psychoanalytic theories of personality, personality traits and subjective disturbances (i.e., the descriptive aspects of personality) are conceptualized as structures that are observable, sometimes referred to as "surface" structures. Surface structures, in turn, reflect the nature of underlying psychological structures, along with the degree of integration and organization of these structures. These underlying psychological structures, sometimes referred to as "deep" structures, cannot be directly observed. Rather, the presence and organization of deep structures is inferred from the observable features of personality, which are understood as organized by, and reflecting of, underlying deep structures.

Internal Object Relations

In psychoanalytic object relations theory, "internal object relations" are the basic building blocks of psychological structures and are the organizers of motivations and related behavioral patterns. An internalized object relation consists of a particular affect state linked to an image of a specific interaction between the self and another person (e.g., fear, linked to the image of a small, terrified self and a powerful, threatening authority figure). From the first days of life, internal object relations are derived from the integration of inborn affect dispositions and interactions with caretakers. When an affect is repeatedly experienced in the context of a particular kind of interaction, affective memories are organized to form enduring, affectively charged representations or memory structures, which we refer to as internal object relations. Internal object relations have a complex relationship to their developmental origins, reflecting a combination of actual and fantasied interactions with others as well as defenses in relation to both. The most basic internal object relations are dyadic, by which we mean they consist of two representations, a representation of the self, and the representation of another person, in interaction. As internal object relations become more highly integrated and organized in relation to one another, they may become triadic, or triangular. Triadic internal object relations consist of a self- representation interacting with two object representations. The prototype of the triadic internal object relation is an image of a sexual or loving couple and a third party who is excluded.

Identity Consolidation and Internal Object Relations

Internal object relations are integrated and hierarchically organized to form the higher-order structures that organize personality and psychological functioning. At the core of our model of personality and personality disorders is the psychological structure or organization we refer to as "identity." A normal, consolidated identity corresponds with the subjective experience of a stable and realistic sense of self and others. In contrast, pathological identity formation corresponds with an unstable, polarized, and unrealistic sense of self and others. From the perspective of motivational systems, normal identity is associated with a broad array of affect dispositions, with the predominance of positive affect states, reflecting the preponderance of loving, affiliative motivations, and the predominance of defensive operations based on repression. In contrast, pathological identity formation is associated with affects that are crude, intense, and poorly modulated, with the predominance of negative affect states, reflecting the preponderance of pathological aggression and the predominance of defensive operations based on primitive dissociation, or splitting.

Fully consolidated identity is the hallmark of the normal personality, as well as the higher-level (or "neurotic") personality disorders (the hysterical, obsessive, and depressive–masochistic personalities). Pathology of identity formation is the hallmark of the severe personality disorders. (We include here all the DSM-IV personality disorders, save the obsessive–compulsive personality). This approach has been developed by Kernberg (1976), incorporating significant contributions from other psychoanalytic researchers and theoreticians, notably, Akhtar (1989, 1992), Krause (1988; Krause & Lutolf, 1988), Stone (1980, 1990, 1993a), and Volkan (1976, 1987).

PROBLEMS WITH EXISTING APPROACHES TO CLASSIFICATION OF PERSONALITY DISORDERS

A major question in personality disorder theory and research is how the various behavioral characteristics of any particular personality disorder relate to each another and to their particular predisposing and causative factors. Research efforts have repeatedly found that multiple factors appear to combine in the background of any particular personality disorder, without a clear answer to how these factors relate to each other in co-determining a specific type of psychopathology (Marziali, 1992; Paris, 1994; Steinberg, Trestman, & Siever, 1994; Stone, 1993a, 1993b).

Researchers proceeding with a dimensional model usually carry out complex factor analyses of a great number of behavioral traits. These studies lead to specific factors or a few overriding behavioral characteristics that, in different combinations, would seem to characterize the particular personality disorders described by clinicians (Benjamin 1992, 19936 Clark, 1993; Cloninger, Svrakic, & Przybeck, 1993; Costa & Widiger, 1994, 2002; Widiger & Frances, 1994; Widiger, Trull, Clarkin, Sanderson, & Costa, 1994; Livesley, 1998; Millon, 1981; Wiggins, 1982). This approach links particular behaviors and lends itself to establishing a general theory that could integrate the major dimensions arrived at by statistical analyses. These dimensions, however, tend to have only a rather general relation to any specific personality disorder, thus limiting their clinical utility. The clinical utility of this approach is further limited by failure to account for the specific contexts within which a given trait is expressed. (One notable exception may prove to be Benjamin's [1992, 1996] "Structural Analysis of Social Behavior [SASB]," a model strongly influenced by contemporary psychoanalytic thinking.)

A currently well-known dimensional model, the five-factor model, has proposed that neuroticism, extroversion, openness, agreeableness, and conscientiousness constitute basic factors that describe the core dimensions of normal personality, and that personality disorders may be seen as extremes of these basic dimensions (Costa & Widiger, 1994; Widiger et al., 1994). However, there are limited data to substantiate that these five dimensions developed in studies of normal personality can be meaningfully applied to classification of personality disorders. From the perspective of the clinical treatment of personality disorders, it is difficult to imagine that these five general traits can capture the subtleties of the clinical features of specific personality constellations.

Those researchers who are inclined to maintain a categorical approach to personality disorders, usually clinical psychiatrists motivated to find specific disease entities, tend to proceed differently. They study the clinically prevalent constellations of pathological personality traits, carry out empirical research regarding the validity and reliability of the corresponding clinical diagnoses, and attempt to achieve a clear differentiation between personality disorders, keeping in mind the clinical relevance of their approaches (Akhtar, 1992; Stone, 1993a; Westen & Schedler, 1999a, 1999b). This approach, pursued in DSM-III (American Psychiatri Association, 1980) and DSM-IV (American Psychiatric Association, 1994), has had the benefits of better acquainting clinical psychiatrist with some frequently seen personality disorders and facilitating psychiatric research in the area of the personality disorders. However, this approach has been plagued by the high degree of comorbidity among the severe personality disorders (Livesley, 2001) as well as low test–retest reliability (Perry, 1992; Zimmerman, 1994) and, in some instances, poor stability over time (Zanarini, Frankenburg, Hennen, & Silk, 2003). In addition, the DSM system has omitted the less severe personality disorders, which are those most commonly seen in clinical practice, and it is perhaps for this reason that the DSM-IV Axis II system is rarely seen as useful by clinicians (Westen & Arkowitz-Westen, 1998).

Many of these problems with DSM classification reflect the weaknesses of a categorical system in which the "menu" of listed criteria include a mixture of symptoms, behaviors, subjective experiences, and affective states, all of which are equally weighted. Thus, for example, in the diagnosis of borderline personality disorder, suicidal behavior (behaviors that are often episodic) and chronic feelings of emptiness (a subjective inner state that is characteristic of the individual) are both included as criteria and equally weighted. To further complicate matters, in the absence of sufficient empirical data to guide decision making, political factors have unduly influenced decisions about what personality disorders to include and exclude in the official DSM system and under what labels (Jonas & Pope, 1992; Kernberg, 1992; Oldham, 1994). In this setting, the hysterical personality disorder, a common personality disorder with a long historical tradition, has remained excluded. Similarly, the depressive–masochistic personality disorder, excluded under DSM-III, has now reemerged under the heading "depressive personality disorder" in the appendix of DSM-IV, shorn of controversial references to "masochism" (Kernberg, 1992).

A major factor underlying problematic aspects of both existing classification systems, be they categorical or dimensional, is the tendency to anchor diagnostic criteria and, as a result, empirical research predominantly in reference to observable behaviors. The problem here is that the same behaviors can serve very different functions depending on the underlying personality structure. For example, behaviors related to what is seen as social timidity or inhibition may contribute to a diagnosis of either a schizoid or an avoidant personality. However, these same behaviors may in fact reflect the cautiousness of a deeply paranoid individual, or the fear of exposure of a narcissistically grandiose individual, or a reaction formation against exhibitionistic tendencies in a hysterical individual. A related problem is the necessary dependence, in large-scale research efforts, on standardized inquiries or questionnaires, assessment instruments that are known to be relatively poor measures of personality pathology (Torgerson & Ainaeus, 1990). Patients with personality disorders may not be sufficiently aware of certain pathological personality traits to report on them.

Further, even when patients are aware of their personality traits, responses to questionnaires and standard interviews will be influenced by the social desirability of particular traits.

PERSONALITY: CONSTITUTIONAL FACTORS, CHARACTER, AND INTERNALIZED VALUE SYSTEMS

From a psychoanalytic perspective, personality represents the dynamic integration of behavior patterns derived from temperament, constitutionally determined cognitive capacities, character (and its subjective correlate, identity), and internalized value systems (Kernberg, 1976, 1980). Though we discuss them separately, from both a developmental and a functional perspective, these four dimensions of personality are intricately intertwined with one another.

Temperament refers to the constitutionally given and largely genetically determined, inborn disposition to particular reactions to environmental stimuli, particularly the intensity, rhythm, and thresholds of affective responses. In our model, affective responses, particularly affective responses under conditions of peak affect arousal, are crucial determinants of the organization of the personality. Thus, inborn thresholds for activation of both positive, pleasurable, and rewarding affects and negative, painful, and aggressive affects represent the most important bridge between biological and psychological determinants of the personality (Kernberg, 1994). In addition to affect disposition, temperament also includes inborn dispositions to perceptual organization, to motor reactivity, and to control over motor reactivity.

Constitutionally determined aspects of cognition, especially as they interact with affect dispositions, also pay an important role in personality. At the most basic level, cognitive processes play a crucial role in the development and modulation of affective responses by providing the representational aspects of affect activation. It is by way of representation that primitive affect states are transformed into complex emotional experiences. At a higher level of integration, the capacity for "effortful control" is closely linked to constitutionally determined aspects of cognition. Here we refer to the individual's capacity to focus on certain cognitively relevant stimuli in the face of distracting affective stimulation, as well as the capacity to establish priority among various affective stimuli (Posner & Rothbart, 2000; Posner et al., 2002). Effortful control appears to play an important role in the severe personality disorders (Depue & Lenzenweger, 2001; Lenzenweger, Clarkin, Kernberg, & Foelsch, 2001; Posner et al., 2002).

Character refers to the dynamic organization of enduring behavior patterns, including ways of perceiving and relating to the world, that are characteristic of the individual. A description of character includes the level of organization of these patterns of behavior, the degree of flexibility or rigidity with which the observed behaviors are activated across situations, and the extent to which the observed behaviors are adaptive or interfere with psychosocial functioning. From a psychoanalytic perspective, the structured behaviors constituting character traits, and their overall organization into what is referred to as "character," reflect the organization of underlying psychological structures. In particular, "character" refers to the behavioral manifestations of identity. Conversely, the subjective aspects of identity, notably an integrated and crystalized self-concept and concept of significant others (or the lack thereof), are the psychological structures that determine the dynamic organization of character.

The third determinant of personality within a psychoanalytic frame of reference is the system of internalized values. The degree of integration of value systems, in essence, the moral and ethical dimension of the personality, is an important component of the total personality.

Normal Personality: Descriptive Features

The normal personality is characterized, first of all, by an integrated concept of the self and an integrated concept of significant others. These structural characteristics, jointly referred to as identity or "ego identity" (Erikson, 1950, 1956; Jacobson, 1964), are reflected in an internal sense and an external appearance of self-coherence and are a fundamental precondition for normal self-esteem, self-enjoyment, the capacity to derive pleasure from work and values, and an overall zest for life. An integrated view of one's self ensures the capacity for a realization of one's desires, capacities, and long-range commitments. An integrated view of significant others guarantees the capacity for an appropriate evaluation of others, empathy, and social tact. An integrated view of self and others implies the capacity for mature dependency—that is, the capacity to make an emotional investment in others while maintaining a consistent sense of autonomy, as well the capacity to experience concern for others.

A second structural characteristic of the normal personality, largely derived from and an expression of an integrated identity, is the presence of a capacity for a broad spectrum of affect dispositions. In the normal personality affects are complex and well modulated, and even relatively intense affective experiences do not lead to loss of impulse control. Consistency, persistence, and creativity in work and interpersonal relations are also largely derived from normal ego identity, as are the capacity for trust, reciprocity, and commitment to others, which are codetermined by internalized value systems (Kernberg, 1975).

A third aspect of the normal personality is an integrated and mature system of internalized values. Though the system of internalized values is developmentally derived from parental prohibitions and values, in the normal personality moral behaviors and values are no longer closely connected to parental prohibitions. Rather, the mature system of internalized values associated with the normal personality is stable, "depersonified," relatively independent of external relations with others, and individualized. Such a mature system of internalized values is reflected in a sense of personal responsibility, a capacity for realistic self-criticism, integrity as well as flexibility in dealing with the ethical aspects of decision making, and a commitment to standards, values, and ideals.

A fourth structural aspect of the normal personality is an appropriate and satisfactory management of sexual, dependent, and aggressive motivations, which may be experienced subjectively as needs, fears, wishes, or impulses. Appropriate expression of sexual, dependent, and aggressive strivings are fully integrated with normal ego identity. In the sexual sphere, we see the capacity for a full expression of sensual and sexual needs integrated with tenderness and emotional commitment to a loved other. With regard to dependency needs, the normal integration of dependent motivations is expressed in the capacity for interdependence and enjoyment of both caretaking and dependent roles. Finally, a normal personality structure includes the capacity to successfully channel aggressive impulses into expressions of healthy self-assertion, to withstand attacks without excessive reaction, to react protectively, and to avoid turning aggression against the self. Internalized value systems contribute to the normal integration and successful management of the motivational structures we describe.

Normal Personality: Structural and Developmental Factors

The structural conditions that characterize normal identity represent the completion of a series of successive steps leading to progressive integration and organization of internalized object relations. The steps we describe represent a hypothesized (but yet to be validated) developmental model. At the same time, this model corresponds closely with clinical observations emerging from the psychodynamic treatments of patients with severe personality disorders and atypical psychoses.

A basic assumption of our developmental model is that psychological structures derived from interactions associated with high affect activation will have different characteristics from those derived from interactions under conditions of low affect activation. Under conditions of low affect activation, reality-oriented, perception-controlled cognitive learning takes place, leading to the formation of differentiated, gradually evolving definitions of self and others. These definitions start out from the perception of bodily functions, the position of the self in space and time, and the permanent characteristics of others. As these perceptions are integrated and become more complex, and interactions with others are cognitively registered and evaluated, working models of the self in relation to others are established. Inborn capacities to differentiate self from nonself and the capacity for cross-modal transfer of sensorial experience play an important part in the construction of the model of self and the surrounding world.

In contrast, interactions associated with high affect arousal lead to the establishment of specific affective memory structures, framed by the nature of the interaction between baby and caretaker. These structures, which we have referred to as internal object relations, are constituted, essentially, by a representation of the self interacting with a representation of a significant other under the dominance of a peak affect state. The importance of these affective memory structures lies in their constituting the basis of the primary psychological motivational system, directing efforts to approach, maintain, or increase the conditions that generate peak positive affect states and to decrease, avoid, and escape from conditions of peak negative affect states.

In the early organization of these affective memory structures, the structures associated with positive affects and affiliative behaviors are built up separately from those associated with negative affects and aversive behaviors. With time, positive and negatively charged affective experiences come to be actively dissociated from each other. The result is the development of two major domains of early psychological experience. An idealized, or "all good," sector is characterized by purely positive representations of self and other associated with positive affect states. A persecutory or "all bad" sector is characterized by purely negative representations of other and threatened representations of self associated with negative affect states. These representations of negatively charged, painful, and dangerous relationships tend to be projected, leading to a fear of painful and dangerous relationships with people in the environment.

The active dissociation of positive and negatively charged experiences we have described is referred to as splitting. Splitting of positive and negative sectors of experience is a motivated mental operation, often described as a "defensive operation," representing an effort to maintain an ideal domain of experience characterized by the gratifying and pleasurable relation between self and others, while escaping from the frightening experiences of negative affect states. Splitting of experience into "all-good" and "all-bad" sectors protects the idealized experiences from "contamination" with bad ones, until a time when a higher degree of tolerance of pain and a more realistic assessment of external reality under painful conditions have evolved. Defensive operations based on splitting are sometimes referred to as primitive defenses.

This rudimentary stage of development of mental representations of self and other, with primary motivational implications of "move toward pleasure and away from pain," eventually evolves toward the integration of the positive and negative sectors of experience. An important outcome of this process is that the intensity of negative affects and persecutory experiences is significantly diminished, as a result of integration with more positive affective relational experience. Integration is facilitated by the development of cognitive capacities and ongoing learning regarding realistic aspects of the interactions between self and others under circumstances of low affect activation. In simple terms, during this stage of psychological development, the child recognizes that he has both "good' and "bad" aspects, and he also recognizes that so does mother, and so do the significant others in the immediate family circle. It is the predominance of "good," pleasurable affective experiences, intimately linked with positive interactions with mother and other caretakers, that makes it possible to tolerate and organize an integrated view of self and others. That is, the normal predominance of positively charged or "idealized" experiences with caretakers is a prerequisite for the normal integration of positively and negatively charged sectors of mental experience.

The better integrated (neither "all-good" nor "all-bad"), more realistic, and affectively toned down representations of self are organized to form a complex and realistic self-concept that includes a view of the self as potentially imbued with both loving and hating impulses. A parallel integration occurs in the representations of significant others. These developments correspond to the consolidation of normal identity and determine the capacity for experiencing stable, coherent, and ambivalent relationships with others. Identity consolidation, associated with the capacity for ambivalent relations with others, thus marks the stage of "whole" (in contrast to "split") or total internalized object relations.

Erik Erikson (1950, 1956) first formulated the concept of normal ego identity and pathological identity formation, which he referred to as identity diffusion. Erikson proposed that normal ego identity is derived, developmentally, from early internalizations of affectively invested representations of significant others as they are integrated with later identifications that take into account the status and roles of the various members of the family. Erikson stressed that ego identity develops gradually, until a final consolidation of its structure in adolescence. For Erikson, identity included identification with aspects of significant others along with an integration of the individual's view of his position in society and his awareness of society's acknowledgment of his characteristics. Insofar as Erikson considered the confirmation of the self by the representations of significant others as an aspect of normal identity, he already stressed the intimate link between the self-concept and the concept of significant others. However, it was the work of Edith Jacobson (1964) in the United States, powerfully influencing Margaret Mahler's conceptualizations, and the work of Ronald Fairbairn

(1954) in Great Britain, that pointed to the dyadic nature of early internalizations and created the basis for contemporary psychoanalytic object relations theory.

The stage of identity consolidation, corresponding with the integration and crystalization of the experience of self and others, is equivalent to the phase of "object constancy" described by Mahler (Mahler & Furer, 1968; Mahler, Pine, & Bergman, 1975), characterized by the child's developing capacity to maintain a continuous and integrated (in terms of "bad" aspects being part of an overall, integrated, predominantly positive) mental representation of mother, even in the face of frustration and/or physical separation. In Mahler's developmental framework, the achievement of object constancy is hypothesized to take place somewhere between the end of the first year of life and the end of the third year of life.

Mahler's research points to the gradual nature of the integration of the experience of self in relation to others over the first 3 years of life, a process she referred to as "separation–individuation." In this regard, Mahler's framework is consistent with current developmental research. However, Mahler also assumed the existence of earlier phases of development marked by a mental organization corresponding to a "symbiotic" state in which the boundaries between self and other were not clearly established. This assumption is not consistent with more recent infant research, which suggests that infants have the capacity to distinguish self from other from the earliest days of life. As a result, rather than a symbiotic phase, we hypothesize a tendency very early in life to experience "symbiotic" moments of fantasized fusion between self-representation and object representation under peak affect conditions. These momentary fusions are counteracted by the inborn capacity to differentiate self from nonself, and the real and fantasized experience of third parties disrupting the states of momentary symbiotic unity between infant and mother.

The achievement of object constancy coincides with two additional changes in mental organization, the formation of an integrated system of internalized values and the formation of an unconscious system of highly affectively charged motivational structures.

Coinciding with identity formation, the mental structures derived from early prohibitions and later internalized value systems are organized into an integrated system of internalized morals and values, often referred to as the "superego." The superego is seen as constituted by successive layers of internalized self and object representations (Jacobson, 1964; Kernberg, 1984). A first layer of negatively affectively charged, persecutory split representations reflects a demanding and prohibitive, primitive morality as experienced by the child when environmental demands and prohibitions run against the expression of aggressive, dependent, and sexual impulses. A second layer of organization is constituted by ideal representations of self and others reflecting early childhood ideals that promise the assurance of love and dependency if the child lives up to them. The integration of the earliest, persecutory and the later, idealizing representations tones down and modulates the intensity of both. In this process, a new level of organization is introduced into the system of internalized values, corresponding with decrease in the tendency to reproject these representations. This level of organization also brings about the capacity for internalizing more realistic, toned-down demands and prohibitions from the parental figures, leading to a third layer of integration of internalized value systems. This final stage corresponds with the formation of normal identity. Integration and consolidation of the structures that comprise identity facilitate this parallel development in the system of internalized values.

Finally, as part of the process of identity formation and formation of an internalized value system, those representations that are least well integrated and most highly affectively charged are dissociated from the representations that comprise the integrated, conscious sense of self and are eliminated from consciousness. These "high affect" mental structures are often referred to as a group as the dynamic unconscious or the id. The mental structures of the dynamic unconscious serve as an unconscious motivational system, corresponding with extreme manifestations of sexual, aggressive, and dependent impulses, needs, and wishes. The internalized system of values, in conjunction with the dominant sense of self that crystalizes with identity formation, is responsible for rejecting these highly charged and relatively poorly integrated mental structures from the conscious sense of self.

The capacity to reject threatening, painful, or anxiety-provoking aspects of mental experience and to eliminate them from consciousness is referred to as repression. The capacity for repression both reflects and facilitates the progressive integration and organization of psychological structures. As we have described, defensive operations based on splitting involve mutual dissociation of positive and negative sectors of experience to avoid anxiety, and, as a result, splitting-based defenses interfere with the normal integration of these sectors. In contrast, defenses based on repression ("neurotic defenses") do not interfere with the integration of persecutory and idealized structures. As a result, the emergence of defensive operations based on repression reflects some degree of integration of persecutory and idealized sectors and, at the same time, facilitates further integration of persecutory and idealized structures. Repressive defenses do, however, introduce a degree of rigidity into personality organization that is not seen in the normal personality.

Thus far we have focused on the shift from defenses based on splitting to those based on repression from the perspective of psychological structures and personality organization. We would like at this point to comment briefly on this shift from the perspective of the psychological anxieties that motivate defense. We have already described how splitting is motivated by the need to protect the idealized sector of experience from contamination or destruction by the persecutory sector. Further, when splitting predominates, persecutory aspects of experience tend to be projected, leading to typically paranoid fears associated with the predominance of splitting-based defenses. In contrast, with repression, threatening aspects of the inner world are less likely to be projected and are more likely to be experienced as potentially dangerous or destructive aspects *of* the self, rather than dangers coming *toward* the self. In this setting, the dominant sources of anxiety are of doing harm and of being unable to protect the loved and vulnerable parts of the self and others from harm. Kleinian psychoanalysts refer to this dynamic situation as depressive anxiety (Klein, 1935). It is depressive anxiety that motivates repression of threatening internal object relations, relegating them to the dynamic unconscious. Depressive anxieties typically become organized around internal object relations that are derivatives of sexual, dependent, or aggressive needs and wishes.

MOTIVATIONAL ASPECTS
OF PERSONALITY ORGANIZATION:
AFFECTS AND INTERNAL OBJECT RELATIONS

At the core of our model of personality and personality disorders is the development, progressive integration, and hierarchical organization of motivational systems. We stress the importance of the structural organization of motivational systems because the exploration of severe personality disorders consistently finds the presence of pathological aggression predominating. In contrast, a key dynamic feature of the normal personality is the full integration of erotic, dependent, and aggressive needs and wishes, under the dominance of loving, affiliative strivings. Finally, it is predominantly sexual conflicts, in the setting of failure to complete the normal integration of erotic, dependent, and aggressive strivings, that underlie the psychopathological features of the higher-level, neurotic personality disorders.

The developmental sequence of motivational structures begins with affects, which we consider to be the primary motivational system. Affects are instinctive components of human behavior common to all individuals of the human species. Affects are inborn, constitutionally and genetically determined modes of reaction triggered first by physiological and bodily experiences. Almost immediately, affects are activated in relation to, regulated by, and cognitively linked to interactions with caretakers. As we have described, over time, early interactions between children and their caretakers are internalized and gradually organized to form internal object relations. Internal object relations are psychological structures with motivational implications. Because internal object relations are the basic building blocks of all psychological structures, in our model, affects, motivational systems, and psychological structures are intricately related.

Our model is consistent with the work of Krause (1988), who has proposed that affects constitute a phylogenetically recent biological system evolved in mammals to signal the infant animal's emergency needs to its mother. Further, Krause proposes that there exists a corresponding inborn capacity in mother to read and respond to the infant's affective signals, thus protecting the early development of the dependent infant mammal. Using videotapes, Beebe (Beebe & Lachman 2002) has studied the ways in which the baby's affects are shaped by early interactions with mother. In her interactions with her baby and her reactions to baby's affect states, mother helps to regulate and organize the baby's affect arousal. Beebe demonstrates how mother's acknowledgement of the infant's affect state can function to modulate the baby's affects and organize baby's behavior, whereas interactions in which mother fails to acknowledge the baby's affect state can lead to the disorganization of the baby's affective experience and behavior.

Fonagy and Target (Target & Fonagy, 1996; Fonagy & Target, 2003), have taken a similar approach, emphasizing the role of mother–child interactions in the child's developing capacity to reflect on his own emotional states and on the emotional states of others. Specifically, Fonagy and Target suggest that mother, in activating her normal capacity to respond to her infant and young child by "marking" (i.e., signaling that she can empathize with the child's affect state without sharing it), permits the child to internalize her contingent, accurate, and differentiated emotional experience. The child thus becomes able to reflect on his own affective experience. Mother's incapacity to mark her responses to the young child and her incapacity to accurately mirror her child's affective state are hypothesized to increase the dominance of the negative segment of experience for the child.

As we described, in the early life of the human baby, two series of mental structures are developed, one associated with highly charged positive affect states motivating "approach" behaviors and another associated with highly charged negative affect states motivating aversive behaviors. This level of mental organization corresponds with the predominance of two central motivational systems, one associated with positive affective reinforcement and motivating affiliative behaviors and the other associated with negative affective reinforcement and motivating aversive behaviors. Psychoanalysts often refer to these two, overarching motivational systems as the drives, libido, and aggression, respectively.

Rage represents the core affect of aggressive internal object relations, and the vicissitudes of rage explain the origins of hatred and envy, the dominant affects in severe personality disorders. Similarly, the affect of sexual excitement constitutes the core affect of the sexual series of internal object relations. Sensual responses to intimate bodily contact dominate the development of the erotic impulses, and sexual excitement slowly and gradually crystalizes from the primitive affect of elation. Early experiences of pleasurable gratification crystalize to organize dependency needs, which evolve from infantile demands for perfect caretaking to longings for mutually dependent relations.

As mental development leads to the progressive integration of idealized and persecutory internal object relations, affect dispositions become increasingly complex and well modulated. These relatively well-integrated structures, associated with relatively well-modulated affect dispositions, are organized to form conscious motivational systems. With identity formation, these motivational systems are further integrated and become part of normal identity and the mature system of internalized values. At the same time, a subgroup of internal object relations, as a result of constitutional and environmental factors, remains poorly integrated and highly affectively charged. With the achievement of identity formation, object constancy, and the capacity for repression, these psychological structures and associated affect dispositions are repressed and become part of the dynamic unconscious, or the id. The dynamic unconscious contains internal object relations that are relatively extreme manifestations of erotic, dependent, and aggressive impulses.

Ultimately, what emerges from the initial series of mental structures associated with highly charged positive affect states motivating "approach" behaviors on the one hand and highly charged negative affect states motivating aversive behaviors on the other are three distinct motivational systems associated with erotic, dependent, and aggressive strivings, respectively. The erotic and the dependent motivational systems both emerge from the initial series of positively charged mental structures, sharing a common origin in highly charged wishes for physical closeness and fusion, and subsequently differentiate from one another. The aggressive motivational system emerges from the initial series of highly negatively charged mental structures. Each motivational system is associated with specific wishes and fears, organized as fantasies, some of which are conscious and some of which are unconscious. In the normal personality, the three motivational systems are flexibly integrated with one another and with the conscious sense of self, allowing for appropriate and satisfying expression of sexual, dependent, and aggressive needs, wishes, and impulses. In the higher-level, or neurotic, personality disorders we see the predominance of pathology of sexual motivations, in conjunction with anxiety pertaining to integrating sexual, dependent, and aggressive strivings. In contrast, in severe personality disorders, we see the predominance of a very intense, poorly integrated, and poorly modulated form of aggression.

Aggression and the Severe Personality Disorders

We propose that the pathology of aggression seen in patients with severe personality disorders reflects the confluence of constitutional and environmental factors. The theory of development we have presented permits us to account for the concept of inborn dispositions to excessive or inadequate affect activation, thereby doing justice to the genetic and constitutional variations in the intensity, rhythm, and thresholds of activation of aggression. This theory equally permits us to incorporate the role of physical pain, psychic trauma, and severe disturbances in early interactions with caretakers in intensifying aggression as a motivational system by triggering intense negative affects.

A review of the recent literature on alteration in neurotransmitter systems in severe personality disorders, particularly in the borderline and antisocial personality disorders, although still tentative, points to the possibility that neurotransmitters are related to specific distortions in affect activation associated with severe personality disorders (Stone, 1993a, 1993b). Abnormalities in the adrenergic and cholinergic systems, for example, may be related to general affective instability. Deficits in the dopaminergic system may be related to a disposition toward transient psychotic symptoms in borderline patients. Impulsive, aggressive, self-destructive behavior may be facilitated by a lowered function of the serotonergic system (deVagvar, Siever, & Trestman, 1994; Steinberg, Trestman, & Siever, 1994; Stone, 1993a, 1993b; van Reekum, Links, & Federov, 1994; Yehuda et al., 1994). In general, genetic dispositions to temperamental variations in affect activation would seem to be mediated by alterations in neurotransmitter systems, providing a potential link between the biological determinants of affective response and the psychological triggers of specific affects.

The genetic disposition to affect activation, at the level of serotonergic, noradrenergic, and dopaminergic neurotransmitter systems, may determine an organismic hyperreactivity to painful stimuli. This hyperreactivity may be expressed first in an inborn vulnerability to the development of excessive aggressive affect and, secondarily, to the development of severe personality disorders. Genetically determined hyperactivity of the areas of the brain that involve affect activation, particularly hyperactivity of the amygdala in relation to negative affect activation, presumably also play a role in this process. A genetic disposition to the development of severe personality disorders may also involve inborn inhibition of areas of the brain involved in cognitive control, particularly the prefrontal and preorbital cortex and the anterior portion of the cingulum, the areas involved in determining the capacity for "effortful control" (Posner & Rothbart, 2000; Posner et al., 2002). Silbersweig et al. (2001), in a collaborative neuroimaging study with our Personality Disorders Institute, found that patients with borderline personality disorder presented decreased activity in dorsolateral prefrontal and orbitofrontal cortex when compared with normal control subjects during inhibitory conditions. In addition, these patients demonstrated an inappropriate increase in amygdalar activity in neutral word conditions relative to controls. These genetic and constitutional dispositions to excessive aggressive affect activation and lack of cognitive control would result in an inborn, temperamentally given predominance of the negative domain of early experience.

These findings with regard to inborn dispositions to the activation of aggressive affect states are complemented by well-established findings relating structured aggressive behavior in infants to early experience. Specifically, early, severe, chronic physical pain in the first year of life (Grossman, 1991; Zanarini, 2000) and habitual aggressive teasing interactions with mother (Galenson, 1986; Fraiberg, 1983) are related to the accentuation of aggressive behaviors of infants. Grossman's (1986, 1991) convincing arguments in favor of the direct transformation of chronic intense pain into aggression provides a theoretical context for the earlier observations of the battered-child syndrome. The impressive findings of the prevalence of physical and sexual abuse in the history of borderline patients, confirmed by investigators both here and abroad, (Marziali, 1992; Perry & Herman, 1993; Stone, 1993a; van der Kolk, Hostetler, Herron, & Fisler, 1994; Zanarini, 2000) provide additional evidence of the influence of trauma on the development of severe manifestations of aggression.

Further, even in less extreme circumstances, early experiences with caretakers appear to play a crucial function in facilitating affect modulation and regulating the domain of negative affective experience. In particular, Wilfred Bion (1962, 1967, 1970) and after him Fonagy and Target (Target & Fonagy, 1996; Fonagy & Target, 2003) have stressed the function of mother in transforming the infant's poorly defined and highly charged affect states into more highly integrated levels of experience. Conversely, mother's failure to function in this way will intensify the child's anxiety and anger, perhaps functioning as a risk factor for the development of pathological aggression.

Regardless of etiology, we propose that it is the developmental impact of pathological aggression that is responsible for the formation and perpetuation of the personality organization characteristic of patients with severe personality disorders and for the familiar constellation of personality traits that characterize the severe personality disorders. The predominance of pathological aggression reinforces splitting and related defensive operations and interferes with the normal integration of idealized and persecutory mental structures. Failure to integrate the rudimentary psychological structures (i.e., to integrate aggression and transform idealization into reality assessment) fixes personality organization at a stage preceding normal identity formation. This fixation of psychological structures and affects at a relatively poorly integrated level of organization is sometimes referred to as identity diffusion.

Sexuality and the Personality Disorders

While the central motivational feature of the severe personality disorders is the development of pathological aggression, the dominant pathology of the higher-level, or "neurotic," personality disorders (Kernberg, 1975, 1976, 1980, 1984, 1995) is pathology of sexuality. The group of neurotic personality disorders includes particularly the hysterical, the obsessive–compulsive, and the depressive–masochistic personalities, although the centrality of sexual conflicts is most evident in the hysterical personality disorder (Kernberg, 1984). These disorders all present with some form of sexual inhibition related to Oedipal conflicts, and pathological personality traits are dominated by acting out of unconscious guilt over childhood sexual impulses. These Oedipal dynamics reflect the activation of internal object relations unconsciously linked to childhood fantasies of sexual conquest and triumph in relation to one or both parents. Sexual impulses directed toward the parents of childhood, along with related wishes and fantasies, are considered unacceptable and so remain repressed, introducing both sexual inhibition and character rigidity into the neurotic personality. Because, for the neurotic, enjoying sexual pleasure with a partner who is loved (combining erotic and loving strivings) is unconsciously linked to these repressed object relations and related fantasies, neurotics in one way or another avoid the integration of passion and tenderness. Primary conflicts in relation to sexuality are often associated with conflicts around dependency and/or expression of aggression in the neurotic personality.

In contrast to the situation we describe in relation to the neurotic personality disorders, in the severe personality disorders where primary conflicts are in relation to pathological aggression, sexuality is usually "co-opted" by aggression. For the severe personality disorders, sexual behavior is intimately condensed with aggressive aims, a situation that severely limits or distorts sexual intimacy and love relations. In addition, it is common to see the development of paraphilias, which invariably reflect the condensation of sexual and aggressive aims.

Higher-Order Organization of Motivational Systems

The construct of the "drives," aggression and libido, viewed as the basic motivational systems in classical psychoanalysis, has had a long and problematic history. In presenting our model, we have focused on affects and motivational structures, sidestepping the question of whether or not to retain the term "drive." The motivational systems we have described are fundamentally different from the original construct of drives, insofar as drives were considered to be inborn motivational systems, whereas we view affects as the inborn component of motivation. In our view, internal object relations, derived from the interplay of affects and interactions with caretakers, serve as the fundamental structures in the psychological development of motivational systems. However, we remain consistent with classical psychoanalytic approaches to motivation insofar as we do maintain that a theory of motivation based on affects or even on internal object relations alone is not sufficient.

It is our position that despite the problematic nature of the "drives" as a construct, a superordinate integration of motivational structures, organized around particular impulses, fears, and wishes, and associated with specific fantasies, is needed to account for clinical observations and to facilitate clinical work. There are always multiple positive and negative affects expressed toward the same significant other. What emerge in treatment, however, are organized psychological motivational systems, each with its own developmental history and associated with specific wishes, fears, and fantasies, that are characteristic of the individual. A psychological theory that links motives to affects only, without linking affects to integrated motivational systems, does not account for the organized series of mental structures associated with expression of a particular impulse that consistently emerge in the clinical setting. Specifically, hierarchically organized motivational systems corresponding to sexual, dependent, and aggressive strivings consistently emerge in the clinical setting, especially in the treatments of better integrated patients. These motivational systems are organized as integrated systems of internal object relations and are subjectively experienced as conscious and unconscious needs and wishes, linked to unconscious fantasies, that can be seen to have organized the patient's history of past internal object relations. In sum, although we do not retain the original psychoanalytic theory with regard to the origin of the drives, we do endorse a higher-order organization of motivations around aggressive, dependent and sexual strivings.[1] These motivational systems are not inborn but crystalize during psychological development as a result of the interaction of temperamental factors and experiences with significant others. In essence, within a contemporary psychoanalytic frame of reference, drives are the organizational consequence of the activation of inborn affective dispositions under the influence of environmental stimuli.

A PSYCHOANALYTIC MODEL OF NOSOLOGY

The classification of personality disorders we describe in this section was first presented by Kernberg, in 1976. This classification system is organized around the dimension of severity, paying particular attention to identity consolidation, defensive operations, and reality testing. Severity ranges from (1) psychotic personality organization, through (2) borderline personality organization, to (3) neurotic personality organization (see Figure 3.1).

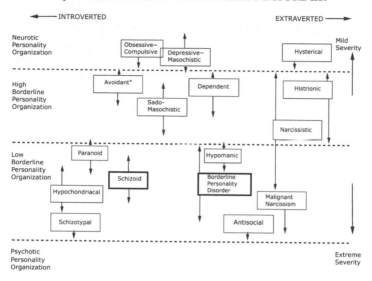

FIGURE 3.1. Relationship between familiar, prototypic personality types and structural diagnosis. Severity ranges from mildest, at the top of the page, to extremely severe at the bottom. Arrows indicate range of severity. *We include avoidant personality disorder in deference to the DSM. However, in our clinical experience, patients who have been diagnosed with avoidant personality disorder ultimately prove to have another personality disorder that accounts for avoidant pathology. As a result, we question the existence of avoidant personality as a clinical entity. This is a controversial question deserving further study.

Psychotic Personality Organization

"Psychotic personality organization" is characterized by lack of integration of the concept of self and significant others, that is, failure to attain normal identity formation ("identity diffusion"), a predominance of defensive operations centering around splitting ("primitive defenses"), and loss of reality testing. Within a psychoanalytic frame of reference, reality testing refers to the capacity to differentiate self from nonself, to distinguish intrapsychic from external sources of stimuli, and to maintain empathy with ordinary social criteria of reality. All these functions are typically lost in the psychoses and are manifested particularly in hallucinations and delusions (Kernberg 1976, 1984). The loss of reality testing reflects the loss of differentiation between representations of self and other, especially under conditions of peak affect activation. All patients with psychotic personality organization really represent atypical forms of psychosis. Therefore, strictly speaking, psychotic personality organization represents an exclusion criterion for the personality disorders in the clinical setting.

Borderline Personality Organization

"Borderline personality organization" is characterized by pathological identity formation (identity diffusion), primitive defensive operations, and varying degrees of pathology of internalized value systems in the setting of maintained but somewhat reduced reality testing marked by a decreased capacity for subtle and tactful evaluation of interpersonal processes, particularly in the setting of more intimate relations. This level of personality organization includes all the severe personality disorders seen in clinical practice. Typical personality disorders included here are the borderline personality disorder, the schizoid and schizotypal personality disorders, the paranoid personality disorder, the hypomanic personality disorder, hypochondriasis (a syndrome which has many characteristics of a personality disorder proper), the narcissistic personality disorder (including the malignant narcissism syndrome [Kernberg, 1992]), and the antisocial personality disorder. The antisocial personality, the syndrome of malignant narcissism, and many of the narcissistic personalities are characterized in addition by significant pathology of internalized value systems (Kernberg, 1989, 1992).

From a clinical standpoint, the syndrome of identity diffusion represents the dominant characteristic of borderline personality organization and, thus, of the severe personality disorders as a group. In particular, in the context of pathological aggression we see a poorly integrated, superficial, and unstable sense of self and others and limited affect dispositions marked by a combination of intensity and superficiality in the setting of the predominance of negative affects. These core features of the severe personality disorders reflect the splitting of the idealized segment of experience from the paranoid. Splitting mechanisms are naturally reinforced by other primitive defensive operations intimately connected with splitting (projective identification, denial, primitive idealization, devaluation, omnipotence, and omnipotent control). This entire constellation of defensive operations serves to distort interpersonal interactions, to create chronic disturbances in interpersonal relations, and to interfere with the capacity to assess other people's behavior and motivations in depth, particularly under the impact of intense affect activation. The lack of integration of the concept of the self interferes with a comprehensive integration of one's past and present into a capacity to predict one's future behavior and decreases the capacity for commitment to professional goals, personal interests, work and social functions, and intimate relationships.

The lack of integration of the concept of significant others interferes with the capacity for realistic assessment of others, for selecting partners harmonious with the individual's actual expectations, and for investment in others. The predominance of negative affect dispositions leads to an infiltration of sexual intimacy by excessive aggressive components. The outcome is, frequently, an exaggerated and chaotic interest in polymorphous perverse sexual practices as part of the individual's sexual repertoire. In more severe cases, we see a primary inhibition of the capacity for sensual responsiveness and erotic enjoyment. Under these latter circumstances, overwhelming negative affect states eliminate the very capacity for erotic response, leading to the severe types of sexual inhibition that are to be found in the most severe personality disorders.

The lack of integration of the concept of self and of significant others also interferes with the internalization of the early layers of the system of internalized values. This leads to a particularly exaggerated quality of the idealization of positive values and ideals, and to an extremely persecutory quality of prohibitions. These developments lead, in turn, to a predominance of splitting mechanisms at the level of internalized value systems, with excessive projection of internalized prohibitions. At the same time, excessive, idealized demands for perfection further interfere with the integration of a normal superego. Under these conditions, antisocial behavior may emerge as an important aspect of severe personality disorders, particularly in the syndrome of malignant narcissism and in the antisocial personality. Of note, the antisocial personality, the most severe of the personality disorders, is characterized not only by the lack of any internalized system of values but also by the greatest severity of identity diffusion seen among the personality disorders (Kernberg, 1984, 1992). In general, consolidation of a normal system of internalized morals and values is a consequence of identity integration, and, in turn, protects normal identity. Severe disorganization of the system of internalized values, in contrast, worsens the effects of identity diffusion.

A particular group of personality disorders presents the characteristics of borderline personality organization while maintaining more satisfactory social adaptation, including the capacity to obtain some degree of intimacy and some degree of satisfaction from work. These patients have relatively good impulse control, relatively little overtly aggressive behavior, some capacity for a benign cycle of intimate involvements along with a capacity for dependency gratification, and a better adaptation to work. These features clearly differentiate this group from the group presenting with more severe pathology. This group constitutes "high borderline" level of personality organization. The high-borderline group includes the cyclothymic personality, the sadomasochistic personality, the histrionic or infantile personality, and the dependent personalities, as well as some better-functioning narcissistic personality disorders.

Neurotic Personality Organization

The next level of personality disorder, "neurotic personality organization," is characterized by normal identity consolidation, the predominance of defenses based on repression, and stable reality testing. This level of psychological organization is associated with a capacity for deep and caring relationships with others and a fully integrated system of internal values. The neurotic personality organization is associated with good anxiety tolerance, impulse control, effectiveness and creativity in work, and a capacity for sexual love and emotional intimacy disrupted only by unconscious guilt feelings reflected in specific pathological patterns of interaction in relation to sexual intimacy. The neurotic personality organization includes the hysterical personality, the depressive–masochistic personality, the obsessive personality, and many so-called avoidant personality disorders, in other words, the "phobic character" of psychoanalytic literature (which, in our view, remains a problematic entity).

The neurotic personality organization is distinguished from the normal personality on the basis of character rigidity. Character rigidity can be defined as the automatic activation of organized constellations of personality traits that are more or less maladaptive and not subject to voluntary control. In the neurotic personality disorders, internal object relations that are threatening are split off from the integrated representations that comprise normal identity. The repression-based defensive operations that ensure that these particular internal object relations remain apart from the dominant, conscious sense of self introduce rigidity into the neurotic personality organization and are responsible ultimately, for neurotic character traits. As we have already described, internal object relations that are rejected from the dominant sense of self are especially highly charged and poorly integrated manifestations of sexual, dependent, and aggressive impulses, wishes, and fears, with conflicts over sexuality predominating.

DEVELOPMENTAL, STRUCTURAL, AND MOTIVATIONAL CONTINUITIES

Having thus classified personality disorders in terms of their severity, we now examine particular continuities that establish a psychopathologically linked network of apparently related personality disorders (see Figure 3.1).

The Borderline and Schizoid Personality Disorders

The borderline personality disorder and the schizoid personality disorder may be described as the simplest forms of severe personality disorders. These disorders reflect identity diffusion in the setting of the predominance of splitting mechanisms and can be seen as the "purest" expression of the general characteristics of borderline personality organization.

Fairbairn (1954) described the schizoid personality as the prototype of all personality disorders and provided an understanding of the psychodynamics of these patients unsurpassed to this day. He described the splitting operations separating "good" and "bad" internalized object relations, the motivated self and object representations that comprise the split-off object relations, the consequent impoverishment of interpersonal relations, and their replacement by a defensive hypertrophy of fantasy life. In fact, in the course of psychoanalytic exploration, the apparent lack of affect display seen in the schizoid personality turns out to reflect severe splitting operations; extreme splitting leads to a fragmentation of affective experience, which "empties out" interpersonal experience. At the same time, the internalized object relations of the schizoid personality have the split, persecutory, and idealized characteristics typical of the borderline personality disorder (Kernberg, 1975). While the schizotypal personality disorder as listed in DSM-IV appears to be a more severe form of schizoid personality, it appears increasingly likely that schizotypal personality is not a personality disorder at all but, rather, a variant of schizophrenia, characterized by a mild thought disorder and a family history of psychotic illness (Lenzenweger, 1998).

The borderline personality disorder presents structural and dynamic features similar to those seen in the schizoid personality, but in the borderline personality we see expression of this pathology predominantly in impulsive interactions in the interpersonal field (Akhtar, 1992; Stone, 1994). In contrast to the schizoid personality, where internal object relations are expressed in conscious fantasy life in the setting of social withdrawal, in the borderline personality disorder the same widely split, internalized object relations are enacted in the interpersonal field. In fact, in the borderline personality disorder, repetitive, powerfully motivated interpersonal behaviors often replace self-awareness. Episodic, intense, overwhelming affect states ("affect storms") and poor impulse control in the setting of identity diffusion are typical of the borderline personality disorder, in marked contrast with the schizoid personality where we see apparent lack of affect and good impulse control.

It may well be that the descriptive differences between the schizoid and borderline disorders reflect temperamental differences. In particular, the borderline and schizoid personalities appear to differ across the dimension of extroversion and introversion, one of the important temperamental factors that emerges under different names in various models of classification.

Pathology of Aggression and the Personality Disorders

Extreme pathology of aggression is characteristic of the paranoid personality disorder, the syndrome of hypochondriasis, the sadomasochistic personality disorder, the syndrome of malignant narcissism, and the antisocial personality. The paranoid personality reflects an increase of aggression relative to the schizoid personality disorder. In the paranoid personality, the projection of aggressive internal object relations creates an external world populated by persecutory figures. Defensive idealization of the self is related to efforts to control this overwhelmingly dangerous external world. Thus, where splitting per se predominates in the borderline and schizoid personality disorders, in the paranoid personality we see the predominance of defenses related to splitting but that rely heavily on the projection of persecutory experiences while trying to control them as they are embodied in the external world. The hypochondriacal syndrome reflects a projection of persecutory objects onto the interior of the body; hypochondriacal personalities usually also show strong paranoid and schizoid characteristics.

Affect Regulation and the Personality Disorders

The intensity of affect activation and the lack of affect control seen in the borderline personality, along with the high incidence of affective illness that characterizes this group, suggest the presence of a temperamental factor relating to affect regulation as a predisposing factor for development of borderline personality disorder. At the same time, it is impressive the degree to which the integration of negative and positive affect states obtained in the course of psychodynamic treatments brings about a marked toning down and modulation of affect response. The increase of impulse control and affect tolerance in the borderline personality seen as a result of successful treatment illustrates that splitting mechanisms play a central role in the pathology of affects seen in borderline personality. In contrast, in the hypomanic and cyclothymic personalities, pathology of affect activation appears to reflect a temperamental disposition in the area of affect regulation.

The borderline personality disorder, when characterized by especially prominent and intense aggression, may evolve into the sadomasochistic personality disorder. With the achievement of identity consolidation, the disposition to strong sadomasochism may become incorporated into or controlled by a relatively well integrated superego structure, establishing the conditions for the depressive masochistic personality disorder. The depressive–masochistic personality may be considered the highest level of two lines that go from the borderline personality through the sadomasochistic to the depressive masochistic on the one hand, and from the hypomanic to the depressive masochistic, on the other. This entire spectrum of personality disorders appears to reflect the internalization of object relations under conditions of abnormal affective development or affect control.

Pathological Identity Formation and the Personality Disorders

In contrast to the clear indication of identity pathology seen in all the other personality disorders included in borderline personality organization, in the narcissistic personality a lack of integration of the concept of significant others goes hand in hand with an integrated, but pathological, sense of self. This structure is sometimes referred to as a pathological grandiose self or pathological identity formation. The pathological grandiose self replaces the underlying lack of integration of a normal self and is responsible for the appearance of better surface adaptation seen in the narcissistic personality disorders relative to the other severe personality disorders (Akhtar, 1989; Plakun, 1989; Ronningstam & Gunderson, 1989). In the course of psychodynamic treatment we may observe the dissolution of this pathological grandiose self and the reemergence of the typical structure of identity diffusion of borderline personality organization before a new integration of normal identity can take place.

In the narcissistic personality the pathological self absorbs both real and idealized self and object representations into an unrealistically idealized concept of self. This structural development leads to a parallel impoverishment of the system of internalized values, where we see a predominance of persecutory superego precursors over idealized structures. In this setting, persecutory structures tend to be projected, interfering with the later development of more integrated superego functions (Kernberg, 1975, 1984, 1992). As a result, the narcissistic personality often presents some degree of antisocial behavior.

When intense pathology of aggression dominates in a narcissistic personality structure we see the development of especially malignant forms of psychopathology. In this setting, the pathological sense of self becomes infiltrated by aggression in such a way that expression of aggression in various forms is perfectly acceptable ("ego syntonic") and also pleasurable. The result is the development of grandiosity combined with ruthlessness, sadism, or hatred. The constellation of narcissistic personality, antisocial behavior, ego syntonic aggression, and paranoid tendencies constitutes the syndrome of malignant narcissism. Kernberg (1992) has proposed that this syndrome is intermediate between the narcissistic personality disorder and the antisocial personality disorder proper, in which a total absence or deterioration of superego functioning has occurred.

The antisocial personality disorder (Akhtar, 1992; Bursten, 1989; Hare, 1986; Kernberg, 1984) usually reveals, in psychoanalytic exploration, severe underlying paranoid trends together with a total incapacity for any nonexploitive investment in significant others. The total absence of a capacity for guilt feelings, or of any concern for self and others, an incapacity to identify with any moral or ethical value in self or others, and an incapacity to project a dimension of personal future characterize the antisocial personality disorder. The less severe syndrome of malignant narcissism is distinguished from the antisocial personality insofar as there is some capacity for commitment to others and for experiencing authentic feelings of guilt. The most important prognostic indicators for any psychotherapeutic approach to the personality disorders are the capacity for nonexploitive object relations (i.e., the capacity for significant investment in others) and the extent to which antisocial behaviors predominate (Kernberg, 1975; Stone, 1990).

The Higher-Level or Neurotic Personality Disorders

At a higher level of personality organization we see the "neurotic" personality disorders, the obsessive–compulsive, hysterical, and depressive–masochistic personalities. The obsessive–compulsive personality can be characterized by the absorption of aggression into a well-integrated but excessively demanding and self-critical superego. This internal situation is expressed in the familiar features of perfectionism, self-doubts, and chronic need to control the environment and the self that are characteristic of this personality disorder.

While the histrionic, or infantile, personality is a milder form of the borderline personality disorder, though still within the borderline spectrum, the hysterical personality disorder represents a higher level of personality, falling in the neurotic spectrum of personality organization. In the hysterical personality, emotional lability, extroversion, and dependent and exhibitionistic traits of the histrionic personality are restricted to the sexual realm. In contrast to the histrionic personality, the hysteric is able to have normally deep, mature, committed, and differentiated relationships outside the sexual realm. Further, in contrast to the sexual "freedom" of the typical infantile personality, the hysterical personality often presents a combination of pseudo-hypersexuality and sexual inhibition.

The depressive–masochistic personality disorder (Kernberg, 1992), the highest-level outcome of the pathology of depressive affect as well as that of sadomasochism, presents not only a well-integrated superego (as do all other personalities with neurotic personality organization) but also an extremely punitive set of internal values. This predisposes the patient to self-defeating behavior, reflecting an unconscious need to suffer as an expiation for guilt feelings or as a precondition for sexual pleasure, reflecting the Oedipal dynamics characterizing the neurotic spectrum of personality disorders. The excessive dependency and easy sense of frustration seen in these patients goes hand in hand with their "faulty metabolism" of aggression. Where an aggressive response is called for, the depressive–masochistic personality is more likely to feel depressed. As a result, a typically excessively aggressive response to the frustration of dependency needs may rapidly turn into a renewed depressive response, as a consequence of excessive guilt feelings over aggression.

Implications of This Classification System

The classification system we have outlined combines structural and developmental approaches to psychological organization, based on a theory of internal object relations. Personality disorders are classified, first and foremost, according to severity of pathology, which mirrors the presence or absence and also the severity of pathology of identity. Level of personality organization is the most powerful "first pass" predictor of prognosis and will guide treatment planning as well. A combined analysis of reality testing, identity, the predominant level of defensive operations, the system of internalized values, quality of object relations, and the degree of integration and organization of motivational structures, as well as their accessibility to consciousness, permits us to characterize severity of psychopathology. In addition, at any level of severity or level of personality organization, we can distinguish among the personality disorders across several dimensions. Specifically, we consider the extent to which pathology is dominated by aggression, the extent to which pathological affective dispositions influence personality development, the effect of the development of a pathological grandiose self, and the potential influence of a temperamental disposition to extroversion/introversion distinguish among the various personality disorders. This classification illustrates the advantages of combining categorical and dimensional criteria for classifying personality disorders.

There are clinically observable affective–developmental lines that link several of the personality disorders to one another, particularly along an axis of severity. Figure 3.2 summarizes the relationships we have outlined that can be seen among the various personality disorders.

PSYCHOANALYTIC AND PSYCHOTHERAPEUTIC TREAMENTS FOR PERSONALITY DISORDERS

A General Therapeutic Frame

The treatments we describe here are long-term psychodynamic psychotherapies and psychoanalytic treatments designed to treat personality disorders. Psychotherapy sessions meet twice weekly and treatments typically last between 2 and 4 years. Psychoanalysands attend sessions three or four times a week, and treatment typically lasts between 4 and 6 years. The amount of time and effort required reflects the ambitious nature of these treatments. The goals of psychoanalytic psychotherapy and psychoanalysis

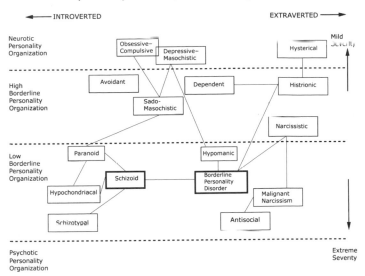

FIGURE 3.2. Continuities and clinically relevant relationships among the personality disorders. Connecting lines indicate clinically relevant relationships among disorders.

are to modify personality organization and the quality of the internal object relations associated with symptoms and pathological character traits.

For patients organized at a borderline level, treatment is organized around the goal of resolving or ameliorating identity diffusion and promoting normal identity consolidation. For patients organized at a neurotic level, treatment is organized around the goal of reducing character rigidity. Our therapeutic approach reflects our understanding of the structural and dynamic features underlying identity diffusion and character rigidity. To resolve identity diffusion, we promote integration of split, mutually dissociated idealized and persecutory internal object relations. To resolve character rigidity, we promote integration of conflictual, unconscious internal object relations into the dominant sense of self. These changes in personality organization correspond with changes in the maladaptive character traits and subjective disturbances characteristic of the various personality disorders.

With all the personality disorders, our technical approach is organized around exploration of the patient's internal object relations. Predictably, conflictual, or pathogenic, internal object relations tend to be played out, and in the process to distort current interpersonal relationships. As a result, in the psychotherapeutic treatment of patients with personality disorders we focus on the patient's internal object relations as they are played out in the patient's current relationships; in our approach, the patient's current interpersonal relationships serve as a window into the patient's inner world. In psychotherapy and psychoanalysis the patient's relationship with the therapist offers a special opportunity for the patient and therapist to explore, in their immediate here-and-now interactions, the ways in which the patient's conflictual internal object relations are enacted in his interpersonal relationships. The tendency for patients in psychodynamic therapies to experience and enact aspects of their pathogenic, conflictual, internal object relations in their interactions with the therapist is referred to as transference. Transference manifestations differ according to the nature of the patient's psychopathology and, in particular, the patient's level of personality organization.

In patients with neurotic level of personality organization, transferences tend to be relatively stable, well organized, and realistic and are associated with complex, relatively well modulated affect states. These internal object relations can be relatively easily understood in terms of an unconscious relationship between the patient's childhood self and the parents of the past. When activated in the transference, these unconscious relationships can be interpreted as reflections of both realistic and fantasied aspects of childhood relationships with the parents, as well as defenses against the reactivation of these unconscious relationships in the present. Neurotic transferences emerge gradually and evolve slowly during the course of treatment, and the internal object relations activated in the transference unfold systematically.

The situation is quite different when it comes to the treatment of patients with severe personality disorders. When treating patients with poorly consolidated identity (borderline level of personality organization), transferences are poorly organized, unstable, and unrealistic. They are associated with affects that are intense, poorly differentiated, and poorly modulated. Although derived from aspects of past relationships, these internal object relations cannot be easily linked to actual or fantasied relationships with the parents of the past. In treatment, internal object relations of this kind are typically activated in the transference immediately and chaotically, often during the first contact between patient and therapist. An additional complication, adding further confusion and instability to the treatment situation, is that in borderline transferences, we see not only shifts among different internal object relations activated in the transference, but also typically rapid shifting of roles within any given internal object relation. Thus, we see a rapid interchange of roles, such as that at one moment the patient will identify with one half of an object relational dyad and, at the next moment, with the other half of the dyad, while attributing the complementary role to the therapist.

Our model of personality disorders, embedded in an object relational frame of reference, permits the therapist to understand and to work therapeutically with what often appears to be complete chaos in the treatment of patients organized at a borderline level. At the same time, our model guides the clinician treating the neurotic patient, helping the therapist to negotiate the different challenges presented by this patient population.

The Treatment of Patients with Borderline Personality Organization

The treatment approach we present has been designed specifically to treat patients with severe personality disorders. This treatment, "transference-focused psychotherapy" for patients with borderline personality organization (TFP-B), is a twice-weekly psychodynamic treatment based on principles derived from psychoanalysis. TFP-B has been systematically described in a treatment manual (Clarkin et al., 1999) and is the basis of an empirical research program that is presently in progress (Clarkin et al., 2001; Clarkin et al., 2004). The treatment is organized around the goals of promoting identity consolidation while containing the destructive acting out that typically characterizes the treatments of patients organized at a borderline level. The basic strategy of TFP-B is to promote integration of "split" persecutory and idealized internal object relations to form better-integrated representations of self and other, while decreasing reliance on splitting-based defenses.

Strategies of Transference-Focused Psychotherapy for Patients with Borderline Level of Personality Organization

The overall psychotherapeutic strategy of TFP for the treatment of patients with severe personality disorders can be conceptualized in terms of three sequential tasks:

Step 1 is to diagnose the idealized or persecutory internal object relation that is apparently dominant within the overall chaotic transference situation and to describe in as much detail and as accurately as possible the representations involved. For example, the therapist might point out to the patient that their momentary relationship resembles that of a sadistic prison guard with a paralyzed, frightened victim.

Step 2 of this strategy is to clarify which is the self-representation and which is the object representation in this internal object relation at the moment and what is the dominant affect linking them. For example, the therapist might point out, in expanding the previous intervention, that it is as if the patient experienced himself as a frightened, paralyzed victim while attributing to the therapist the behavior of a sadistic prison guard. Because of the typical oscillating or alternating attribution of self and object representations seen in the borderline patient, the patient's identification with either half of the dyad is unstable. As a result, later in the same session the therapist might point out to the patient that, now, the situation has become reversed in that the patient behaves like a sadistic prison guard while the therapist has been placed in the role of the frightened victim.

Step 3 of this interpretive strategy is to link the particular internal object relation currently dominant in the transference with the entirely opposite transference, activated at other times in the treatment, that constitutes the split-off counterpart to the object relation currently active. For example, the therapist might remind the patient that even though he presently feels himself to be in the hands of a sadistic prison guard, at other times the patient has experienced the therapist as a perfect, all-giving mother. The therapist would go on to point out that this other experience of the therapist is associated with the patient's experiencing himself as a satisfied, happy, loved baby who is the exclusive object of mother's attention. The therapist might, in addition, suggest that the persecutory prison guard is in fact a frustrating, teasing, and rejecting mother, while the victim is an enraged baby who wants to take revenge but is afraid of being destroyed if he does so. The therapist might further add that this terrible mother–infant relationship is kept completely separate from the idealized relationship. A complete interpretation would also establish a hypothesis as to the meaning of or motivation for the patient's dissociating the persecutory and idealized transferences. For example, the therapist might interpret that the patient feels he needs to do this out of fear that if he allows the idealized relationship with the therapist to be contaminated by the persecutory relationship, the ideal relationship might be permanently destroyed, taking with it all hope.

This approach will lead to the gradual integration of persecutory and idealized internal object relations to form the more realistic transferences typical of patients organized at a neurotic level. The successful integration of mutually dissociated idealized and persecutory internal object relations in the transference results in the integration not only of the corresponding self and object representations but also of primitive affects. The integration of intense, polarized affects leads, over time, to affect modulation, an increase in the capacity for affect control, and a corresponding decrease in impulsive behaviors, as well as a heightened capacity for empathy with both self and others and a corresponding deepening and maturing of interpersonal relations.

The three-part strategy we have outlined relies on three basic tools of psychoanalytic technique, all modified to meet the clinical demands of patients with severe personality disorders. We refer to interpretation of unconscious conflict, systematic transference analysis, and technical neutrality. We define each of these terms and then explain how each has been modified for TFP-B.

Interpretation. Interpretation is a three-step process, beginning with clarification, followed by confrontation, and leading finally to interpretation proper. Clarification entails systematic exploration of the details of the patient's subjective experience. Confrontation involves pointing out contradictions, inconsistencies, and omissions in the patient's verbal and nonverbal communications. Interpretation entails establishing hypotheses about the unconscious determinants of the patient's behavior. In contrast to standard psychoanalysis, in TFP the emphasis is on clarification and confrontation rather than on interpretation proper. To the degree that unconscious meanings are interpreted in TFP, this is done in a restricted fashion, limited largely to the unconscious meanings of the patient's behavior in the "here and now."

Systematic Transference Analysis. In TFP-B, as in psychoanalysis, the therapist focuses his attention on the patient's internal object relations as they are activated in the treatment. However, in TFP-B the therapist cannot afford to focus his attention entirely on transference developments. Instead, in each session, the therapist must also maintain ongoing attention to the patient's long-range treatment goals and to the dominant, current conflicts in the patient's life outside the sessions. This is necessary because when borderline patients are in psychotherapy they tend to lose sight of treatment goals and to neglect the demands of external reality. This propensity on the part of borderline patients reflects the activation of defensive operations that lead to dissociation between external reality and treatment hours.

Technical Neutrality. Technical neutrality is central to the strategy of TFP-B. When we describe the TFP therapist as maintaining a "neutral" stance, we mean that he or she makes an effort to avoid taking sides in the patient's inner struggles. This does not imply that neutral therapist is in any way detached from the patient. Rather, the neutral therapist is actively engaged with the patient and maintains an attitude of concern for the patient's best interests. The hallmark of the neutral therapist is his or her capacity to reflect on the ways in which the patient is affecting the therapist and to use his or her reactions to the patient to deepen understanding of the patient's conflicts. In contrast to treatments for neurotic patients, in which the therapist can maintain a neutral stance relatively consistently throughout the treatment, in TFP-B, technical neutrality is an ideal position from which the therapist repeatedly deviates and then returns. The impossibility of consistently maintaining technical neutrality reflects the severe acting-out characteristic of borderline patients, inside and outside the treatment hours, which often requires limit setting and structuring of the treatment situation. Every time the therapist intervenes in this way he or she is deviating from technical neutrality. After doing so, the therapist will reinstate technical neutrality by reviewing and interpreting the reasons for having moved away from a position of technical neutrality.

Given the strong tendencies toward acting out on the part of borderline patients, dangerous complications of treatment are common and pose a chronic threat to the treatment. Specifically, characterologically based (i.e., not linked to affective illness) suicide attempts, drug abuse, self-mutilation and other self-destructive behaviors, and aggressive behaviors that may be life threatening to the patient and to others are all typical features of the psychotherapeutic treatments of many patients with severe personality disorders. As a result, the assessment of whether there are emergency situations that require immediate intervention is an important aspect of each session. On the basis of our general treatment strategy and experience in the treatment of severely ill borderline patients, we have constructed the following set of priorities of intervention that reflect the need to assess, diagnose, and treat these and other complications.

A threat of imminent suicidal or homicidal behavior has the highest priority in each session. If there seem to be immediate threats to the continuity of the treatment, these constitute the second highest priority that needs to be taken up by the therapist. If the patient appears to be communicating in deceptive or dishonest ways, this constitutes the third highest priority; psychodynamic psychotherapy demands honest communication between patient and therapist and the meanings that underlie the patient's dishonesty or deceptiveness must be interpreted. Acting out in the sessions as well as outside the session constitutes the next highest priority. With these priorities considered, the therapist is free to concentrate fully on the analysis of the patient's internal object relations as they are being enacted in his current life, with special attention to the transference.

The Treatment of Patients with Neurotic Personality Organization

Transference-focused psychotherapy for patients with neurotic personality organization (TFP-N) has been designed specifically to treat patients with neurotic personality organization (Caligor, Clarkin, & Kernberg, 2004). In contrast to TFP-B, the clinical technique of TFP-N is very similar to the technique employed in psychoanalysis, with few modifications. The main difference between TFP-N and psychoanalysis is that TFP-N is more focal and less ambitious in its goals. The goal of psychoanalysis is reduction of character rigidity across all affected areas of functioning. In contrast, the goal of TFP-N is reduction of character rigidity in a specific area of functioning, manifested in the patient's presenting complaints and designated in the mutually agreed on treatment goals. In keeping with the more limited goals of TFP-N relative to psychoanalysis, in developing TFP-B, we have modified analytic technique to focus on particular areas of conflict rather than endorsing the less selective attitude of "evenly hovering attention" assumed by the psychoanalyst. The basic strategies of TFP-N and psychoanalysis are to promote integration into the dominant sense of self of conflictual internal object relations that have been split off and repressed, while decreasing reliance on neurotic defenses relative to healthy or mature defenses. The overall approach is to bring repressed and dissociated internal object relations into consciousness where the underlying conflicts can be explored and worked through. The outcome of this process is that previously conflictual internal object relations become better integrated and less affectively charged and, as a result, are assimilated into the dominant sense of self.

Strategies of Transference-Focused Psychotherapy for Patients with Neurotic Level of Personality Organization

The overall psychotherapeutic strategy of TFP for the treatment of patients with neurotic personality organization can be conceptualized in terms of five sequential tasks, described below. In TFP-N, implementation of these tasks is restricted to circumscribed areas of character rigidity. Specifically, the treatment focuses on areas of character rigidity tied to the patient's dominant symptoms and the problems that have been agreed upon as the targets of the treatment, as well as on those character defenses that interfere with exploration of these specific areas.

Step 1 is to facilitate activation of conflictual representations of self and others and associated affects in the treatment. This is accomplished by the therapist's maintaining a neutral stance while systematically exploring the internal object relations enacted in the session, beginning with defensively activated representations and moving toward those more closely associated with impulse expression. The process of clarifying, exploring, and ultimately interpreting the functions of the patient's defensively activated internal object relations is referred to as analysis of resistance.

Step 2 of this strategy is to diagnose the affectively dominant internal object relation that is being enacted in the treatment and to describe in as much detail and as accurately as possible the representations involved. For example, the therapist might point out to the patient that his discomfort with regard to speaking openly with the therapist appears connected to an experience of himself as a self-conscious child in the presence of an admired but potentially disapproving parent.

Step 3 of this strategy is to clarify and ultimately interpret the conflict embedded in the affectively dominant object relation activated in the treatment. For example, the therapist might point out, in expanding the previous intervention, that it is as if the patient experienced himself as entirely free of disapproving and critical impulses, feeling only self-conscious and admiring. The therapist would suggest that it might make the patient feel anxious to experience himself as at all critical of the therapist or of the other important people in his life. This is an example of analysis of resistance, in which the patient's defensively activated internal object relations are identified, explored, and ultimately interpreted. In this example, the therapist's interpreting, over time, the patient's defensive use of attributing all critical feeling to an object representation while dissociating himself from these feelings will pave the way to uncovering the impulse underlying the patient's defensive self-representation, along with the anxiety associated with expression of that impulse.

Step 4 of this interpretive strategy is to explore the repressed and dissociated, impulsive, internal object relations that underlie the defensively activated internal object relations, along with the anxiety associated with impulse expression. For example what might emerge in the foregoing example is that the self-conscious child self and the admired but potentially disapproving parent defends against activation of the experience of a hurt and angry child who wants revenge in relation to a critical, derisive, and rejecting parent. The patient avoids consciously experiencing this internal object relation because feeling angry and vengeful, as well as critical and derisive, are unacceptable feelings, associated with guilt, depression, anxiety, and fear. During the course of the treatment, the patient will become aware of his unconscious identification with both halves of the impulsive dyad, both the angry and vengeful child and the critical, derisive, and rejecting parent.

Step 5 is to work through the guilt and regret associated with acknowledging and taking responsibility for formerly unconscious impulses, represented as affectively charged internal object relations. In this process, the patient will make amends, in fantasy and reality, for the potential harm to others associated with the expression of his conflictual impulses. For example, the patient we have been describing, now aware of his potential hostility and derision as well as his anger and wishes for revenge, might experience a new level of concern for the important people in his life. He might pay special attention to the needs of his employees or his children or his parents, and he might demonstrate similar feelings and efforts in relation to the therapist in the transference. The outcome of this process of uncovering unacceptable impulses, taking responsibility for them and making reparation, repeated over time, is that representations associated with expression of hostile, derisive impulses become more complex and differentiated and associated affects become less intense and less anxiety provoking. As the internal object relations associated with expression of hostile and derisive impulses become better integrated, they will become part of the patient's dominant sense of self. These changes in psychological structures correspond with a decrease in character rigidity in relation to the expression of hostility and greater freedom to enjoy intimacy and interdependence.

The strategy we have outlined relies on the same three basic tools of psychoanalytic technique—interpretation, systematic transference analysis, and technical neutrality—described in relation to TFP-B but without the modifications introduced for the severe personality disorders.

NOTE

1. These strivings are best synthesized in the concepts of libido and aggression: the intimate connection between sexual and dependent strivings warrants their condensation as libido.

REFERENCES

Akhtar, S. (1989). Narcissistic personality disorder: Descriptive features and differential diagnosis. In O. F. Kernberg (Ed.), *Narcissistic personality disorder: Psychiatric Clinics of North America* (pp. 505–530). Philadelphia: Saunders.

Akhtar, S. (1992). *Broken structures*. Northvale, NJ: Jason Aronson.

American Psychiatric Association. (1980). *Diagnostic and statistical manual of mental disorders* (3rd ed.). Washington, DC: Author.

American Psychiatric Association. (1994). *Diagnostic and statistical manual of mental disorders* (4th ed.). Washington, DC: Author.

Bateman, A. W., & Fonagy, P. (2004). *Intensive multi-context intensive psychotherapy for severe personality disorders: A manualized application of a psychoanalytic attachment theory model*. Oxford, UK: Oxford University Press.

Beebe, B., & Lachman, F. M. (2002). *Infant research and adult treatment: Co-constructing interactions*. Hillsdale, NJ: Analytic Press.

Benjamin, L. S. (1992). An interpersonal approach to the diagnosis of borderline personality disorder. In J. F. Clarkin, E. Marziali, & H. Munroe-Blum (Eds.), *Borderline personality disorder: Clinical and empirical perspectives* (pp. 161–198). New York: Guilford Press.

Benjamin, L. S. (1996). *Interpersonal diagnosis and treatment of personality disorders* (2nd ed.). New York: Guilford Press.

Bion, W. (1962). *Learning from experience*. London: Heinemann.

Bion, W. (1967). *Second thoughts*. London: Heinemann

Bion, W. (1970). *Attention and interpretation*. New York: Basic Books.

Bursten, B. (1989). The relationship between narcissistic and antisocial personalities. In O. F. Kernberg (Ed.), *Narcissistic personality disorder: Psychiatric clinics of North America* (pp. 571–584). Philadelphia: Saunders.

Caligor, E., Clarkin, J. F., & Kernberg, O. K. (2004). *Psychotherapy for neurotic personality*. Unpublished manuscript.

Clark, L. A. (1993). *Manual for the Schedule for Nonadaptive and Adaptive Personality (SNAP)*. Minneapolis: University of Minnesota Press.

Clarkin, J. F., Yeomans, F., & Kernberg, O. F. (1999). *Psychotherapy for borderline personality*. New York: Wiley.

Clarkin, J. F., Foelsch, P. A., Levy, K. N., Hull, J. W., Delaney, J. C., & Kernberg, O. F. (2001). The development of a psychodynamic treatment for patients with borderline personality disorder: A preliminary study of behavioral control. *Journal of Personality Disorders, 15*(6), 487–495.

Clarkin, J. F., Levy, K. N., Lenzenweger M., & Kernberg, O. F. (2004). The Personality Disorders Institute/Borderline Personality Research Foundation randomized control trial for borderline personality disorder: Rationale, methods, and patient characteristics. *Journal of Personality Disorders, 18*(1), 51–71.

Cloninger, C. R., Svrakic, D. M., & Przybeck, T. R. (1993). A psychobiological model temperament and character. *Archives of General Psychiatry, 50,* 975–990.

Costa, P. T., & Widiger, T. A. (1994). Introduction. In P. T. Costa & T. Widiger (Eds.), *Personality disorders and the five-factor model of personality* (pp. 1–10). Washington, DC: American Psychological Association.

Costa, P. T., & Widiger, T. A. (2002). *Personality disorders and the five-factor model of personality* (2nd ed.). Washington, DC: American Psychological Association.

Depue, R. A., & Lenzenweger, M. F. (2001). A neurobehavioral dimensional model. In W. J. Livesley (Ed.), *Handbook of personality disorders* (pp. 136–176). New York: Guilford Press.

deVagvar, M. L., Siever, L. J., & Trestman, R. (1994). Impulsivity and serotonin in borderline personality disorder. In K. R. Silk (Ed.), *Biological and neurobehavioral studies of borderline personality disorder* (pp. 23–40). Washington, DC: American Psychiatric Press.

Erikson, E. H. (1950). Growth and crises of the healthy personality. In *Identity and the lifecycle* (pp. 50–100). New York: International Universities Press.

Erikson, E. H. (1956). The problem of ego identity. *Journal of the American Psychoanalytic Association, 4,* 56–121.

Fairbairn, W. (1954). *An object-relations theory of the personality*. New York: Basic Books.

Fenichel, O. (1945). *The psychoanalytic theory of neurosis*. New York: Norton.

Fonagy, P., & Target, M. (2003). *Psychoanalytic theories: Perspectives from developmental psychopathology*. London: Whurr.

Fraiberg, A. (1983). Pathological defenses in infancy. *Psychoanalytic Quarterly, 60,* 612–635.

Galenson, E. (1986). Some thoughts about infant psychopathology and aggressive development. *International Review of Psychoanalysis, 13,* 349–354.

Grossman, W. (1986). Notes on masochism: A discussion of the history and development of a psychoanalytic concept. *Psychoanalytic Quarterly, 55,* 379–413.

Grossman, W. (1991). Pain, aggression, fantasy, and concepts of sadomasochism. *Psychoanalytic Quarterly, 60,* 22–52.

Hare, R. D. (1986). Twenty years of experience with the Cleckley psychopath. In W. H. Reid, D. Dorr, J. I. Walker, & J. W. Bonner III (Eds.), *Unmasking the psychopath* (pp. 3–27). New York: Norton.

Jacobson, E. (1964). *The self and object world.* New York: International Universities Press.

Jonas, J. M., & Pope, H. G. (1992). Axis I comorbidity of borderline personality disorder: Clinical implications. In J. F. Clarkin, E. Marziali, & H. Munroe-Blum (Eds.), *Borderline personality disorder* (pp. 149–160). New York: Guilford Press.

Kernberg, O. F. (1975). *Borderline conditions and pathological narcissism.* New York: Jason Aronson.

Kernberg, O. F. (1976). *Object relations theory and clinical psychoanalysis.* New York: Jason Aronson.

Kernberg, O. F. (1980). *Internal world and external reality: Object relations theory applied.* New York: Jason Aronson.

Kernberg, O. F. (1984). *Severe personality disorders: Psychotherapeutic strategies.* New Haven: Yale University Press.

Kernberg, O. F. (1989). The narcissistic personality disorder and the differential diagnosis of antisocial behavior. In O. F. Kernberg (Ed.), *Narcissistic personality disorder: Psychiatric clinics of North America* (pp. 553–570). Philadelphia: Saunders.

Kernberg, O. F. (1992). *Aggression in personality disorder and perversions.* New Haven: Yale University Press.

Kernberg, O. F. (1994). Aggression, trauma, and hatred in the treatment of borderline patients. In I. Share (Ed.), *Borderline personality disorder: The psychiatric clinics of North America* (pp. 701–714). Philadelphia: Saunders.

Kernberg, O. F. (1995). *Love relations: Normality and pathology.* New Haven: Yale University Press.

Klein, M. (1935). A contribution to the psycho-genesis of manic depressive states. *International Journal of Psycho-analysis, 16,* 145–174.

Krause, R. (1988). Eine Taxonomie der Affekte und ihre Anwendung auf das Verständnis der frühen Störungen. *Psychotherapie und Medizinische Psychologie, 38,* 77–86.

Krause, R., & Lutolf, P. (1988). Facial indicators of transference processes in psychoanalytical treatment. In H. Dahl & H. Kachele (eds.), *Psychoanalytic process research strategies* (pp. 257–272). Heidelberg, Germany: Springer.

Lenzenweger, M. F. (1998). Schizotypy and schizotypic psychopathology: Mapping an alternative expression of schizophrenia liability. In M. F. Lenzenweger & R. H. Dworkin (Eds.), *Origins and development of schizophrenia: Advances in experimental psychopathology* (pp. 93–121).Washington, DC: American Psychological Association.

Lenzenweger, M. F., Clarkin, J. F., Kernberg, O. F., & Foelsch, P. (2001). The Inventory of Personality Organization: Psychometric properties, factorial composition and criterion relations with affect, aggressive dyscontrol, psychosis-proneness, and self domains. *Psychological Assessment, 4,* 577–591.

Livesley, W. J. (1998). Suggestions for a framework for an empirically based classification of personality disorder. *Canadian Journal of Psychiatry, 43,* 137–147.

Livesley, W. J. (2001). Conceptual and taxonomic issues. In J. W. Livesley (Ed.), *Handbook of personality disorder* (pp. 3–38). New York: Guilford Press.

Mahler, M., & Furer, M. (1968). *On human symbiosis and the vicissitudes of individuation*. New York: International Universities Press.

Mahler, M., Pine, F., & Bergman, A. (1975). *The psychological birth of the human infant*. New York: Basic Books.

Marziali, E. (1992). The etiology of borderline personality disorder: Developmental factors. In J. F. Clarkin, E. Marziali, & H. Munroe-Blum (Eds.), *Borderline personality disorder* (pp. 27–44). New York: Guilford Press.

Millon, T. (1981). *Disorders of personality. DSM III: Axis II*. New York: Wiley.

Oldham, J. M. (1994). Personality disorders. *Journal of the American Medical Association, 272*, 1770–1776.

Paris, J. (1994). *Borderline personality disorder*. Washington, DC: American Psychiatric Press.

Perry, J. C. (1992). Problems and considerations in the valid assessment of personality disorders. *American Journal of Psychiatry, 149*(19), 1645–1653.

Perry, J. C., & Herman, J. L. (1993). Trauma and defense in the etiology of borderline personality disorder. In J. Paris (Ed.), *Borderline personality disorder* (pp. 123–140). Washington, DC: American Psychiatric Press.

Plakun, E. (1989). Narcissistic personality disorder: A validity study and comparison to borderline personality disorder. In O. F. Kernberg (Ed.), *Narcissistic personality disorder: Psychiatric clinics of North America* (pp. 603–620). Philadelphia: Saunders.

Posner, M. I., & Rothbart, M. K. (2000). Developing mechanisms of self-regulation. *Developmental Psychopathology, 12*, 427–441.

Posner, M. I., Rothbart, M. K., Vizueta, N., Levy, K., Thomas, K. M., & Clarkin, J. (2002). Attentional mechanisms of borderline personality disorder. *Proceedings of the National Academy of Sciences USA, 99*, 16366–16370.

Ronningstam, E., & Gunderson, J. (1989). Descriptive studies on narcissistic personality disorder. In O. F. Kernberg (Ed.), *Narcissistic personality disorder: Psychiatric clinics of North America* (pp. 585–602). Philadelphia: Saunders.

Silbersweig, D. A., Pan, H., Beutel, M., Epstein, J., Goldstein, M., Thomas, K., Posner, M., Hochberg, H., Brendel, G., Yang, Y., Kernberg, O., Clarkin, J., & Stern, E. (2001, January). *Neuroimaging of inhibitory and emotional function in borderline personality disorder*. Paper presented the meeting of American College of Neuropsychopharmacology.

Steinberg, B. J., Trestman, R. L., & Siever, L. J. (1994). The cholinergic and noradrenergic neurotransmitter systems and affective instability in borderline personality disorder. In K. R. Silk (Ed.), *Biological and neurobehavioral studies of borderline personality disorder* (pp. 41–62). Washington, DC: American Psychiatric Press.

Stone, M. (1980). *The borderline syndromes*. New York: McGraw-Hill.

Stone, M. (1990). *The fate of borderline patients*. New York: Guilford Press.

Stone, M. (1993a). *Abnormalities of personality*. New York: Norton.

Stone, M. (1993b). Etiology of borderline personality disorder: Psychobiological factors contributing to an underlying irritability. In J. Paris (Ed.), *Borderline personality disorder* (pp. 87–102). Washington, DC: American Psychiatric Press.

Stone, M. (1994). Characterologic subtypes of the borderline personality disorder: With a note on prognostic factors. In I. Share (Ed.), *Borderline personality disorder: Psychiatric clinics of North America* (pp. 773–784). Philadelphia: Saunders.

Target, M., & Fonagy, P (1996). Playing with reality II: The development of psychic reality from a theoretical perspective. *International Journal of Psychoanalysis, 77*(3), 459–479.

Torgerson, A. M., & Ainaeus, R. (1990). The relationship between MCMI personality scales and DSM III, axis II. *Journal of Personality Assessment, 55,* 698–707.

van der Kolk, B. A., Hostetler, A., Herron, N., & Fislea, R. (1994). Trauma and the development of borderline personality disorder. In I. Share (Ed.), *Borderline personality disorder: Psychiatric clinics of North America* (pp. 715–730). Philadelphia: Saunders.

van Reekum, R., Links, P. S., & Federov, C. (1994). Impulsivity in borderline personality disorder. In K. Silk (Ed.), *Biological and neurobehavioral studies of borderline personality disorder* (pp. 1–22). Washington, DC: American Psychiatric Press.

Volkan, V. (1976). *Primitive internalized object relations.* New York: International Universities Press.

Volkan, V. (1987). *Six steps in the treatment of borderline personality organization.* Northvale, NJ: Jason Aronson.

Westen, D., & Arkowitz-Westen, L. (1998). Limitations of Axis II in diagnosing personality pathology in clinical practice. *American Journal of Psychiatry, 155,* 1767–1771.

Westen, D., & Schedler, J. (1999a). Revising and assessing Axis II, Part I: Developing a clinically and empirically valid assessment method. *American Journal of Psychiatry 156,* 258–272.

Westen, D., & Schedler, J. (1999b). Revising and assessing Axis II, Part II: Toward an empirically based and clinically useful classification of personality disorders. *American Journal of Psychiatry, 156,* 273–285.

Widiger, T. A., & Frances, A. J. (1994). Toward a dimensional model for the personality disorders. In P. T. Costa & T. Widiger (Eds.), *Personality disorders and the five-factor model of personality* (pp. 19–40). Washington, DC: American Psychological Association.

Widiger, T. A., Trull, T. J., Clarkin, J. F., Sanderson, C., & Costa, P. T. (1994). A description of the DSM-III-R and DSM-IV personality disorders with the five-factor model of personality. In P. T. Costa & T. Widiger (Eds.), *Personality disorders and the five-factor model of personality* (pp. 41–56). Washington, DC: American Psychological Association.

Wiggins, J. S. (1982). Circumplex models of interpersonal behavior in clinical psychology. In P. Kendall & J. Butcher (Eds.), *Handbook of research methods in clinical psychology* (pp. 183–221). New York: Wiley.

Yehuda, R., Southwick, S. M., Perry, B. D., & Giller, E. L. (1994). Peripheral catecholamine alterations in borderline personality disorder. In K. Silk (Ed.), *Biological and neurobehavioral studies of borderline personality disorder* (pp. 63–90). Washington, DC: American Psychiatric Press.

Zanarini, M. C. (2000). Childhood experiences associated with the development of borderline personality disorder. *Psychiatric Clinics of North America, 23*(1), 89–101.

Zanarini, M. C., Frankenburg, F., Hennen, J., & Silk, K. (2003). The longitudinal course of borderline personality pathology: 6-year prospective follow-up of the phenomenology of borderline personality disorder. *American Journal of Psychiatry, 160,* 274–283.

Zimmerman, M. (1994). Diagnosing personality disorders: A review of issues and research methods. *Archives of General Psychiatry, 51,* 225–245.

CHAPTER 4

■ ■ ■

Interpersonal Theory
of Personality Disorders
The Structural Analysis of Social Behavior
and Interpersonal Reconstructive Therapy

LORNA SMITH BENJAMIN

Annie's first overdose occurred when she was 18, and she has had been hospitalized at least once for suicidality after that. At this time, at age 30, she has been hospitalized again for suicidal thoughts, this time centering around messages from a voice that often tells her that somebody in her family will be seriously harmed or killed. She says: "Somebody in my family will die, and I want to be the first. I cannot deal with the thought of losing a loved one." Annie is so upset by these thoughts that she does little but cry all day long. She has been diagnosed with major depression with psychotic features and generalized anxiety disorder. Whenever she tries to concentrate, she depersonalizes: "I leave my body, go off somewhere. I don't know what I am doing. Everything is dark. My body feels numb. I am aware I don't feel. I space out in my own little world." This depersonatization began in grade school, whenever teachers would call on her. Conflict about school continues to be manifested as a constant battle in her head. One side says: "I will go back to school. I can do this." The other side says: "No you can't. You are stupid. No way. You have problems." Then she panics and says: "I must be stupid." She has been treated with various antidepressants, anxiolytics, and antipsychotics and has had several psychotherapies. There, she has learned: "I have mood swings, and have to deal with it." Presently she feels safe when with her husband and parents, but they are getting tired of hearing about her worries and depression.

How can a theory of personality help us to understand Annie in ways that psychosocially oriented clinicians can use to direct effective treatment? This chapter sketches one such possibility: interpersonal reconstructive psychotherapy (IRT; Benjamin, 2003).

I saw Annie for consultation and after discharge her from this hospitalization, she was treated for 1½ years by two successive IRT trainees. When the second IRT therapist had to leave to go on internship, Annie continued in therapy for a while in another agency in consultation with IRT advisers. She made no more suicide attempts and had no further hospitalizations. Two years after the main IRT treatment ended, Annie wrote to the second IRT trainee and, along with personal information not included here, said:

> I actually am enjoying life! A lot has happened since I last talked with you but I (thanks to you) have learned how to deal with all the challenges that life throws my way! I have learned a lot. I really do appreciate all that you and Dr. B did for me. I hate to think of where I would be if Dr. B would not have accepted me in her program.

One such "testimonial" does not comprise empirical validation of the IRT treatment, but such radical changes are not unusual, even in the nonresponder population that forms the data base. Benjamin (2003, Chap. 10) describes a pilot outcome study. In this chapter, Annie's case illustrates how IRT explains and directs the psychosocial aspects of treatment. Because Annie agreed to be in the pilot research program, data are available to illustrate how the technology associated with Structural Analysis of Social Behavior (SASB; Benjamin, 1978, 1987, 1996a) can be used to operationalize many of the concepts associated with IRT.

OVERVIEW

In addition to this overview and concluding remarks, this chapter has three main sections:

1. A description of IRT theory, with applications to Annie.
2. A description of the SASB model, the method used to operationalize the case formulation, the therapy process, and interpersonal and intrapsychic aspects of outcome in IRT. SASB predictive principles are illustrated by Annie's case. This section includes reference to formal validity studies of SASB models and predictive principles.
3. Illustrative applications of both IRT and SASB to Axis II personality disorders with emphasis on those that best characterized Annie according to the Wisconsin Personality Inventory (WISPI), an SASB-based instrument of DSM Axis II disorders.

The first section describes IRT, an attachment-based theory of psychopathology that provides a framework to help treating clinicians draw on interventions from any school of psychotherapy in optimally effective ways. Although almost any intervention is acceptable if it is consistent with the case formulation, IRT draws most frequently on client-centered, psychodynamic, and cognitive-behavioral perspectives.

The description of IRT is followed by an exposition of the SASB model and selected aspects of its technology. These, too, are illustrated using Annie's data. When applied to IRT, SASB methods are central in assessing reliability of case formulations, adherence to recommended treatment processes, and outcome in terms of expected changes in relevant internalizations as well as in interpersonal patterns with current important figures.

Although my own interest has been in applying the SASB model to IRT, the SASB model is theory neutral. Because its concepts are operationalized in objective terms, the SASB model can be used to study any theory of personality that involves interactions (e.g., patient and therapists; patient and God; cocaine and the patient; patient and his or her wishes; and child and mother, mother and father, and employee and peers)

Acknowledgment of selected historical antecedents to IRT and to SASB appear sometimes in context but usually at the end of each topical section rather than at the beginning. Throughout the chapter, there is an emphasis on references to more recent studies that have found the SASB model and technology to be useful in a wide variety of contexts not necessarily related to IRT. The middle section of the chapter concludes with a sketch of tests of validity of the SASB model and of IRT.

The third section reviews applications of the SASB model and IRT theory to personality disorder as described in DSM-IV (Benjamin, 1996a). That book suggested prototypical developmental histories for individuals with each of the DSM Axis II disorders, along with associated treatment recommendations. The interpersonal translations of the DSM definitions of personality disorder offered there were formalized in a self-rating instrument, the WISPI (Klein et al., 1993; Smith, Klein, & Benjamin, 2003). Annie provided WISPI data at the beginning and end of her IRT treatment, and her profiles are used to relate her progress to DSM-IV measures as well as in other ways of describing dysfunction. For example, features of the two Axis II disorders ranking highest in Annie's profile (schizotypal and avoidant personality disorder) and disorders related to her presenting symptoms (anxiety, depression, thought disorder) are explored in a sample of 139 psychiatric inpatients. The purpose is to show how some of the SASB parameters perform in relation to measures of personality disorder and of other symptoms in larger-scale studies, with Annie providing a concrete clinical context.

IRT THEORY OF PERSONALITY PSYCHOPATHOLOGY AND PSYCHOTHERAPY

IRT Case Formulation

IRT begins and ends with the presenting problems described in terms of DSM. They are considered to be the tip of the psychological iceberg and to organize the clinician's thinking about which social relationships are relevant to the presenting problems and how. In addition to initializing the case formulation, presenting problems provide a major target in assessment of treatment outcome. The IRT theory of psychopathology attempts to account for the presenting symptoms in terms that can be understood *by the patient* and reliably agreed on by participating clinicians as well as by observer researchers. Moreover, the theory attempts to maximize parsimony, observability, and testability. These principles of good behavioral science are central to IRT as well as to the SASB model and technology.

Annie's Presenting Problems and Key Figures

Annie presented with high anxiety, despair and depression, depersonalization, and severely compromised function. The flow diagrams specify that after identifying such presenting problems, the IRT case formulation moves to a survey of current stresses, responses to them, and their impact on the conscious self-concept. Annie's medical record described her continual financial stress and worry about being scrutinized. During the IRT consultation, Annie also showed concern about whether God would forgive suicide; she had concluded that the severity of her pain would justify it. She had been unable to hold a job for very long during the past year or so. There were no acute precipitating events noted in the record.

    Before the present-day return to Kraepelinian brain disease-based psychiatry, there was strong pressure for the clinician to answer the question: Why is there an exacerbation now? IRT adheres to that older tradition. If we correctly understand the current presentation, we can understand why things are worse now. The answer according to contemporary brain disorder theories would likely invoke the diathesis stress model and conclude that cumulative financial stress had finally surpassed Annie's threshold for triggering her genetically based vulnerabilities, and thus she collapsed psychologically. The explanation is not very specific, and somewhat circular in its identification of the threshold at which stress precipitates exacerbation (if Annie is in exacerbation, the threshold must have been exceeded; "therefore," her threshold was exceeded). By contrast, toward the end of the 90-minute IRT consultative interview, a highly specific and reasonable hypothesis emerged to explain why Annie's despair and fear had become so acute. The relevant event is mentioned later, after describing details of Annie's psychosocial history that help us understand her catastrophic reaction to the event.

Annie's diagnoses, treatments, and current living conditions, all a formal part of the IRT case formulation method (Benjamin, 2003, Chap. 2), were described at the beginning of this chapter. The interviewing method (described in Benjamin, 1996a, Chap. 3) that leads to identification of psychosocial contributions to her symptoms follows a free associative path, a method believed to track patient concerns that are not necessarily conscious. Chaotic as the IRT interview may seem because of its free associative structure, the information that emerges can be collected in a highly organized flow diagrams (Benjamin, 2003, Figs. 2.1, 2.2). These provide the structure necessary to construct a well organized case formulation.

In Annie's case, the free associative path went to her current husband, a kind but somewhat irresponsible man who left the jobs of earning, cooking, cleaning, and so on to Annie; an ex-husband who was an extremely abusive and possessive man who also held Annie responsible for everything; to her mother; and finally, to her mother's youngest brother. This uncle was 2 years older than Annie and lived with the family. The young uncle functioned as a brother, as Annie's mother was also serving as his mother. Annie's mother was very busy with her community service activities and most of the housework was left to the children. All but Annie were remiss in their assignments. Her mother, who was quite demanding and perfectionistic about how housework should be done, would frequently get upset when things were not done properly. To keep her mother from getting upset, Annie, the oldest female child, tried to get her siblings to do their jobs. Her mother disapproved of Annie's attempts to take control, and so, after several reprimands from her mother, Annie settled on just doing their jobs for them. Her mother subsequently came to expect that Annie would take care of things. Moreover, her mother would punish her if she did not complete additional household tasks (e.g., clean the inside of all the cupboards) before she could enjoy privileges granted to others without such conditions (e.g., go to the mall on Saturday). Annie wet the bed until she was 9, and was waked, spanked by her mother, and forced to wash and change the linen in the middle of the night. Her father, who was kind to her when he was not depressed but markedly absent otherwise, administered spankings for instances of disobedience and failure to please. After each spanking, Annie was so ashamed, she crawled under her bed.

The young uncle was a central figure in Annie's development. In the family, he was seen as perfect. "He could do no wrong." He would intimidate Annie with extreme violence, and no matter what the circumstances, her mother would support him. For example, he once bashed Annie in the head with a brick when he wanted something she had. Another time, he broke down the bathroom door "because" Annie was in there ahead of him. In all such exchanges, her mother's response was to ask Annie what she had done to provoke him. On a daily basis, Annie's uncle would taunt her with questions from his current lessons in school, and when she understandably did not know the answers because she was 2 years behind him, he would call her stupid. If she ever did better than he did in anything (e.g., in a board game), he would violently attack her, again, without consequence for him. Annie learned that she could not excel, that she had to let him be the best and to win.

Copy Processes Link Problem Personality Patterns to Key Figures

Key figures are those people in relation to whom the patient developed problem patterns—that is, the patterns clearly associated with presenting symptoms. According to IRT theory, presenting symptoms can be linked to patterns practiced with key figures via one or more of three copy processes. These are (1) be like him or her; (2) act as if he or she is still there and in control; and (3) treat yourself as he or she treated you. They are, respectively, named identification, recapitulation, and introjection. Copy processes can appear in negative image, but because opposites are precisely defined in terms of the SASB model, they are not described until the SASB model has been presented.

In Annie's case, the following copy processes were observed: With her two husbands, she recapitulated early patterns practiced with her mother. The most important recapitulations included *taking inordinate amounts of responsibility while trying to avert disaster by keeping everything in order.* Annie also had introjected her mother's reprimands about trying to boss siblings and about wetting the bed. The result was deep *feelings of shame and unacceptability.* In relation to her father and uncle, Annie recapitulated the pattern of *obey or suffer severe punishment.* In the triangle among Annie, her mother, and her uncle, Annie learned that if she failed to obey an aggressor, *there would be nobody to see her side and protect her.* She recapitulated the pattern of obey or suffer extreme punishment with her first husband. She repeated the pattern of accepting/taking excessive amounts of responsibility with both husbands. For example, at the time of the IRT inpatient consultation, Annie had been trying to hold various odd jobs in order to meet expenses, which included perceived responsibility to make payments on her first husband's expensive truck and on an earlier (also abusive) boyfriend's luxury car.

The *conflict reified by the chronic version of her voice* literally recapitulated what her uncle always told her (you are stupid; you can't do anything in school) versus what she knew to be true (I can do it. I am smart. Doing well in school was highly valued in the family, and the uncle reaped many rewards on that account.). This aspect of the voice was shaped by the copy process "introjection." The voice's threats to Annie and her family are discussed below. Her *depersonalization* experiences seemed to reflect a strong conflict between her wish to answer questions in school and do well versus her uncle's "mandate" that she not do well or else she would be attacked. As is often the case with people who are subjected on a long-term basis to severe trauma in inescapable situations, Annie learned to solve the problem by leaving her body, losing sensation, and escaping mentally. She also adapted by not excelling in school despite her ability to do so

Copy Processes Also Link Problem Patterns to Axis I Symptoms

There were good reasons for Annie's *acute despair and anxiety* at the time of her hospitalization, as well as the *voice's message that she and someone dear to her were going to die soon.* Her first husband, who once committed her and told the neighbors not to talk to her because she was crazy, had repeatedly threatened to kill both her and members of her family if she ever left him. After several years of enduring his violent attacks, she decided she could stand it no longer, and filed for divorce. As he promised, he actually did try at that time to kill her and her sister. After some chase scenes, there was an encounter between her ex-husband, Annie, and her sister. Annie managed to wrestle the gun away, delaying the seemingly inevitable disaster just long enough for a SWAT team to come and rescue Annie and her sister. As he was taken away, the ex-husband said: "Just remember, I'll be back to get you and your family some day." Shortly before the voice recently began telling her that family members would be killed, the ex-husband, then a miner in another state, had telephoned explaining he had just been laid off and was on his way to get her. Annie, believing that she was the one who would be responsible for whatever happened, that she was sure to be attacked for displeasing an aggressor, and that there was nobody to protect her, was totally overwhelmed. Because she "obviously" was the one responsible for this, the best thing would be for her to die first.

Copy processes of recapitulation and introjection provide working hypotheses for why Annie's voice said what it said, why she would choose a violent first husband, and why she would assume in marriage that it was her job to be responsible for everything. Anxiety and depression can be explained in part by clinical and laboratory studies that suggest that depression and anxiety can be precipitated by perception of *overwhelming demand.* Anxiety and depression triggered by overwhelming conditions are distinguished by action tendencies (Benjamin, 2003, Chap. 2; Zinbarg, Barlow, Brown, & Hertz, 1992). *Anxiety is a natural correlate of a tendency to try to cope* with the overwhelm, while *depression is a natural correlate of a tendency to give up* in face of overwhelm. *Comorbidity between anxiety and depression is frequently a result of vascillation between these two ways of reacting* to perceived overwhelming demand. Self-criticism and loss are two additional possible psychosocial antecedents of depression (Benjamin, 2003; Blatt, 1974). Annie had introjected criticism from both her mother and her uncle. Her sense of being alone to cope and her shame about her alleged flaws was a very long-standing belief that had its roots in her early interpersonal learning.

In sum, Annie's acute depression and anxiety were understandable correlates of the interaction between her presumed inherited temperament and her learned interpersonal patterns (personality). IRT focuses mostly on the learning aspect of personality development. The immobilizing exacerbation prior to hospitalization stemmed from the possibility that her ex-husband might reappear with violence directed toward her and/or family members as before.

With respect to psychotic processes, IRT theory presumes there is a predisposition to retreat to imagination as a solution to interpersonal dilemmas but holds that the content of imagination is very much affected by the copy processes. This idea that psychotic process reflects social order has been supported in a study that asked approximately 30 inpatients to rate their hallucinations on the SASB questionnaires (described later). Results indicated that individuals with different psychotic disorders have qualitatively distinct "relationships" with their hallucinations (Benjamin, 1988b). For example, manic individuals have hallucinations that are affirming and empowering; individuals with borderline personality disorder have hallucinations that are attacking. Moreover, patients have internally consistent, orderly, and complementary relationships with their hallucinations (Benjamin, 1997). Annie accepted the hypothesis that her voice represented her uncle, and her awareness of that connection subsequently proved useful in treatment whenever the voice reappeared. She also agreed that her "inability to concentrate" in school and her tendency to leave her body (consistent with the features of depersonalization described in DSM-IV) were related to her fear of what her uncle would do if she did well, and to her belief that he was right when he called her stupid.

In sum, Annie's Axis I symptoms have been framed in terms of copy processes and a list of clinically (and to a limited extent, experimentally) observed connections between psychosocial perceptions and symptoms of depression and anxiety. They also help account for her depersonalization experiences in school throughout childhood, as well as the content of her threatening voice. Benjamin (2003, Chap. 2) lists these and other frequently observed links between problem patterns (e.g., Axis II disorders) and Axis I symptoms. The exposition there is brief. A book that is devoted to providing further detail and illustrations of comorbidity between personality patterns and Axis I symptoms in terms of IRT is under contract (Benjamin, 2004).

In the third section of this chapter, I offer illustrative empirical data that support the IRT proposals that key figures can be specifically linked to problem patterns and to presenting symptoms.

Psychic Proximity and the Gift of Love to Key Figures

The problem of nonresponders is not new. To be sure, their current situations may be quite stressful, but experienced clinicians know that even if current situations improve, nonresponders are highly likely to find themselves repeating the same scenario all over again. Hence it is foolish to think that getting rid of current problem situations will solve the many problems typically faced by nonresponders. A widely recognized example is for abuser and abusees to repeat their respective "roles" in successive relationships. Moreover, their maladaptive responses are not necessarily connected to current relations with the original key people or events. For example, Annie's uncle was no longer in her life, and her contemporary relationship with her mother was quite good. Because Annie's mother had acknowledged and apologized for earlier treatment, they had become quite close.

From the fact that so many patients seem devoted to destruction of themselves and loved ones regardless of reality, Freud concluded that there must be a fundamental "death instinct." Freud named this force that holds people in destructive positions Thanatos. Subsequent analysts invoked the concept of repetition compulsion to explain this force (Fenichel, 1945). Another explanation for nonresponsiveness might be that patients are showing what Allport (1937) called "functional autonomy." That might suggest that once patterns are set ("hardwired"), they become habitual and are unaffected by their results. The idea is interesting but seems to contradict the well-established learning principle of "extinction," and it does not provide effective clinical guidance. The very existence of the nonresponder category (not responsive to medications or psychosocial interventions) establishes that the problem of relentless self-destruction cannot be remedied simply by helping with relearning. Even the latest theories of brain disorder and the associated treatments with medications likewise have not yet mastered the problem of how to help nonresponders (Thase, Friedman, & Howland, 2001; Rueck et al., 2003; Cassano et al., 2003).

According to IRT, nonresponsiveness is organized by internal templates associated with key figures called Important People and their Internalized Representations (IPIRs). Nonresponder patients are understood to be more concerned with their relationships with these IPIRs than with what is going on in their contemporary world. It is likely that such organizing internalized representations of loved ones have been encoded neurologically according to principles of learning. The internal "programs" for how to relate to self and others are not easy to change, either by chemistry or by talking. For example, Annie's major key figures were her abusive uncle, her punitive father, her neglectful mother, and her first husband. The section on copy processes sketched how each of her presenting symptoms involved problem patterns directly associated with these key figures. Attempts to help her get free of her depression, anxiety, voice, and abusive relationships using medications and talking therapy had not yet succeeded in providing relief.

The concepts of psychic proximity and gifts of love (Benjamin, 1993) attempt to explain why concern with her internalized representations (IPIRs) had so much power over Annie. The explanation rests on the suggestion that the copy processes were continually reinforced by positive motivation in relation to the IPIRs. Love, not hate (as in Thanatos), supports copy process learning. IRT explains the phenonmenon of nonresponders by suggesting that they are following the perceived rules and values of their internalized representations. Reality is not important compared to the perceived need of nonresponders to receive affirmation and love from the IPIRs. Their behavioral testimony to the views, rules, and values of the IPIRs represents a gift of love. Very briefly, a gift of love is given in order to receive love. "Here, you think I am trash? I am proving to you that I agree with you as I treat myself like trash. Surely this is what you want, so please say I am OK, and love me."

For example, Annie took an impossible amount of responsibility in the first place because she wanted to please and be affirmed, even protected, by her mother. One of her gifts of love to her mother is that she continues to try to receive approval by taking on everything that needs doing. As another example, it may be presumed that good realistic sense initially led Annie to accept her uncle's rule: Obey or be severely attacked. But Annie then chose men who continued to abuse her in the same ways (ex-husband and a relationship before that). Thus the gift of love to her uncle may have been that she repeated this pattern out of loyalty to his view of her. Preserving his role as star scholar in the family, Annie accepted his idea that she was stupid. With her mother's apparent support for him, Annie also held that it was his right to intimidate her to have his needs met at her expense. In her choice of men like her uncle, Annie showed that she accepted the rules for her that he represented and that were endorsed by her mother.

Gifts of love enable psychic proximity, which is perceived closeness to the internalized representations of the relevant key figures. Annie accepted these horrible rules because she wished to be closer to and have more affection from her mother, who so clearly communicated support and affirmation for the uncle. As mentioned previously, perhaps Annie also wished for affirmation from the uncle himself, even though her narrative was much more focused on her mother. By acting according to the rules and values of her mother and uncle, Annie derived the only security she knew: psychic proximity to the internalized representations of these key figures.

Some patients may declare that they hate a given key figure, but more often than not, all the fury is about a wish for reconciliation and love in the end. No matter how badly abused they have been, people hang on (usually without being aware of it) to the hope that if they do "right," the IPIR ultimately will relent, apologize, and show approval, acceptance, and love. Wishes for psychic proximity to IPIRs also can explain how wishes for revenge, punishment, hostile triumph, and restitution can persist. To be sure, aggression is hardwired in the primate. But according to IRT, hostility is better dealt with as a moderator of intimacy and distance than as a primary energy. If the patient is angry, it is important to learn the interpersonal purposes of the anger and to address those purposes directly. For example, if the anger is to enhance hostile enmeshment with a destructive IPIR, it is not a good idea for the therapist to facilitate that anger. The better alternative is to address grief about wishes that cannot be met and to gain some psychological distance from the internalization. On the other hand, if the anger represents outrage and a wish to distance from a destructive internalization (e.g., if he wants me to hurt myself, I am not doing it), enhancing it can be very therapeutic. Anger is not a source of energy that must be disposed of one way or another. According to IRT, if there is no perceived need for control or distance, there is no anger.

Some readers may say that the gift-of-love interpretation is not parsimonious. Why bring in an hypothesis about underlying motivation that sustains the patterns? Originally the rewards for Annie's patterns were negative. She avoided harsh punishment by obedience and self-negation. If simple learning accounts for Annie's persistence, her behavior might be compared to that of traumatized dogs, which, after being given severe inescapable shock, would give up and passively accept shock when later given an opportunity to escape (Solomon & Wynne, 1953). These experiments and naturalistic observations suggest that learning involving avoidance of extremely aversive situations is very resistant to extinction. Moreover, the learner need not be a victim. Merely sensing strong negative affect in the caregiver suffices. For example, a baby monkey needs only to observe the mother's fear of a specific venomous snake once and he or she has the avoidance lesson for a lifetime (Jay, 1965). Survival is assisted if the developing primate is greatly affected by negative affect in a key caregiver. Thus it should be no surprise that traumatized people find it difficult to extinguish their adaptations.

That sensible analysis and correct observation that patterns learned in traumatic situations are difficult to extinguish do not address the puzzle posed by nonresponders such as Annie. She, and they, repeatedly end up in situations that present the same challenges. Obviously they do not say: I am going to pick a new partner who will repeat the same problem patterns. Nor do they "want" to have financial stress, or repeated loss, or whatever else is at issue. They are unlikely to be aware of the mechanisms of copy processes, principles of complementarity (explained in the section on SASB) that facilitate repetitions of patterns, or gifts of love in relation to IPIRs. Nonetheless, these behavioral principles do lead them, in effect, to *seek out repetitions* of the problem situations. Returning now to the analogy to traumatized animals, it is clear that it would be highly unlikely to see any of Solomon's dogs find and reenter cages similar to those in which they were severely shocked. Ordinary examples belie that idea. Consider the cat that ran and hid every time a man in any kind of uniform entered the house; a horse that avoided males in cowboy garb if possible and aggressed against them if not; and a dog that disappeared whenever anyone in hunting apparel and a gun showed up. In each case the animals avoid people who resemble situations in which they have been abused. On the strength of many such observations of traumatized animals, it is safe to conclude that animals are not attracted to situations in which they have been abused. But people like Annie are. The difference between these simple examples with animals and the puzzle of nonresponders lies in the fantasy life of humans—in the persistent wish to love and be loved by IPIRs. The final argument in support of the idea that gifts of love motivate "repetition compulsions" is that consistent focus on it in IRT is able to free patients such as Annie of their repetitions of self-destructive patterns.

While behavioral psychologists might wish IRT to be simpler, psychoanalysts might feel it oversimplifies. They might be particularly concerned about whether IRT accommodates the central analytic concepts of conflict and defenses. Yet conflict is central to every intervention in IRT. Each step in IRT should address a conflict between the Regressive Loyalist (Red) and the Growth Collaborator (Green). The term "Regressive Loyalist" describes all behaviors associated with copy processes and gifts of love that have been linked to presenting symptoms. The term "Growth Collaborator" describes behaviors associated with a normative thrust toward healthy independence. The Red/Green conflict and the IRT definition of normality are discussed in the SASB section of this chapter and in the treatment segment of this section.

Defenses protect the person from having to give up the wishes associated with gifts of love and all the behaviors, affects, and cognitions associated with them. Nonresponders are terrified and grief stricken as they contemplate letting go of the impossible wishes associated with the gifts of love. To protect themselves from these painful realizations, they can distort perceptions (e.g., projection, splitting, idealization, and devaluation) and ways of responding to those perceptions (e.g., displacement, acting out, sublimation, compensation, regression, and undoing). They also can block awareness of the wishes and related links among the parallel domains of affect, behavior, and cognition (e.g., repression, somatization, denial, intellectualization, lying, dissociation, and isolation.) Defenses were discussed in more detail by Benjamin in 1995 and, to a lesser extent by Benjamin in 2003. No formal validating data have yet been developed for this view of defenses.

There also are no published empirical data that test the IRT concepts of gift of love or psychic proximity (or their equivalent as described by Fairbairn, 1952). However, the SASB methodology, described in the next section, provides a means to do so. Moore (1998) clearly established that male alcoholics begin to drink when they *wish for more love* from their significant other person. Sandor (1996), showed that heroin addicts feel that their *drug of choice nurtures them*. These are two examples of how behaviors that are recognized as being destructive in reality are sustained by wishes for love.

Historical Background on the Role of Internalizations in Psychopathology

The IRT developmental model draws heavily on the work of Bowlby (1969) and Harlow (1958). Both showed that attachment is primary in the organization of behavior. Bowlby's method of exploring attachment was to use compelling clinical observation and data on children separated from parents. Harlow's method was to conduct laboratory experiments on baby monkeys whose attachment had been disrupted by removal from their mothers at birth. The impact of Bowlby's attachment theory and the research it has inspired cannot be overstated. Cassidy and Shaver (1999) offer an informative summary. Attachment has been shown to be involved in personality disturbance and many forms of psychopathology.

Bowlby (1969) suggested that attachment experiences shape personality as the child takes in representations of the caregivers. The child retains them as "internal working models" (p. 81). These working models organize the child's social perceptions and responses. Bowlby (1969, pp. 179–180) also proposed that attachment in the infant, a need for proximity to a parent, takes precedence even over "biological drives" such as food and drink. The idea is both surprising and powerful and does have sensible biological meaning. Young primates must stay close to a protective mother or else they are left behind in the forest. They must return to her when danger threatens, so they can be carried to safety (plus access to food, water, warmth, and whatever biological drives can be named).

If a developing primate is able to retain proximity to a reliable caregiver, the primate becomes secure. Secure attachments are strongly associated with normal behaviors, whereas insecure attachments of various types are associated with different forms of psychopathology (surveyed in Cassidy & Shaver, 1999). Bowlby noted that secure attachment, a comfortable dependency on a reliable home base, is required for a child to be able to develop stable independence. He described this tension between attachment to a secure base and the natural tendency to separate from it as the "dance between dependence and independence." The reliable parent is consistently protective but also permits exploration of the world and the development of competence. "The child takes in the experience with the parent and develops an internal working model of the relationship. The model provides the security *and permission* [italics added] needed to reach out" (Bowlby, 1977, p. 204). The idea of psychic proximity in IRT provides an intrapsychic analogue to the experimental model of a secure base. By behaving according to the rules and values of internalized representations, patients such as Annie reach for security, just as the frightened child goes back to his or her mother, regardless of the history of interactions with mothers. Harlow and Harlow (1962) showed that even if the laboratory mother monkey (defined as a huggable, very familiar figure) abused the baby, the baby would return to her when challenged or frightened. Baby monkeys were more likely to explore a new, even mildly frightening situation if their "mothers" were present in the room. The "mothers" provided security adequate to support steps toward independence.

In the psychoanalytic literature a secure person is said to have a strong ego, and he or she may be described as showing "basic trust" (Erikson, 1950) or "mature dependence" (Fairbairn, 1952) or as having "introjected a good object" (Klein, 1948/1975). Based on conversations with adults, the psychoanalyst Fairbairn (1952) had predated Bowlby with the suggestion that psychopathology stems directly from the quest to renew ties to an early loved one. But Bowlby's compelling descriptions of children with impaired attachments, and the research it inspired, make the power of attachment easier to see. Still, Bretherton (1985) noted that Bowlby had not clearly delineated exactly *how* attachment affects working models and personality. The IRT version of internal working models is quite specific about the nature of the internal working model for each individual—about its links to specific key persons, personality, and the presenting symptoms. Further discussion of the nature of IPIRs and additional connections to the literature appears in Benjamin (2003, Chap. 2).

Treatment in IRT

IRT proposes that the reason it has been clinically successful in encouraging constructive change in patients such as Annie is that it directly addresses the underlying motivation for the problem patterns. This motivation is the desire for psychic proximity which is to be achieved via gifts of love. In Annie's case, her relationship with the internalizations of her uncle and mother were the prime targets of the treatment. After she became less enmeshed with them and their rules and values for her, she was then able to use her previous learning in parent training, assertiveness training, relationship skills, and the like to develop a new and better life for herself. Therapeutic change rested on the acquisition of a secure base (which probably included the IRT therapist and other as well as new, more loving relationships in her life) and insight into the meaning and purposes of her relationship with her internalizations. *The insight helps mobilize the will to change and to learn new ways of doing things, while the security of the therapy relationship strengthens the courage needed to make a profound change in one's ways of seeing oneself in relation to others.*

The Core Algorithm in IRT

The IRT manual sumarizes principles of IRT treatment. IRT draws on any and all schools of therapy with restriction that choices must be likely to invoke the core algorithm. Its components (rules) are (1) accurate empathy; (2) maximal support for the Growth Collaborator (Green) and minimal support for the Regressive Loyalist (Red); (3) focus on key aspects of the case formulation; (4) articulation of detail about input, response, and impact on the self for any given interpersonal episode; (5) exploration of any episode in terms of affect, behavior, and cognition (the ABCs); and (6) implementation of one or more of the five steps from the learning hierarchy.

The Five Steps in IRT

1. With accurate empathy, consistently implement a pattern of collaboration between the therapist and the patient against "it," the maladaptive patterns.

2. Help the patient learn about intrapsychic patterns along with their associated affects and cognitions. Help the patient learn about where the patterns came from and what they are for (how they were adaptive at one time).

3. Block maladaptive patterns (especially life-threatening and other seriously damaging actions).

4. Enable the will to change (help change the relationship with the IPIR). If there is to be behavior change during psychotherapy, the individual's relationship with the unconscious organizers must be brought to light and renegotiated. This is accomplished by recognizing one's patterns and their relationship to the early key figures (insight). Then the person must in one way or another *decide* whether to detach (give up old wishes and fears)

in favor of new and better attachments and ways of being. Differentiation from and letting go of the IPIRs often involve grief. In effect, there has to be a psychological funeral for the patient's hopes that the IPIR will start providing unadulterated affirmation and love. Differentiation does not mean that the IPIR is "exorcised." That is probably not possible. Differentiation means that the enmeshment with the IPIR is terminated and a contract for peaceful coexistence is signed. In reality, relationships with key figures (if they are still living and available) can improve greatly once old expectations have been given up and the idea of friendly independence is better understood.

5. Learn new more adaptive and appropriate patterns. Usual and customary therapy techniques, especially behavior therapy, work very well with individuals with personality disorder after differentiation has taken place. The "now what?" phase opens the patient to new ideas on how to do things differently and better. The therapy relationship offers some better ways of relating, but that must be supplanted by other alliances in the patient's environment (marital, filial, collegial).

Benjamin (2003), divides interventions at each step into those that are motivational (self-discovery) and those that build new patterns (self-management). The summary appears here as Figure 4.1. Inspection of the figure reveals the wide variety of techniques that are acceptable in IRT.

At each step, the clinician remains aware of the conflict between loyalty to old rules and values (Red) and the wish to become more functional and achieve therapy goals (Green). As specified by the core algorithm, the clinician works from an empathic baseline and tries to enhance Green and minimize Red.

At each step as the Red/Green conflict is addressed, both self-discovery and self-management interventions are used. Typically (but not exclusively), psychodynamic (self discovery) techniques serve to enhance motivation to do things differently, whereas cognitive-behavioral techniques are used to build new patterns. In IRT, insight into where patterns came from and what they are for serves no purpose other than to encourage the person to reconsider his or her goals and to start the relearning process. Telling stories and reliving problem events in words is a very important part of IRT because it facilitates the grieving that accompanies successful relinquishing of wishes that have been desperately held for so long. Usually (but not always), behavioral (self-management) techniques serve to provide positive alternatives to problem behaviors. Nonresponders, by definition, have been unable to take advantage of them and learn more adaptive ways of being. According to IRT, the reason for the nonresponsiveness is that these patients are motivated to continue doing things as they always have in order to receive affirmation from their internalized key figures. If that ori-

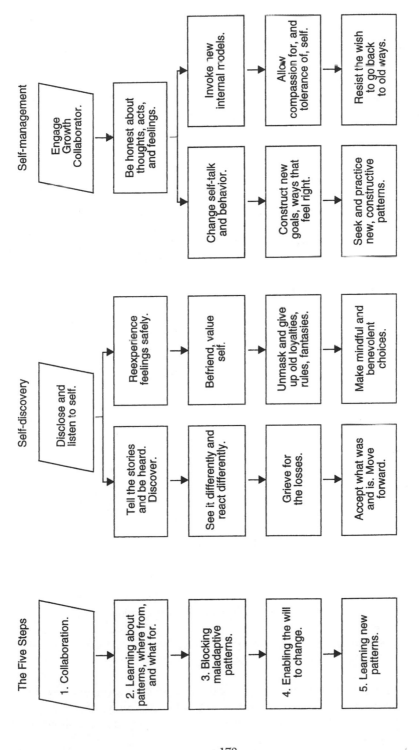

FIGURE 4.1. Therapy steps and tasks. From Benjamin (2003). Copyright 2003 by The Guilford Press. Reprinted by permission.

entation can be changed by effective grieving of the relevant wishes, then the learning technology can become more effective.

The five steps generally occur in sequence, but not always. As is true for many descriptions of stages, there is considerable overlap among them, and their chronological order is only approximate. Therapists are encouraged to choose interventions that invoke more than one stage at a time. For example, later in this section I describe an intervention that involved telling Annie to let her voice speak only between 8 and 9 A.M. This procedure invoked collaboration and blocked a problem pattern. Adding the shared understanding that the voice represented her uncle involved insight and very much mobilized the will to change. Helping Annie see that she could control the voice taught her a new pattern, namely, that she could control the voice. Hence the intervention that might sound preposterous to some, invoked all five steps at once and was an optimal, highly adherent IRT intervention. It was effective in controlling the voice, her despair, and her anxiety and would therefore, if included in formal study, contribute to a finding of an association between adherence and outcome.

Data on the Five Steps

Although there have not yet been randomized controlled studies of the effectiveness of IRT, the approach is based on principles well established in empirical research as well as good clinical practice. Benjamin and Pugh (2001, pp. 429–432) provided a survey of empirical literature that establish the contribution of each of the five steps to better outcome in therapy.

1. Formal studies consistently show that collaboration is vital to good outcome.
2. Insight (variously defined within different schools of therapy) contributes as well as, but less consistently than, collaboration.
3. Blocking maladaptive patterns naturally is an important component of effective therapy.
4. Stages of the will to change (e.g., Prochaska, DiClemente, & Norcross, 1992) have strong correlations with outcome, but better definition and more documentation of effective ways of moving people through stages (e.g., from precontemplation to action) are needed.
5. Techniques that help patients learn new patterns comprise the bulk of modern empirically supported therapies.

Cognitive-behavioral therapy, perhaps the most widely studied and empirically supported psychotherapy approach, teaches new ways of thinking and behaving. IRT draws heavily on these well-established technologies but

holds that they can only be effective with nonresponders after the supporting motivations, the gifts of love, have been let go. For example, a suicidal/
homicidal young man, hospitalized for 2 weeks, was sent home on a trial
basis armed with instructions on coping skills in relation to his struggles
with family members. Within 2 hours of arriving home, he had overdosed
and stolen and crashed his grandfather's car. According to IRT, his desperate behaviors were to force family members to change their ways and, surprisingly, bring them together. He had no interest in using his coping skills.
Until and if his fantasy that his destructive behaviors would solve the family problems was successfully addressed, he could not change and remained
a danger to himself and others.

Flow Diagrams Give Quite Specific Instructions for What to Try to Do

Several flow diagrams explain what to do at key junctures in IRT. Perhaps
the most important, reproduced in Figure 4.2, is "coming to terms." It provides directions for how to take a current episode in therapy and focus on
exploring and relinquishing the gifts of love in favor of implementing more
adaptive new responses. Coming to terms is closely related to what is
known in psychodynamic approaches as working through. It addresses the
heart of reconstructive change: giving up the motives that have been sustaining the problem patterns.

Figure 4.2 reminds the clinician that any episode can potentially result
in coming to terms if the clinician helps the patient clearly delineate an episode in terms of input, response, and impact on self; by making sure that
affect, behavior, and cognition associated with that social episode are
heightened; and by tracking via copy process links to origins and the associated wishes and looking forward to better alternatives.

For example, suppose Annie is allowing her children to fail to complete their reasonably assigned household duties and that they attack and
denigrate her until she just completes the tasks for them. The children are
learning to be hostile and disrespectful, and they are not learning to be
responsible. Their uncooperative hostility demoralizes Annie further, and
she becomes even more convinced she is a bad mother. Review of input,
response, and impact on self in this situation includes exploration of the
ABCs: How does she feel about it? What does she say and do? What and
how does she thinks about it?

With the ABCs clearly in mind, Annie is invited to reflect on whether
she has felt this way before, and that naturally will take her back to when
her uncle did little to help in the house and trashed Annie while her mother
blamed and punished her for upsetting her uncle and for the house being
out of order. No wonder Annie would scramble so hard to please others.

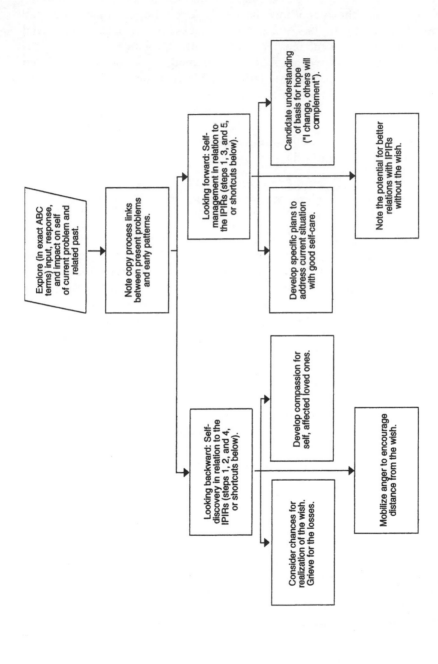

FIGURE 4.2. Coming to terms. From Benjamin (2003). Copyright 2003 by The Guilford Press. Reprinted by permission.

Now that Annie is no longer in that particular situation, Figure 4.2 suggests that to get free of these old interpersonal reflexes, she needs to consider whether her mother will ever affirm her in the way she wants. She also needs support in coming to realize how tragic her situation was back then and to have compassion for herself in that long past setting. It might be helpful for Annie to explore whether she is angry enough about all of her losses then and now to break up this repeating pattern: serve others and get beat up in the process.

Moving to self-management activities, Annie might be helped via role play to explain to the children that they need to learn to be responsible and to treat Annie and others respectfully. Annie needs help in understanding that the children likely will act more appropriately as she makes it clear that she expects them to do their jobs and to speak to her in a decent manner. She is no longer just going to do their work for them if they fail to perform, and there will be additional consequences if they treat her badly. Finally, Annie can be encouraged to try these new ways by noting that although they never would have worked with her uncle and her mother, they very much can work now. In fact, everyone will feel much better about themselves and each other if they all start relating in more friendly and cooperative ways.

In sum, the combination of looking backward and forward in terms of the case formulation is effective. First Annie is helped to want to change by understanding how and why her problem interactions with the children have evolved (self-discovery; looking backward). Then she is helped to change once she is ready to (self-management; looking forward). The procedures in Figure 4.2 were used with Annie and were very helpful. Each component was difficult for her and took many sessions over many months. Ultimately she did manage to do it all, and relations with her self and her children improved.

Figures 4.1 and 4.2 show that IRT is explicit about how to select interventions at different moments in therapy. It is important to note that even though IRT is highly structured, and therefore might seem too "intellectualized" to some, equal weight is given to the domains of affect, behavior, and cognition (ABCs). It is also important to note that the language used by IRT therapists is jargon free. Even though adherent therapists constantly keep the case formulation in mind, it is unusual for them to rely on IRT-specific words such as "copy process" or "gift of love." Rather the language is everyday, clear, and "earthy" and uses the patient's own language whenever possible. IRT encourages imaginary scenarios that apply the case formulation. For example, when Annie would become troubled by the voice telling her she was stupid and could not do something, the IRT therapist might say something like the following: "Is your uncle at it again?" This would bring her attention to her uncle, the architect of the voice. In so doing, the intervention would engage her will to be free of his tyranny and help her dare to take on the new challenge of believing in herself and expecting to be treated decently.

While getting ready for termination from the second IRT therapist and to transfer to a new agency (with IRT consultative follow-up for the first few months), Annie's voice became extremely active and, despite having been given appropriate antipsychotic medication, she was filled with anxiety and despair about messages of failure coming from the voice. Annie and the second IRT therapist had many conversations about termination and concentrated on transitioning and how to maintain coping mechanisms. But the voice was "winning." After a while, the IRT therapist told Annie: "Please tell the voice he can only have his say for an hour a day: how about 8 A.M. to 9 A.M.? Annie agreed to this and was able to do it. After a week of successful containing of the voice to one specified hour per day, Annie observed: "Why, I can control the voice." That experience appears to have given her much more courage to take control of her own mind, and to continue—slowly—on her path to freedom from the voice, better functionality, and enhanced inner peace. Again, it is vital to note that progress was not sudden or smooth. Annie would move ahead with the tasks of resisting her voice and managing the children better, and then she would slip backward. But the general progression was forward, and gradually Annie was able to maintain her new patterns with greater consistency. Annie's spontaneously written follow-up note, quoted at the beginning of this chapter, suggests that after termination from her work with the second IRT trainee, she was able to continue to apply IRT principles and, once released from Red instructions, actively pursue new Green strengths with continued support from standard therapy approaches.

Data on IRT and Outcome

Benjamin (2003, Chap. 10) describes a minimalist pilot outcome study of effectiveness of IRT. Some patients, including Annie, were treated by graduate students in an IRT practicum; others were from my private practice. Eight volunteered to fill out before-and-after measures (treatments that ranged from 4½ months to 2½ years). A Wilcoxin signed ranks test showed significant improvement on several of the Symptom Checklist—90—Revised (SCL-90-R) scales (Derogatis, 1977), and on the WISPI (Klein et al., 1993). In addition to those patients who completed the before-and-after measures, there were about 20 other patients carried by IRT students learning to treat "difficult cases." From the group of 8 patients who made formal ratings and the 20 who did not, only one from this frequently self-destructive population made a suicide attempt and required rehospitalization. After a second rehospitalization (both rehospitalizations occurred within 3 weeks of discharge), we conducted an IRT family conference, led by me in collaboration with the student IRT therapist. For the rest of that academic year, IRT treatment continued with full support of the family and the primary physician. The patient had no more hospitalizations and made no more suicide attempts. The long-term outcome was very good in the opinion of the patient, her immediate family, her IRT student therapist, and the private long-term therapist who treated her after the IRT student left on internship.

The ongoing IRT clinic at the University of Utah Neuropsychiatric Institute is providing an opportunity for more systematic data collection. Continuing clinical success is suggested by very high service satisfaction ratings in this psychiatrically experienced and disillusioned nonresponder population. Early research efforts are concentrated on developing better methods of implementing (teaching) and assessing IRT. The idea is to be sure there is good adherence to this complex procedure and to see that adherence is relevant to outcome before trying to mount a larger formal study of effectiveness of IRT. The SASB methods described in the next section are important in testing the reliability and validity of case formulations and the adherence of therapists to the treatment model along with assessment of whether adherence relates significantly to outcome. Because IRT draws from so many empirically validated therapy principles, previous published studies of psychotherapy have indirect if not direct relevance to IRT. IRT is empirically informed, and its contribution is mostly to more sharply define which therapy intervention or principle should be applied and when in order to help nonresponders begin to change.

Following are some examples of SASB-based studies or reviews of psychotherapy principles that are relvant to IRT. Constantino (2000) published a particularly helpful review of published studies of psychotherapy that report clinically important findings based on SASB measures. A number of these relate directly to therapy principles shared by IRT—for example, changes in internalizations during therapy as measured by SASB (Greenberg & Foerster, 1996; Hartkamp & Schmitz, 1999), the effect of the therapy relationship (step 1) on outcome (Hilliard, Henry, & Strupp, 2000; Holmqvist & Armelius, 2000); Jorgensen, 2000; Pavio & Bahr, 1998); Safran & Muran, 1996), and the centrality of attachment in pathology targeted for treatment (Pincus, Dickinson, Schut, Castonguary, & Bedics, 1999).

Historical Antecedents to the IRT Treatment Method

The review of the historical antecedents to the case formulation method made it clear that IRT owes much to psychoanalysis, which has split more or less into two camps. On the one hand, there are those who remain loyal to Freud's original drive theory, which sees personality primarily in terms of internal struggles among the id (primary energies such as sexuality and aggression), the superego (the messages from "the dominant mass of ideas" from society), and the ego (the executive within that has the job of negotiating between the irrational demands of the id and the restraints imposed by society). On the other hand, there are object relations theorists and interpersonal theorists who emphasize the impact of social learning on the development of personality. Internal conflict explicitly (but not exclusively) reflects actual or perceived relations with others. Greenberg and Mitchell (1983) offer an informative and highly readable view of the various versions of psychoanalysis, with an emphasis on detailing the object relations and interpersonal components.

With its interventions guided by the belief that problem patterns are implemented via internal models linked by copy process to historical and current relationships, IRT would be classified in the interpersonal branch of the dichotomy. That emphasis stems both from clinical observation and from the hypothesis that attachment (to others) is a primary, not secondary, driver of personality. Not a variant of psychoanalysis, IRT nonetheless borrows heavily from psychoanalysis for decisions concerning intervention (e.g., impact of early development; vital role of conflict in psychopathology; relevance of the unconscious and its direct, if not recognized links to behavior and awareness; the wisdom of tracking free associations and recognizing patterns in dreams; and much more).

As already noted, IRT also draws heavily on Skinner's (1990) fundamental theorem of behavior (what works is what is repeated) and, hence, on much of cognitive-behavioral therapy. IRT diverges from traditional behavioral therapies primarily in its definition of what is reinforcing. Everyday "rewards" such as getting attention, getting control, and being taken care of are "reinforcing" according to IRT if and only if they are experienced as likely to bring affirmation and love from the internalized representations.

Still other therapy schools are a part of IRT (see Benjamin, 2003, Chap. 10, for further detail). Selection from all perspectives is unified by the requirement that interventions need to be chosen that are consistent with the case formulation, that apply the core algorithm, and that follow the flow diagrams.

THE SASB MODEL

The SASB model is the lens through which patterns can be seen clearly and linked to relationships with key figures. Clinicians familiar with SASB principles are able to see trends that might not be apparent otherwise.

Researchers can use SASB to objectify important aspects of relevant inter-actions, regardless of the school of therapy or context. Although the SASB model itself is theory neutral, its principles operationalize many concepts central to IRT. Hence, for IRT, the SASB model serves as a vital adjunct to teaching, certifying competence, and research.

The Structure of the SASB Model

The Basic Dimensions

The most user-friendly version of SASB, the simplified cluster model, appears in Figure 4.3. The full SASB model, presented in Figure 4.4, is more complex but also more versatile.

There are three surfaces or sections in all versions of the SASB model, and each represents a different attentional focus. In Figure 4.3, the different foci appear as different types of print (bold, underlined, italicized). In Fig-ure 4.4, the different foci are represented in different locations (top, middle,

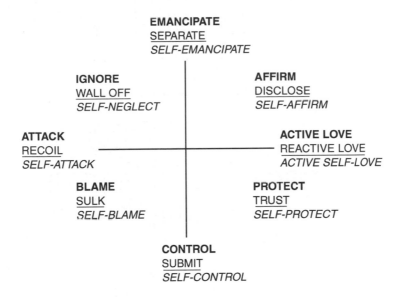

FIGURE 4.3. The simplified cluster SASB model. The points shown on the full model in Figure 4.4 can be grouped to provide a simpler version. The horizon-tal axis runs from hate to love, and the vertical axis from enmeshment to differ-entiation. The three types of focus are represented by different styles of print. Complementarity is shown by adjacent **BOLD** and <u>UNDERLINED</u> points. Intro-jection is shown by adjacent **BOLD** and *ITALICIZED* points. From Benjamin (1996a). Copyright 1996 by The Guilford Press. Reprinted by permission.

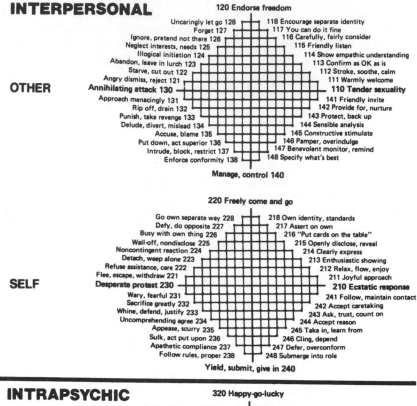

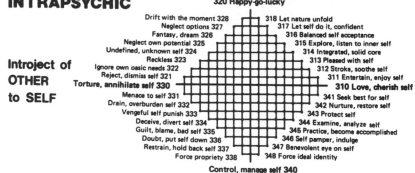

FIGURE 4.4. The full SASB model. From Benjamin (1979). Copyright 1979 by the William Alanson White Psychiatric Foundation. Reprinted by permission.

bottom). Parent-like behavior, which describes transitive actions focused on others, is shown by the bold print in the simplified model (Figure 4.3). In the full model, parent-like behavior appears in the top section (Figure 4.4). These prototypical parent-like behaviors are matched by child-like behaviors, which describe intransitive states focused on self. Child-like behaviors are shown by the *underlined* print in the simplified model (Figure 4.3), and by the middle surface on the full model (Figure 4.4). Finally, introjected behaviors, transitive actions directed inward, are shown by the *italicized* print in the simplified model (Figure 4.3) and by the bottom section of the full model (Figure 4.4).

On the horizontal axes of all versions, maximal hostility appears on the left-hand side, while maximal affiliation is represented on the right-hand side. The vertical axes differ for the three types of focus. On the simplified model (Figure 4.3), when focus is on other, the vertical axis runs from CONTROL to EMANCIPATE. If the focus is on self, the vertical axis in the simplified model ranges from SUBMIT to SEPARATE. And if introjection is the domain, the vertical axis goes from *SELF-CONTROL* to *SELF-EMANCIPATE*. On the full model (Figure 4.4), when the focus is on other, the vertical axis runs from 140 Manage, control to 120 Endorse freedom. When the focus is on self, the vertical axis goes from 240 Yield, submit, give in to 220 Freely come and go. If the focus is Introjected, the vertical model ranges between 340 Control, manage self and 320 Happy go lucky.

The vertical axes describe enmeshment at the bottom sections of the model and differentiation and the top sections of the model. In quadrant form, the SASB models describe friendly differentiation in the upper-right-hand quadrant (AFFIRM/DISCLOSE/SELF-AFFIRM); hostile differentiation in the top left (IGNORE/WALL OFF/SELF-NEGLECT); hostile enmeshment in the lower left (BLAME/SULK/SELF BLAME); and friendly enmeshment in the lower right (PROTECT/TRUST/SELF-PROTECT). The ability of the SASB model to define friendly and hostile versions of enmeshment and differentiation is very important when distinguishing normal and psychopathological patterns in personality. Examples related to Annie follow.

Coding an Event or Situation

To understand how a psychosocial event can be characterized by codes based on the SASB model, consider how to quantify the responses of Annie's mother when the uncle attacked Annie and the mother asked: "What did you do to provoke him?"

The first step in SASB coding is to identify two interacting components, or referents. The *referents* here, respectively, X and Y, would be mother to Annie. SASB coding is from the perspective of X. SASB-based descriptions are always interactional and can apply to parent–child interactions; to therapy process in individual, group, or marital settings; to peer–peer interactions; to boss–employee interactions; to between-group interactions (e.g., physicians and nurses); and more. This review is confined primarily to applications relevant to the study of psychopathology and psychotherapy.

The second step in SASB coding is to assess X's focus. At the moments in question, Annie's mother was focused on other (Annie), and hence the mother's behavior would be described by a point in the parent-like domains (bold print in Figure 4.3 or top section of Figure 4.4). The mother's message was clearly hostile, and it was controlling. The decision that the event was hostile places it on the left-hand side of the models, and the decision that it was controlling places it in the lower half of the models. Altogether, the three decisions regarding Annie's mother were focus on other, hostile, and controlling. Those judgments place the event in the lower-left-hand corner of the models, the region of hostile controlling focus on another person. This means that on the simple model, Annie's mother is described by the point: BLAME. Judging that the behavior has approximately equal amounts of CONTROL and BLAME, on the full model, she is described by the point, 135 Accuse, Blame. The quadrant for hostile control is summarized in the simplified model as BLAME.

Important Differences between the Simplified Cluster and the Full Model

The full model and the simplified cluster model are identical conceptually, but the full model provides greater articulation of subdivisions within quadrants. On the simplified model, there is only one midpoint in each quadrant. By contrast, in the full model, there are eight subdivisions that define each quadrant. For example, the quadrant for hostile control is located between the poles of pure control and pure attack. On the simple model, the midpoint is BLAME. On the full model there are eight points in this quadrant for hostile control. Moving counterclockwise from the control pole toward the attack pole, the successive points contain proportionately less control and more attack. For example, 138 Enforce conformity, located next to the control pole, consists of 8/9 Control and 1/9 Attack. Moving through the quadrant counterclockwise, the Point 131 Approach menacingly appears just prior to the attack pole and contains 1/9 control and 8/9 attack.

The richness of descriptions based on the full model helps us to understand complex communications. In some situations, that enhanced descriptive power fully justifies the extra intellectual effort required to master the full model. As just mentioned, the full model identifies eight varieties of hostile control, beginning with <u>138 Enforce conformity</u> at the control pole and ending with <u>131 Approach menacingly</u> at the attack pole. Clearly, use of the "average" name, BLAME in the simplified model for this whole quadrant loses considerable information. Yet in many situations, the average descriptions based on the simplified cluster model (Figure 4.3) are quite adequate, as analyses in the third section of this chapter demonstrate. Meanwhile, the next section continues the exposition of the models by discussing a unique and conceptually important feature of full model.

Tracks within the Full Model

The numbers that accompany each point on the full model (Figure 4.4) describe their exact locations. All parent-like points are represented by the 100s series; all child-like points, by 200s; and all introjective points, by 300s. The middle, or 10s, digits describe quadrants according to the Cartesian convention: 1 = upper-right-hand section, 2 = upper-left-hand section; 3 = lower-left-hand section, and 4 = lower-right-hand section. The last, or 1s, digit represents the subdivision of the respective quadrants. These range between 1 and 8. Hence, the point 135 represents focus on other (100s), region of hostile control (30), the fifth subdivision starting from the horizontal axis (5/9 control and 4/9 attack).

The numbers for full model points have interesting properties. For example, all points ending in 0 describe poles of the model, or the "primitive basics"; all points ending in the digit 1 describe approach–avoidance; all points ending in 2 describe nurturance and needs fulfillment; all points ending in 3 describe attachment and security-related behaviors; all points ending in 4 describe logic and reason; all points ending in 5 describe communication and learning; all points ending in 6 describe balance in relationship; all points ending in 7 refer to struggles for identity; all points ending in 8 describe intimacy/distance. All points ending with the same digit are said to belong to the same *track*.

The eight tracks describe developmental stages that articulate varying positions with respect to the basic developmental tasks of attachment and separation. Life begins and ends with the primitive basics, and development progresses more or less regularly through the behaviors marked on the full model by successive numbers 1–8. The poles are based on assumed biological givens: <u>sexuality</u> (right-hand horizontal pole), <u>power</u> (bottom poles), <u>aggression</u> (left-hand poles), and <u>separate territory</u> (top poles). They are always relevant but perhaps more apparent in infancy and adolescence. Learning to strike a balance among these primitive basics to create the more "civilized" behaviors located midway between poles (i.e., tracks 4 and 5: logic and reason and communication and learning) requires socially guided practice in a supportive setting.

Unlike other features of the SASB model, the empirical behavior of tracks has not been evaluated in many contexts. However, in a sample of mothers of 226 pediatric patients (age 0–21 years) rating their focus on their child, there were significant positive correlations between age and tracks 4, 5, 6, 7, 8 and the axes, with the greatest magnitudes appearing for tracks 5, 6, and 7. Correlations between tracks 2 and 3 were negative (but not significant). These trends (negative r for the lower numbers, with increases in magnitude for the mid- and upper-range numbers) are consistent with the hypotheses that the earlier developmental issues are described by tracks 2 (nurturance and needs) and 3 (attachment and security), while focus on the more "civilized" middle tracks (4 = logic and reason; 5 = communication and learning) comes later. Enmeshment and differentiation (track 7) also were significantly associated with parenting the older children.

By definition, the track scores embrace conflict, as each track includes exact opposites for every represented point. It is interesting to find that the SASB model can define so many developmental conflicts and associate them empirically with developmental ages, at least from the perspective of parental focus. The next relevant question is to check for associations between tracks and diagnoses (e.g., personality disorder). Tracks were computed in earlier versions of SASB software but dropped in an effort to simplify and make the output more user-friendly. However, a separate program that yields track scores for long-form data can be prepared on relatively short notice for interested current users of the long form.

Why the SASB Model Is Not Drawn as a Circle

The SASB models are drawn as quadrilateral figures with equal sides rather than as circles, as is the contemporary convention. The reason is that the axes on the SASB model are not relative. The primitive basics are givens. Drawing the model as a quadrilateral makes the pivotal role of the poles of the axes very clear. All other points are composed of components from these axes. For example, 143 Protect, back up on the full model is made of 6/9 love and 3/9 control. Presenting the model as a circle would imply that any set of orthogonal points could serve equally well as bases of remaining points. For example, PROTECT on the simplified model is made of 50% ACTIVE LOVE and 50% CONTROL. This (as well as the location of the other simplified cluster model points) is confirmed by dimensional ratings of SASB items by naïve judges (Benjamin, 2000b; Rothweiler, 2003), and makes inherent sense. Moreover, the names of the poles of the axes of the SASB model correspond in orderly fashion to the names of factors that emerge in principal-components analysis without rotation (Benjamin, 2000b; Rothweiler, 2003).

If the axes were rotated 45 degrees in the clockwise direction, then ACTIVE LOVE would be made of PROTECT and AFFIRM. If these two points serve as "primitive basics," then ACTIVE LOVE would be their derivative rather than an underlying component of each. That perspective could be argued, but it is neither parsimonious nor intuitively correct. Conceptually, such a shift in orientation would be like rotating the axes of geographic maps of the earth 45 degrees off the North and South poles presently anchored in relation to the flow of magnetic fields about the earth. Rotated maps would work, but uses of compasses directed by those magnetic fields would be complicated by the need to translate positions back to those defined in relation to the magnetic poles.

Thus the use of quadrilaterals for the SASB models derives from the concept of primitive basics as biological givens that provide an absolute frame of reference. One of many predictions that stem from that assumption is that there might be neurological nodes for each of the poles of the model, and other behaviors could be implemented via interactions among impulses from these polar nodes. This proposal was developed further by Benjamin and Friedrich (1991).

Intensity on the SASB Model

The primitive basics (track 0) are extreme and intense. Unlike other models based on two axes (e.g., Leary, 1957), intensity is not described in the SASB models by length of a vector from the origin. Rather, intensity in SASB defined interpersonal space is marked by proximity to the primitive basics shown on the axes. The poles of the axes (e.g., ATTACK and CONTROL) are the most intense, and the points midway between axes are the most moderate (e.g., AFFIRM and PROTECT).

Complex Codes

Earlier, Annie's mother was described as <u>135 Accuse, blame</u> on the full model when she demanded to know what Annie had done to provoke her uncle after he attacked her. The fact that Annie's mother would do this even when the uncle's attacks were extreme needs to be recorded along with the fact that Annie got the blame. Annie's mother consistently overlooked the context; Annie's crimes were normative, and her punishments by the uncle were extreme. When Annie's mother failed to take proportionality into account, she defaulted in her parenting role. That aspect of the mother's focus on Annie was hostile and it left Annie on her own (EMANCIPATE). The three components—focus on other, hostile, emancipate—combine to place the transaction in the upper-left-hand corner of the model. On the simple model, the result is IGNORE, and on the full model, the result is 123 Abandon, leave in lurch. This needs to be added to the previous description of Annie's mother as BLAME or 135 Accuse, blame. The two components together comprise a complex code: BLAME + IGNORE, or 135 Accuse, blame + 123 Abandon, leave in lurch. (A variation appropriate to some contexts would be to substitute 133 Punish, take revenge for 135 Accuse, blame in this complex code.) Both elements (one indicating hostile control and the other hostile neglect) are required to describe what Annie's mother was doing. Neither alone would suffice. The two parts of a complex code are inextricably combined.

If BLAME and IGNORE had occurred in sequence rather than inextricably, they would be recorded separately and called multiple codes rather than a complex code. For example, if the uncle had not been so violent but perhaps had mildly teased Annie about something trivial, and Annie had called him an offensive name, the mother might have said: "Annie, you need to learn to take a little bit of teasing and you certainly should not use language like that. This would be coded as a simple BLAME. If Annie then asked for something and mother paid no attention, that would probably be described as IGNORE. The full model equivalents would be 135 Accuse, blame, and 126 Ignore, pretend not there. In this scenario, the messages are not complex. First there is BLAME and then there is IGNORE.

The ability of the SASB model to describe simple events in terms of underlying dimensions marked by the axes (love/hate; enmeshment/differentiation) and complex events by combining simple codes gives it substantial versatility. The SASB model can provide convincing description of complicated clinical events. For example, Humphrey and Benjamin (1986) suggested that complex coding adequately captures the examples of what Bateson, Jackson, Haley, and Weakland, (1956) and Wynne and Singer (1963) called the double bind. Henry, Schacht, and Strupp (1986) reported that therapists who gave complex codes (usually indicating pseudofriendly accepting messages delivered in a condemnatory fashion) had worse outcomes than did therapists who gave clean, simple messages.

Methods of Describing Individuals or Groups in Terms of the SASB Model

This section reviews methods of gathering and analyzing SASB data sets. It includes illustrative tests of the validity of the structure of the SASB models and provides some published examples of how SASB data sets can inform clinical theory and practice, whether or not it is oriented by IRT.

There are two approaches to measurement of a rater's interpersonal behavior or views of self and others in terms of the SASB model: (1) the SASB questionnaires, called the Intrex questionnaires, which provide ratings by self and others and (2) the SASB coding system (Benjamin & Cushing, 2000), which provides objective observer ratings of videotapes of any interactions such as therapist–client, parent child, peer–peer, husband–wife, employer–employee, teacher–student, and so on. SASB codes can even be used to characterize systems themselves, as in family or group therapy (e.g., MacKenzie, 1990; Benjamin, 1996b, 2000a). Software is available to qualified users that generates a number of parameters that summarize and characterize the data gathered by questionnaire and by the coding system.[1] Comprehensive manuals are included that explain the meanings of the various parameters, provide a variety of validity tests, list various possible applications, and more. The manual for questionnaires explains how to set up a battery of ratings, while the coding manual explains how to generate simple and complex codes such as the ones mentioned earlier in the descriptions of Annie and her mother and uncle.

The Intrex long-form questionnaires provide one item for each of the points on the full SASB model. Examples of items that might describe Annie's mother include: 123 Abandon, leave in lurch (Just when P is needed most, P abandons C, leaves C alone with trouble), 124 Illogical initiation (P ignores the facts and offers C unbelievable nonsense and craziness), 125 Neglect interests, needs (P neglects C, C's interests, needs), and 126, Ignore pretend not there (P just doesn't notice or pay any attention to C at all). Such long-form items provide detailed sampling of a given region of interpersonal space. In this example, the region of hostile differentiation describes a critically relevant aspect of Annie's mother in the parent-like role.

In contrast to the richness offered by the full model, the Intrex short forms provide only one item for each of the points on the simplified model. For example, there is only one item to sample the entire region of hostile differentiation involving parent-like focus. For IGNORE, the short-form item is, Without giving it a second thought, P uncaringly ignores, neglects, abandons C. There is a second equivalent short form. The item from Version 2 for the parent-like hostile differentiation, IGNORE, is Without giving it a thought, P carelessly forgets O, leaves him/her out of important things. The medium form combines the alternative versions of the short form to yield two items per model point. The medium form is a good choice because it is moderate in length compared to the long form but does not rely on just one item to represent each model point. Normative mean scores for medium form are close to those obtained by the long form.

Intrex questionnaires can be used to assess views of self and others. Some examples for Annie are given in the third section of this chapter. An important feature of the SASB technology for assessing personality is that the patient's view of important other people is considered as explicitly as are the ratings of the self. Many assessment instruments ask the rater to describe him- or herself (an "I" form). The interpersonal perspective, explicitly included in Intrex assessments, addresses "He and She" or "They" as well as "I." Because there are so many perspectives to be assessed, Intrex ratings invoke four different meanings of the word "self":

1. "Self ratings" is consistent with conventional usage that mean the person being assessed provides the data.

2. There also is a traditional assessment of the rater's view of him- or herself relating to others (the "I forms"). However, the rater's view of others is assessed (the "he/she/they forms") in addition to the traditional "I" perspective.

3. Profiles generated for these various perspectives (he/she/they and me with him/her/them) are based on sets of eight clusters that correspond to one of the three surfaces on the SASB model (Figures 4.3 and 4.4): focus on other, self, and introject. When an eight-cluster profile refers to items assessing the focus on self (middle) surface of the SASB models (Figures 4.3 and 4.4), the language used to label the set of eight clusters is "I/he/she/they react to (person or persons)."

4. When the eight-cluster set refers to items assessing the introject surface of the models, the language used to label the set is "Introject."

To review, the word "self" can mean (1) data are provided by the rater; (2) the "I" forms are being discussed; (3) data were generated by items describing the focus on self surface, in which case the language used is (person or persons) reacts to (person or persons); and (4) data were generated by items describing the introject surface. Here the language used for the set of eight is *introject*. None of these meanings presumes to describe "self-concept" in its entirety, although data assessing the introject surface of the model are most centrally related. A theoretical discussion of the relation between self-concept and the various possible assessments via SASB models appears in Benjamin (2003, p. 139).

For each of the possible sets of eight clusters describing a given surface of the SASB model in Figure 4.4, there are three different ways of summarizing the data. There are (1) profiles based on the eight-cluster scores, (2) pattern coefficients that summarize the relations among the eight-cluster scores, and (3) plots in a two-space with weighted affiliation and autonomy scores for a given set of eight-cluster scores. The third section of this chapter provides examples to demonstrate the uses of the three methods. Each has advantages and disadvantages.

1. Briefly, the profiles based on clusters show most directly how the relationship is experienced. They are easily used for conventional between-group comparisons using repeated-measures multivariate analyses of variance. Such profiles are familiar to most researchers who use profile mea-

sures such as the Minnesota Multiphasic Personality Inventory (MMPI), the Millon Clinical Multiaxial Inventory (MCMI), the SCL-90-R, and the like.

2. The pattern coefficients are especially useful at the level of $N = 1$ because they quantify a relationship in terms that patients and clinicians can understand (attacking, controlling, conflicted). Surprisingly, when processed as patterns (and reflected in the SASB pattern coefficients), interpersonal perceptions may be categorical. Subjects' ratings yield pattern coefficients that are bimodally distributed, whereas randomly generated ratings do not. Unfortunately, there are few familiar statistical procedures for handling data that are so clearly distributed bimodally (see Benjamin & Wonderlich, 1994, and Benjamin, 2000b, for an extended discussion of the bimodality problem/strengths).

3. The weighted affiliation and autonomy scores provide simple, easily understood vectors locating a rating by a single point in intrapersonal space defined by the SASB axes. Each cluster position is weighted according to its distance from the attachment pole (weighted affiliation score, AF), or from the autonomy pole (weighted autonomy score, AU). The AF or AU score is the average of the cross-products of a rater's cluster scores and the weights assigned to the respective cluster scores by location on the model.

Comparison of Data Based on Questionnaires with Data Based on SASB Codes

With the same parameters available for self-ratings (questionnaires) and objective observer ratings (SASB codes), it is possible to assess distortions in perception of others as well as of the self relating to others. Different perspectives can be compared and contrasted by having different raters complete the questionnaires or by comparing questionnaire ratings with observer codes of actual interactions. For example, Humes and Humphrey (1994) showed that parents with a drug-dependent adolescent described themselves as more friendly to this daughter than did objective observers coding videotapes of family interactions. One clinical implication is that the family fight about the daughter needs to be dealt with more explicitly if there is therapeutic value in starting with an accurate understanding of existing patterns.

The Intrex questionnaires are relatively easy to use, but they suffer from the usual problems of measures based on self-ratings. The SASB questions are not at all tricky. They mean what they say, so a rater needs to approach them honestly for results to be valid. This means that SASB questionnaires are probably not appropriate for use in adversarial settings, as in forensics. A highly collaborative relationship is desirable. This is naturally present when giving SASB to patients in one's clinical practice. If the responses to the questionnaire are going to affect the case formulation and the treatment plan, it is in the patient's interest to answer the questions as accurately as possible. Using the SASB Intrex questionnaires to focus the patient's understanding of his or her own interpersonal patterns and links among them can facilitate the therapy process greatly (MacKenzie, 1990). In research studies based on the SASB Intrex questionnaires, giving feedback for purposes of enhancing personal growth of the rater is an optimal incentive, although quite a number of studies with normals have simply offered the traditional course credits for completing the questionnaires. It is not unusual for research participants to comment that they learned a lot just by answering the questions and seeing similarities in their responses to different key people in their lives. Some patients participate in research that offers small amounts of money. Many others make the ratings out of wishes to contribute to understanding of and ability to help people with mental disorders. This is the case for participants in the IRT clinic, who usually are very pleased with their treatment and eager to do whatever they can to help others benefit from IRT.

SASB coding of transcripts of interviews, sessions, or other contexts is more objective and includes the ability to record complex events and to assess sequences of events. However, analyses of data gathered by coding studies are more difficult and time intensive. The investigator must learn to code, and the process of coding is quite slow. SASB coding studies are best designed with the principle of "high quality, low quantity" in mind.

Sequential analysis of a therapy session discussing what happened after a patient's mother telephoned helped explain why she became suicidal after the call. The sequences in the therapy narrative replicated the mental sequences during and after the phone call (Benjamin, 1986). Here is another example of how and why SASB sequential studies can be complex but clinically informative in unique and powerful ways. Karpiac and Benjamin (2004) analyzed a sample of 22 individuals with anxiety disorder treated by cognitive–behavioral therapy (CBT) and a sample of 20 individuals with anxiety treated by time-limited dynamic psychotherapy (TLDP). The first analysis examined whether the topic changed following therapist affirmation. The second assessed whether therapist affirmation was of adaptive or maladaptive content and whether those distinctions related to outcome. Results of the CBT sample "suggest that affirmation sustained conversation on the current topic, but its base rate was not related to outcome. . . . Affirmation of maladaptive content predicted worse outcome at 12 months follow up when the criterion measure was symptom change" (p. 10). In CBT, wherein the discussions often were about symptoms, affirmation sustains attention on the current topic, and if maladaptive content was affirmed, outcome was worsened.

Results in the TLDP sample, wherein symptoms were rarely discussed, suggested that affirmation

> did not increase the likelihood of continuing with the same topic of conversation. Overall base rates of affirmation were unrelated to most outcome measures, but significantly related to poorer relations with a significant other at 12 months follow-up. [Moreover,] predicted therapist affirmation of maladaptive statements was associated with worse outcome when the measure was change in relations with a significant other person. Unexpectedly, therapist affirmation of maladaptive statements was significantly associated with *improvement* in introjected views of the self. . . . This finding . . . may not be so puzzling. Most of the discussion in these TLDP sessions was focused on interpersonal matters. Marital and family therapy researchers have historically been wary of individual treatment for relationship problems because studies indicate that it corresponds with higher rates of deterioration (see Gurman & Kniskern, 1978) than conjoint treatments. Although speculative at this point, we reason people take nonspecific affirmation to mean they are "right," that TLDP patients might have talked a lot about troubles with their significant other and taken therapist affirmation to mean that they were "right" regarding their significant other. Patients might then have become more alienated from their significant other and more affirming of the self. . . . This speculation would need to be confirmed by expanding the 2 × 2 table and examining differential outcomes for affirmation of maladaptive statements in relation to significant other versus relation to introjected feelings about the self. Unfortunately, these data did not permit any finer grained analyses . . . and need to be replicated independently before the interpretation can be taken as definitive. (Karpiac & Benjamin, 2004, pp. 12–14)

The findings suggest that in a technique-oriented therapy such as CBT, therapy process (i.e., when but not how much affirmation is delivered) can have an unrecognized impact on outcome. Attending more systematically to that process could enhance outcomes. The same is true for TLDP, a less specifically focused interpersonal therapy, when the measure is of relations with significant others. However, results may also show that at least for patients with an anxiety disorder, there is an implicit tension between feelings about self and others; if the therapist affirms maladaptive statements about significant others, patients feel better about themselves. This is an undesirable result and could be avoided if therapists address this possible misconstrual and more explicitly pursue the IRT therapy goal of friendly relations with self *and* others. The highly informative finding required combined use of Intrex questionnaire measures of attitudes about self, relations with significant others, and sequential analyses of SASB codes of therapy process.

Validity Tests of the Structure of the SASB Models

An overview of SASB-based studies that have contributed to its construct validity of the SASB model and its predictive principles appeared in Benjamin (1996). Results touch on questions of reliability, content validity, concurrent validity (associations with other measures), and construct validity (significant findings that make clinical sense and/or that confirm predictions).

Some of the major tests of validity are reviewed here, with greater specificity. Formal tests of *content validity* have established that judges unfamiliar with SASB would describe the questionnaire items in terms of the predicted underlying theoretical dimensions. The dimensional ratings procedure (Benjamin, 1988a, 2000b; Rothweiler, 2003) provided that undergraduate students rate each SASB item on scales respectively representing the theoretical underlying dimensions (focus, love–hate, enmeshment–differentiation). Average ratings for each item were then used to reconstruct the model. For example, the items representing the point AFFIRM were assigned values for focus (other, self, introjected) on the affiliation (horizontal) and interdependence (vertical) axes by the naive students. Group results suggested that the items for AFFIRM did reflect focus on another person, moderate degrees of friendliness, and moderate amounts of freedom giving. These judgments placed AFFIRM at approximately 1:30 o'clock on Figure 4.3. The process was repeated for each point of the model. The result was not a "perfect circle" but was a reasonable facsimile of the cluster version of the SASB model. Points appeared in the predicted circular order, and the axes were placed at approximate right angles.

This dimensional ratings procedure formally established the content validity of each of the SASB items on the long, medium, and short forms. Other widely used circumplex personality measures (e.g., Wiggins, 1978) do not report comparable direct assessments by naïve judges of the underlying dimensionality of each of the items on the instrument. In fact, inspection of the eight Interpersonal Adjective Scales (IAS) items in any given cluster does not suggest that they all have the same dimensionality. Rather, somewhat different items are averaged together to create a single point exactly where it "should" be on a "perfect" circle. An in-depth conceptual and empirical comparison of dimensional analyses of SASB and IAS items was offered by Rothweiler (2003). Standard deviations of dimensional ratings of items within IAS clusters were larger than standard deviations within SASB clusters.

For testing construct validity, a frequently used method is factor analyses of subjects' application of items to themselves (Wiggins & Broughton, 1985). Examples of validating factor analyses via self-ratings on Intrex questionnaires appeared in Benjamin (1974, 1994, 2000b). The predicted

underlying factors do consistently emerge, and factor loadings can be used
to generate reasonable facsimiles of the model. Like the dimensional ratings
data, the factor-analytic reconstructions of raters' application of the items
to themselves generally affirm the hypothetical structure of interpersonal
space. Several examples for SASB are given in the Intrex user's manual
(Benjamin, 2000b). Similar published general confirmations of the structure of the SASB models have been offered by Lorr (1991), Lorr and Strack
(1999), Pincus (1998), and Pincus, Newes, Dickinson, and Ruiz (1998).
Some of these papers have suggested that the SASB model might more accurately be represented as an ellipse (with the attachment axis as major, and
the interdependence axis as minor) rather than a circle.

Another and well-replicated SASB-based method of confirming the circular structure of the SASB model is to find circumplex order when data for
a given set of eight model points (e.g., mother focused on me) are correlated with a dependent variable of interest (e.g., depression). Figure 4.5
presents an example of this type of circumplex ordering of results for the
personality diagnosis most relevant to Annie, namely, schizotypal personality disorder (SZT). She also scored high on avoidant personality disorder
(AVD), among others. AVD is included here for purposes of comparison
because it shares the feature of social withdrawal but is not the same as

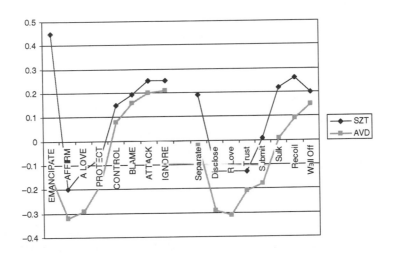

FIGURE 4.5. Correlations between ratings of mother on the Intrex and personality disorder scores based on the Morey (1988) derivations from responses
to MMPI-I. This sample of 136 psychiatric inpatients showed very orderly
(circumplex) relationships between personality disorder scores and views of
their mothers.

SZT from the perspective of DSM. In the figure, which is from a sample of 136 inpatients (the Benjamin inpatient sample, described later) that did not include Annie, it can be seen that patients scoring high on SZT or AVD rated their mothers relatively low on AFFIRM and ACTIVE LOVE items, and progressively higher as the hostile side of the model is approached. The peaks were at ATTACK and IGNORE, features that were salient in Annie's experiences with her uncle–mother dyad. It may be of interest that the SZT ratings showed a stronger association with hostile maternal focus than did AVD ratings, but AVD ratings showed a larger deficit in AFFIRM and ACTIVE LOVE.

Because almost all SASB data sets show such patterns of circumplex order (with shifts in peaks and valleys corresponding sensibly to whatever is being correlated), it is possible, among other things, to identify the contributions of deficits in normative (e.g., friendly) experiences as well as the presence of nonnormative (e.g., hostile) experiences. For example, Goedken (2004), using this same sample of psychiatric inpatients, showed that depression is more strongly associated with deficits in affirm and love, while anxiety is more strongly associated with actively hostile types of maternal focus. Thus, although anxiety and depression are highly comorbid, there are important differences in their interpersonal templates. According to IRT, procedures for repairing deficits in positive interpersonal experience would not be the same as procedures for addressing damages from excessive negative interpersonal experiences.

One of the more compelling published examples of validation by circumplex ordering of results within SASB data sets was offered by Ratti, Humphrey, and Lyons (1996). These investigators found circumplex order in *effect sizes* when contrasting index family (bulimia or polysubstance abuse) SASB coding scores to SASB scores for control groups. The finding was that the magnitude of differences in effect size between clinical and control groups on cluster scores would maximize at a particular point, BLAME, for example, and progressively diminish until reaching the opposite point, AFFIRM; then increase again to complete the circle. This amazing result was presented for both mother focuses on daughter and daughter reacts to mother (Ratti et al., 1996, Figures 1, 2 and 3, pp. 1259–1261). Of course, the investigators were primarily focused on significant effect sizes that distinguished the respective clinical from their control groups. But Ratti et al. (1996) also commented on the aforementioned circumplex ordering of effect sizes: "Using the SASB measures enabled us to examine in depth two key clinical concepts, autonomy and connectedness in a multimethod and multitheoretical context. Analysis of the patterns in effect sizes revealed a basic simplicity underlying a complicated multivariate design" (p. 1263). This kind of order requires that the SASB structure be circular, as claimed.

The Predictive Principles from the SASB Model

The predictive principles can suggest what may have preceded and what may follow a given interpersonal event. The main predictive principles are complementarity, introjection, similarity, opposition, and antithesis.

Complementarity

Two individuals are in complementary positions if their focus is on the same person and if their behaviors can be coded at the same angular location in interpersonal space. The first person must be focused on other while the second person is focused on him- or herself. For example, when Annie's mother engaged in the complex combination of BLAME + IGNORE, the complementary response from Annie would be predicted to be hostile focus on self: SULK + WALL OFF. Annie would give in to mother's view of the situation and not express her own feelings or thoughts. In the language of the full model, Annie's complex complementary response to her mother's complex message would be 235 Appease, scurry + 223 Detach, weep alone.

In IRT, complementarity is most likely to support the principle of recapitulation. Recapitulating raters tend to show the same reactions to their significant other person that they gave to parents. For example, with her ex-husband and an earlier abusive relationship and with her children, Annie recapitulated the appeasing responses she learned in relation to her mother and uncle. According to SASB theory, complementarity is a natural, hardwired propensity. If one is being ATTACKed, one Recoils; If one is being AFFIRMed, one Discloses, and so on. The process is bidirectional. For example, if one Recoils, one is more likely to be ATTACKed. Hence, Annie's compliant willingness to take the blame ("responsibility") led her to find partners who repeated her uncle's abusive ways. Such bidirectionality in complementarity is becoming better recognized in the folk lore. People have begun to recognize that presenting in a fearful manner increases the likelihood of oppression. Presenting in a friendly manner increases the chances things will go well, and so on.

Complementarity recapitulated in subsequent relationships is the principle mechanism for what is otherwise known as the repetition compulsion. As noted in the section "IRT Theory of Personality Psychopathology and Psychotherapy," IRT theory holds that people (including Annie) do not give up their recapitulations of positions that will draw for repetition of the original problem because they seek to present and receive the gift of love.

A rather simple empirical demonstration of complementarity appears in Table 4.1, Where the eight clusters for "Mother focused on me" appear in rows and the eight clusters for "I reacted to mother" appear in columns. There is no matching of complementary items in the Intrex questionnaire

TABLE 4.1. Complementarity between Mother and Rater in a Sample of 184 Psychiatric Inpatients

	Separate	Disclose	Reactive Love	Trust	Submit	Sulk	Recoil	Wall-Off
Emancipate	0.653	0.343	0.287	0.209	-0.044	-0.016	0.206	0.224
Affirm	0.226	0.697	0.737	0.605	-0.088	-0.445	-0.394	-0.387
Active Love	0.159	0.640	0.774	0.645	0.036	-0.263	-0.364	-0.305
Protect	0.061	0.539	0.685	0.642	0.074	-0.321	-0.389	-0.340
Control	-0.143	-0.147	-0.090	0.117	0.571	0.485	0.297	0.256
Blame	0.114	-0.370	-0.467	-0.400	0.232	0.653	0.679	0.617
Attack	0.148	-0.346	-0.421	-0.440	0.149	0.575	0.676	0.596
Ignore	0.182	-0.405	-0.479	-0.435	0.202	0.604	0.662	0.635

Note. Mother focused on me (rows) and I reacted to her (columns). Diagonals = complementary match. All diagonal entries are significant. Six of eight are the maxima for the column, and the remaining two were within .003 of the maximum.

forms. In fact, the items are presented in a randomly determined order (unlike the IAS questionnaires, which arrange items on the page so that opposition and similarity is apparent to the interested rater). Entries on the diagonals of Table 4.1 are all significant, as they should be if complementarity holds. For six of the eight diagonal cells, the entry is the maximum for its column, as it should be. The two "misses" were within .003 of the maximum for the column. Note that the magnitudes of the r tend to decrease with distance from the diagonal until they become negative at the more distant points. The circumplex order in the matrix represented in Table 4.1 is clearly visible but not perfect. The trend is clearest for points nearer the horizontal axis, but it is also discernible for points near the vertical axis. There is no agreed-on method for assessing the degree of circumplex order in such a table. One obvious solution would be to compare the entries in the table to those in a table that describes a perfect circle. However, the nonindependence of the entries precludes any significance testing. The most that can be said for such a result is that the method can report the percent variance shared by the data and a perfectly circumplexial set. For Table 4.1, that r is .636 = 40.45% shared variance between perfect and obtained circumplex values. I have not found in the literature any comparable tests of complementarity for data sets based on the Interpersonal Circle or the IAS. Orford (1986) noted that studies using the single circumplex showed good complementarity on the horizontal (hate to love) dimension, but results for the vertical dimension (dominance to submit) were not very compelling. That same finding was reported by Bluhm, Widiger, and Miele (1990) and interpreted as follows: "affiliative behavior was due largely to situational (complementarity) effects and control behavior was due largely to individual differences (p. 464). By contrast, Table 4.1 suggests that complementarity in SASB data holds for both dimensions regardless of context.

A more complex test of complementarity in a psychiatric sample of SASB data was performed by Gurtman (2001) using a randomized pairing method to control for base rate pairings of complementary points. In comparing the obtained pairings to the randomized pairings, Gurtman reported: "A z test comparing the obtained sample mean of .643 with this mean value yielded a test statistic of 10.58, with a chance probability of occurrence much less than .001. (Indeed, none of the 1,000 random pair sample means exceeded the obtained mean.) Hence, the obtained complementarity result may be regarded as highly significant."

Perhaps it should be noted that the simpler method shown in Table 4.1 does not suffer from a base rate problem because product–moment r computed between subjects naturally includes a correction for base rate (mean) as well as a correction for variations in scale (standard deviations). Karl Pearson addressed the presently relevant version of base rate problem long ago. His between-subjects r simply = the sum of the cross-products of the *standard scores*, divided by n.

Introjection

Introjection is shown whenever an individual treats him- or herself as he or she has been treated by important others. In Annie's example, maternal IGNORE would be predicted to be introjected as *SELF NEGLECT*, while the BLAME would be internalized as *SELF-BLAME*. On the full model, the parental <u>123 Abandon, leave in lurch</u> would be introjected to yield <u>323 Reckless</u>, and <u>135 Blame, accuse</u> would be internalized as <u>335 Guilt, blame, bad self</u>. If the parents do not care about them, children are unlikely to care about themselves. If parents blame them, they blame themselves. Introjection was illustrated by Annie's inability to care about herself and by her sense that she was bad and needed to ignore her own needs in order to serve others.

Results of tests of the principle of introjection using the methods illustrated in Table 4.1, and also Gurtman's method, are comparable to tests of complementarity. For example, Gurtman (2001) wrote:

> As before, a z test was done to compare the obtained sample mean (3.64) with that of the empirical sampling distribution. Gurtman's test of introjection in a sample of psychiatric inpatient (N = 187) gave the following result: A z value of 3.67 was obtained; on the basis of the normal curve, the probability of such a result occurring by chance is $p < .001$. Thus, when compared with an appropriate sampling distribution, the obtained mean for introjection was highly significant.

Showing patients that they are treating themselves as they were treated by important others can help patients control self-destructive urges. For example, when Annie realized that to call herself stupid was to treat herself as her uncle had treated her and to believe it and act upon it (e.g., not go back to school) provided testimony to the validity of his beliefs, she was better able to choose on her own behalf.

Links between perceptions of parents and introject have been reported by many (e.g., Armelius & Granberg, 2000; Friedman, Wilfley, Welch, & Kunce, 1997; Wonderlich, Klein, & Council, 1996). Rudy, McLeore, and Gorsuch (1985) showed that patients' views of their interactions with their therapists on the SASB Intrex questionnaires was significantly correlated with therapy outcome as measured by SASB introject scores. Hilliard et al. (2000) used SASB questionnaire and coding methods to find "a direct effect of patient early parental relations on process and outcome, *a direct effect of therapist early parental relations on process*, and a direct effect of process on outcome–and thus indirect effects of both patient and therapist early parental relations on outcome mediated by the process" (p. 125, italics added). Their startling results suggest, among other things, that the therapist process can reflect the impact of the developmental experiences of *both* the therapist and the patient. This would be expected if the SASB predictive principles are operative within therapist phenomenology as well as in patients

Similarity

Similarity is shown whenever an individual copies or acts like someone else. The child development literature provides reliable testimony to the role of imitation in human development from the earliest days of life (e.g., Meltzoff, & Moore, 1977). A more familiar clinical term, and the IRT term for this pattern, is "identification." If they identify with their parents, children who grew up in an atmosphere characterized by parental IGNORE are more likely to do the same to their own children. Annie did not identify with her mother in this way of relating to children. Annie's departure shows that SASB predictive principles can be disconfirmed as well as confirmed. IRT hypotheses assessed via SASB are concrete and refutable at the level of a single individual. The failure here confirms the objectivity of the tests of the predictions. Then, when predictions fail, it is important to be able to provide an explanation. This problem is discussed further in the section "Predicting Which Principle Will Apply."

A particularly compelling direct test of similarity was offered by Cushing (2003), who asked drug-abusing (cocaine) and matched normal control mothers to rate their memories of their mothers with them and themselves with their own daughters. The measure was the SASB Intrex questionnaires. Using canonical correlations, Cushing found significant associations suggesting that normal mothers identify with their own mothers. The trend was less clear in the cocaine-using mothers (see the section "Predicting Which Principles Will Apply" for further discussion) than in the normal sample. By virtue of the fact that canonical correlations, begin with the computation of cross-products of Z scores, they, like produce–moment correlations, control for base rate effects.

In many SASB data sets, correlations between "Mother focused on father/Father focused on mother" with "Rater focuses on spouse" have behaved as shown in Table 4.1. That table was examined in the section on complementarity for loadings on the diagonal and for systematic decreases in the magnitudes of r when moving away from the diagonal. That discussion of Table 4.1 invoked a harsh test of the predictive principle of complementarity because it required not only that specific predicted pairs match (i.e., the cells on the diagonal) but also that other pairs match in progressively changing degrees depending on their proximity to any given theoretically matched pair. Canonical R offers a softer test of the overall strength of the relationship between rows and columns in matrixes such as the one shown in Table 4.1. Unlike the discussion of Table 4.1 in the complementarity section, use of canonical R does not put restrictions or ordering within rows or columns.

Hence, to assess imitation without regard for whether rows and columns behave according to circumplex order, one could use canonical R to compare, for example, the eight clusters for "Mother focused on father" with the eight clusters for "I focus on my significant other." This would identify general similarity between wife focuses on husband as observed in the parental relationship and the female rater's own behavior as wife focusing on husband. For example, in a sample of 104 normal females included in the Intrex user's manual (Benjamin, 2000b), ratings of "I focus on my significant other at best" showed a significant tendency to imitate fathers' focus on mother (but not fathers' reaction to mother), and mothers' reaction to father (but not mothers' focus on father). Normal females did imitate both parents in most respects as they related directly to the rater (e.g., mother focused on me and I focus on my spouse).

This section suggests that predictive principles can be assessed by different methods (e.g., inspection of matrixes like the one in Table 1; Gurtman's method; and canonical R, followed by inspection of relevant product–moment r). There are advantages and disadvantages to each. All methods show successful predictions and failures of prediction. As has already been mentioned, interpretation of those successes and failures (i.e., of which principles apply and when) is discussed below.

Opposition

Opposition is shown at 180-degree angles on the SASB model. The opposite for IGNORE, shown by Annie's mother when her uncle attacked, would be described by PROTECT on the simplified model. On the full model, the complement of <u>123 Abandon, leave in lurch</u> was <u>223 Detach, weep alone</u>, and that is what Annie did. Its opposite would have been <u>243 Ask, trust, count on</u>. But Annie, could not trust: After she was punished, she crawled under her bed. Annie explained that she did so because she was so ashamed. The image vividly conveys her introjected sense of unacceptablility and also convincingly establishes that she felt utterly alone. One treatment implication is that Annie very much needed to have a protective advocate in order to learn self-care. The IRT therapists did do that at several points. One example was to help her locate a competent but inexpensive lawyer who would help free her of the inappropriate financial obligations that rightfully belonged to others. A test of opposition is also discussed in the section "Predicting Which Principles Will Apply."

Antithesis

The complement of an opposite is an antithesis. The antithesis of IGNORE is TRUST. Through the principle of complementarity, the antithesis pulls for the opposite of any given position. For example, to the extent that children show the sweet dependency marked by the point TRUST, neglectful parents are less likely to IGNORE them and more likely to provide the opposite, namely, PROTECT. The child's friendly dependency "pulls" for caregiving, though success is not guaranteed, as Annie's history suggests. A different predictive principle must have been operative in Annie's mother. For example, her neglect of Annie may have represented identification with her own mother. The grandmother may have neglected Annie's mother while also demanding that Annie's mother take care of her youngest son, Annie's uncle. In that case, it would appear that Annie's mother was more affected by the internalization of her own mother than by any natural draws toward taking care of her own daughter, Annie. At some point, Annie learned not to ask for fair treatment and accepted that she had to do much more to have the same privileges as the others, like go to the mall. An analysis of 41 depressed and 29 control mothers and their toddlers during the second reunion after they had been subjected to the Ainsworth Strange Situation showed antithesis (Cushing & Benjamin, 1999). Mothers universally greeted their babies by picking them up and trying to hug them. Almost all infants initially showed what Bowlby described as "detachment." In terms of SASB codes, mothers showed PROTECT, while the babies showed the antithesis, WALL OFF, or a complex combination of WALL OFF + TRUST. Infants of normal mothers more quickly moved to the complementary position of TRUST and subsequently went off to explore the playroom (SEPARATE). They had more secure attachments (Benjamin, Cushing, Schloredt, Callaway, & Gelfand, 2005) and behaved just as Bowlby would have predicted. Babies of depressed mothers, by contrast, were slower to move back to the complementary position of TRUST, and they tended to remain close to their mothers throughout the rest of the experimental period, unable or unwilling to explore. Results of this study, which was based on a data set provided by Gelfand, Teti, and Fox (1992) and SASB coded by Schloredt and Callaway, are described and discussed in further detail elsewhere. The point here is that antithesis can be observed in defined groups and situations, and that sequential analyses contribute to the understanding of differences between clinical and control groups in those situations.

Predicting Which Principle Will Apply

It is not yet possible to predict exactly when one principle rather than another will be invoked. What is clear is that connections between childhood social learning and adult personality can often be found in terms of just a few of these SASB predictive principles. The copy processes in IRT describe the most commonly observed connections: (1) the adult personality is similar to (IRT identification) the observed parental behaviors, (2) the adult personality continues to show patterns that were complementary to the parental positions (IRT recapitulation), and (3) the adult personality treats the self as did the parents (SASB and IRT introjection).

It is important to know that ratings can vary greatly for the various states and situations in the Intrex series (e.g., my introject, me with spouse at best and at worst; mother with me; father with mother). It also is important to know that there may be strong evidence of copy process within nearly every individual data set, but when averaged across relationships (e.g., across all mothers for all females) the consistency fades. The key figures are not the same for everyone, and this makes it more difficult to find copy process in group analyses. The solution to this problem is to identify variables likely to encourage one copy process more than another and then to create subgroups based on those variables. The subgroup analyses should clearly show the associated copy process.

To date, only a few variables have been identified at the group level that allow prediction of which principle or copy process will apply in a given situation. For example, it appears that imitation and introjection are more likely if the model exhibits warmth and dominance (Mussen, Conger, & Kagan, 1971). When the 133 normal subjects were divided into quadrants on the basis of the SASB-based coordinates of their ratings of their mother during childhood, those in the quadrant of friendly control show the highest correlations between the items representing mother focused on me and the items representing their introject. (Benjamin, 2000b).

Less often, children show the opposite and/or the antithesis of the original positions. Opposition and antitheses are defined as copy processes too, because they are defined precisely at 180 degrees away from the original position. So, there can be identification in reverse, as well as identification. This means the basic three copy processes actually can assume six forms (Benjamin, 2003, Table 6.1). One identified variable that increases the likelihood of opposition is hostility in the parent. Some abused children become loving parents, saying: "I would never treat a child of mine that way." This possibility was suggested in Cushing's data set. She divided her sample into rater mothers whose own mothers were hostile. This subgroup had an elevated tendency to be the opposite of their mother when relating to their own child. A clinically recognized variable that increases likelihood of antithesis is overcontrol by parents in relation to adolescents. That frequently yields <u>227 defy, do opposite</u>.

This list of variables (dominance with warmth; overt and consistent hostility) that affect selection of copy process is short and not well substantiated. Nonetheless, tests of the predictive principles already provide strong support at a statistical level. In addition, the reader may note that many of the reported analyses correspond well with his or her own observations and "folk wisdom." Future work with present data bases, along with new ones, is expected to expand the list and add to understanding of the predictive principles. The astonishingly simple and direct connections suggested by the interpersonal copy processes as defined by the SASB predictive principles, combined with inherited temperament, ensure that personality "runs in families."

Use of SASB to Define Normality and Pathology

Normal Personality

According to IRT, normal personalities are characterized by SASB codes in the so-called attachment group (AG; Benjamin, 1995, 2003). For the parent-like domain, these include AFFIRM, ACTIVE LOVE, and PROTECT. In the child-like domain, they include DISCLOSE, REACTIVE LOVE, and TRUST. Introjected, they become SELF-AFFIRM, SELF-LOVE, and SELF-PROTECT. These normal behaviors reflect clear friendliness and moderate degrees of differentiation and enmeshment. Such normative, "good" internalizations are the expected result of friendly, well-balanced (on the continuum of enmeshment/differentiation) caregiving. The associated behaviors are maintained by wishes to maintain good relations with benign internalizations that may have been modeled by parents, siblings, teachers, coaches, and others.

Normative behaviors are not normative unless they are contextually appropriate. Consistent love regardless of context would be described by a complex code in the SASB coding system. For example, if a parent warmly supports a child who has just hit another on the head with a hard object (as in the case of Annie's uncle), that support of the offender is coded as PROTECT + IGNORE. The offending child's development is not facilitated by failing to address such pathological behavior. A similar complex code would be used to describe a psychotherapist who provides affirmation and noncontingent support of a patient engaging in cutting her arms.

Normality requires balance of focus in addition to requiring baseline friendliness and uncomplicated hostile differentiation or enmeshment. In a mature relationship, one person focuses on another about as often as on him- or herself. If focus in the parent–child relationship is not balanced by the end of adolescence, the child has not learned the skills necessary for mutuality. When the parent focuses exclusively on the child, the parent does not have a self as far as the child knows, and thus the likelihood of narcissism in the form of expecting nearly exclusive focus on self is increased (via recapitulation of the complementary position). On the other hand, when the parent focuses exclusively on him- or herself, the child can become "parentified." Such a parent will elicit caregiving from the child as the principle of complementarity demands. The child, like Annie, is very likely to fail to focus on self adequately (Burkett, 1991).

Pathological Behaviors

Behaviors that are the opposite of normal behaviors are salient in pscho-pathology. In the parent like domain, these include IGNORE, ATTACK, and BLAME. In the child-like domain, disaffilitative behaviors are WALL OFF, PROTEST, and SULK. Pathological introjected behaviors are SELF-NEGLECT, SELF-ATTACK, and SELF-BLAME. Collectively, these are the disaffiliative group (DAG). Patients reliably show far more DAG behaviors than do normals.

This DAG group of behaviors is normal only in limited, highly specific contexts. For example, a normal person could engage in DAG behaviors and perhaps even try to kill someone who is threatening fatal bodily harm. As another example, in extraordinary circumstances, a normal person might utterly neglect self-interests on behalf of others. But, again, such a departure from contextually relevant friendliness should not be a "baseline" position, as it was for Annie.

Contrary to popular clinical beliefs (e.g., controlling mothers create pathological responses), the vertical axis poles of enmeshment (CONTROL/SUBMIT) or differentiation (EMANCIPATE/SEPARATE) do not necessarily correlate either with pathology or normality. Context very much affects the impact of enmeshment or differentiation. The poles of the vertical axis describe behaviors that can be adaptive and appropriate in some contexts and pathological in others. For example, there are situations in which a normal parent tries to exert absolute control (e.g., don't play in the busy street). However, if occupied too often without regard for context, polar behaviors describe and encourage pathology (e.g., As long as you live in this house, you will do everything I say).

Analyses of SASB data bases (e.g., Benjamin, 2000b; Rothweiler, 2003) show that normal samples give greater endorsement to AG behaviors than do patient samples. Patient samples, by contrast, give greater endorsement to DAG behaviors than do normal samples. Exact patterns of different clinical populations vary by diagnosis, and some also are characterized by more extreme scores on the poles (CONTROL/SUBMIT; EMANCIPATE/SEPARATE). Antisocial subjects (ASP), for example, are distinguished from individuals with borderline personality disorder (BPD) by significantly greater tendencies to show autonomy. Both ASP individuals with BPD are more hostile than normals (Benjamin, 1997). More recent comparisons of these groups, using normed rather than raw scores (Benjamin & Critchfield,

2004) clarify that BPD is best described by SASB data in terms of hostile enmeshment (lower-left-hand quadrant of Figures 4.3 and 4.4), whereas ASP is best described by hostile differentiation (upper-left-hand quadrant of Figures 4.3 and 4.4). These examples illustrate the claim that SASB data bases consistently support the IRT interpersonal definitions of normality and pathology.

IRT Therapy Goals

With its clear definition of normality and pathology, the SASB model provides an absolute, nonrelativistic description of changes needed in therapy. There should be a change from frequent hostility; excessive enmeshment, or differentiation to a baseline of uncomplicated friendliness with moderate degrees of enmeshment and differentiation.

If someone places a high value on oppression or annihilation of other persons or groups, he or she would not be acceptable candidates for IRT unless he or she chose to work to modify those rules and values to be consistent with AG behaviors. In IRT, patients are clearly informed about the friendly interpersonal goals at the beginning of treatment and are free to choose not to pursue them (Benjamin, 2003, Chap. 5). The parallel models (Benjamin, 2003, Chap. 4, app.) describe specific affects and cognitions that are expected to accompany AG behaviors, and they are included in the description of IRT goals. Affects parallel to parent-like AG behaviors are accept, love, and nurture. Affects parallel to child-like AG behaviors are be centered, delighted, and hopeful. Cognitions parallel to AG parent-like behaviors are understand, enhance, and concentrate. Cognitions parallel to AG child-like behaviors are expressive, optimistic, and well-directed. These expected affects and cognitions are pleasant and effective and easily embraced as goals by most patients.

By now, it may be clear that IRT, based on principles of the SASB model, proposes that normality and pathology develop in the same way. Maladaptive behavior is not a sign of breakdown. Rather, it is the natural result of attempts (implemented via the SASB predictive principles) to adapt to the perceived rules and values of important other people. *Differences between normality and pathology are found in what is modeled and copied, not in what is intact and what is broken.*

Historical Antecedents to the SASB Model

The geometric emphasis on the axes of SASB is founded in primatology. The extremes represented by clearly marked poles of the SASB model have long been discussed as prime movers in various versions of psychoanalysis. Sexuality and aggression were named primary sources of energy by Freud

(1896/1959). Adler (1955) added the idea that there is a primary drive for power or superiority. Mahler (1968) and others emphasized an inherent thrust toward differentiation—toward separate psychological "territory." In the animal world, the earliest form of differentiation is weaning. Additional underlying givens or drives have been postulated by various personality theorists. Murray (1938, pp. 79–84), for example, posited a hierarchy of 13 primary (e.g., air and water) needs and 28 secondary (e.g., nurturance) needs. He also was one of the earliest theorists who attempted to define and assess psychoanalytic concepts in operational terms, including study of the unconscious.

The Single Circumplex Tradition: The Interpersonal Circle

The SASB model belongs to the circumplex tradition. These comprise a group of interpersonal models based on two axes, and usually appear as a circle. In the later 1930s, among many others, Murray developed instruments to measure human needs (e.g., Thematic Apperception Test), and tried to test his ideas empirically. The secondary needs were primarily interpersonal, and that emphasis was later developed in depth by others, including Sullivan (1953). The interpersonal and empirical emphases by Sullivan and Murray affected the development of the interpersonal circumplex (IPC), which is both interpersonal and devoted to the value of defining and measuring personality in ways that can be tested empirically. The IPC itself was introduced by Freedman, Leary, Ossorio, and Coffey (1951). They explored the clinical implications of the IPC at the Kaiser Foundation Hospital during the 1950s. In 1957, Leary published an extremely important book that described particular personality types that were found in the clinic to be associated with various positions on the IPC. His book, *Interpersonal Diagnosis of Personality*, remains a classic to this day. Leary's circle had many levels; the points on the interpersonal level were managerial–autocratic, responsible–hypernormal, cooperative–overconventional; docile–dependent; self-effacing–masochistic; rebellious–distrustful; aggressive–sadistic; competitive–narcissistic (p. 65).

The idea of using combinations of two dimensions that combine to define points arranged on a circle was named a circumplex by Guttman (1966). The Leary group's circle was developed independently of Guttman. Nonetheless, Guttman is important in the history of circumplex theory because he provided a clear mathematical rationale for it.

Following the publication of Leary's book, there was a spate of variations on his version of a circumplex, some of which were mentioned by Benjamin (1974) and most of which were cited in a comprehensive review by Wiggins (1982). In his summary table (p. 186), Wiggins listed 21 different theorists whose work was based on the idea that personality could be described in terms of two axes given names that corresponded reasonably to the concepts of dominance and love.

Wiggins's own version, the IAS, lists these points: PA, ambitious–dominant; NO, gregarious, extraverted; LM, warm, agreeable; JK, unassuming, ingenuous; HI, lazy, submissive; FG, aloof, introverted; DE: cold, quarrelsome; and BC, arrogant, calculating. Wiggins constructed his IAS by searching dictionaries for trait words that related well to a subgroup of needs selected from Murray's (1938) list (Wiggins & Broughton, 1985, p. 4). The IAS model points are located on a circle on the basis of loadings on the two factors that emerged from the measure he felt sampled selected key needs from Murray's list. Wiggins then compared responses on his IAS to responses on other personality inventories representing a variety of research traditions. These included Stern's activity index; Campbell's Need Scales; Edward's Personal Preference Schedule; Gough and Heibrun's Adjective Check List; and Jackson's Personality Research Form. Finding that they all projected well onto Wiggins's IAS, Wiggins and Boughton concluded the IAS does represent a useful "taxonomic framework" within which to view personality from a variety of traditions. Later Wiggins (1995), refined his measure; presently, it is called the IAS-R.

The single circumplex has been enormously influential in the research traditions of social psychology but has had less impact in clinical psychology and practice. The IAS literature is primarily trait based. Items are endorsed for their general applicability to the rater and not relative to specific interpersonal relationships (e.g., me with spouse, with father, and with mother) which had originally been proposed by Leary (1957). Studies of the IPC usually are in normal populations. Ns are large and the statistical methods impeccable.

Some IPC studies have attempted to use the IPC to characterize personality disorders as represented on Axis II in DSM. For example, in 1982, Wiggins proposed the following arrangement for personality disorder on the IAS: PA, ambitious/dominant = Compulsive; NO = gregarious, extroverted = chronic hypomanic; LM, warm, agreeable = histrionic; JK, unassuming, ingenuous = dependent; HI, lazy, submissive = passive–aggressive; FG, aloof, introverted = schizoid; DE, cold, quarrelsome = paranoid; BC, arrogant, calculating = narcissistic. Sim and Romney (1990) used ratings on the Leary Interpersonal Check List and personality disorder measured by the Millon MCMI-I to test Wiggins's predictions in a sample of 90 patients and 90 students. There was modest support for the predictions when the reconstructed models were compared to predictions in terms of quadrants rather than octants (p. 338). The predictions about relations between SASB measures and DSM are discussed in the section "Application of SASB and IRT to DSM Personality Disorders." Because Benjamin's (1996a) view of personality disorder includes different predictions by state and situation as well as by trait, such simple projections onto a single figure are not appropriate.

The IPC as refined by Wiggins (the IAS-R model) has been adapted to at least one published assessment instrument that is sometimes used in clinical populations: The Inventory of Interpersonal Problems (IIP; Horowitz, 1996) was based on collation of the interpersonal complaints of persons presenting for outpatient treatment that were factor-analyzed and related to the IAS-R. The IIP is popular for measuring pre–post changes during psychotherapy (Gurtman, 1996).

The "circular" measures of personality were compared to alternative assessment systems also based on factor analysis by O'Connor and Dyce (1998). These authors concluded that the circular measures (e.g., IAS-R) were inadequate in describing a clinical and community sample. O'Connor and Dyce reported that better validation was found for Costa and McRae's five factors (N = neuroticism; E = extroversion; O = openness; Conscientiousness; Agreeableness). The universality of the NEO-PI has been further argued by Widiger and Costa (1994). Widiger has proposed that some version of the many available personality trait measures based on factor analysis should be used to define pathology in the official nomenclature of the American psychiatric Association. There is some evidence that they or others like them may be used in the DSM-V (Kupfer et al., 2002).

Major Points of Divergence between SASB and IPC Literature

SASB belongs to the IPC-based group of models of personality. One of the most important differences is in the definition of the vertical axes of the models. Like the IPC models, including Leary's IPC, The SASB model has a horizontal axis that runs from love to hate. However, the vertical dimension is quite different from the IPC. As already noted, the SASB model places EMANICPATE rather than SUBMIT as the opposite of CONTROL. The idea of opposing control with emancipate came directly from Schaefer (1965), who consistently found that result in factor analyses of an instrument that measured parenting behaviors in a number of different cultures. The SASB model places submission at a location complementary to CONTROL on a separate surface or domain. The creation of two surfaces, parent-like and child-like in the SASB model, clearly and sensibly distinguished opposites and complements. Opposites are 180 degrees away from one another, and complements match geometric coordinates but differ in focus. For example, control and emancipate are opposites. Control and submit are complements, not opposites. Emancipate and separate are complements in SASB models and are not represented on a distinct dimension in the various versions of the IPC.

In the octant version of the SASB model, there are eight distinctive sets of complements and eight distinctive sets of opposites. Inspection of complements and opposites in Figures 4.3 and 4.4 give the reader a sense of the content validity of the claims. For a simple example, blame and affirm are opposites. The complement of blame is sulk and the complement of affirm is disclose.

On the IAS, ambitious, dominant is opposed and complemented by lazy, submissive. arrogant, calculating is opposed and complemented by unassuming, ingenuous. Differentiation is either missing or poorly articulated on the IPC models. For example, on the IAS, the point that comes closest to describing differentiation is aloof, introverted. By contrast, on the SASB simplified model, there are six types of differentiation (all interpersonal clusters on the upper half of Figure 4.4). This ability to define and measure differentiation in various forms is vital in assessing progress in therapies that seek to enhance differentiation but not alienation. For example, if Annie had achieved friendly differentiation in relation to internalizations of her uncle and mother, she would no longer be driven by voices and habits that implemented their destructive rules and values for her in her current life. Her follow-up note indicated she had achieved that goal. She also would be able to talk to and correspond with them in person in friendly but separate ways and not become upset by what they did or did not do. Her follow-up note did not mention current relations with these important figures, so it is not clear whether she had differentiated to such a degree that she could actually be in their presence and still maintain friendly differentiation. SASB concepts and methods allow for clear definitions and assessment of such crucial clinical goals.

Another important difference is that the SASB model defines interpersonal focus on other, on self, or other-directed focus turned inward upon the self. This feature has many clinical and theoretical implications. For example, it provides a direct way to assess the copy process principle of introjection, which specifies that people will treat themselves as they have been treated. For another example, the dimension of focus explicitly calls the clinician's attention to whether the patient is talking about him- or herself or someone else. Constant codes of focus on other in the therapy narrative suggests an external orientation that, unless addressed and changed, precludes personal growth. The dimension of focus, in conjunction with the names of the poles on the vertical axes, yields straightforward and unique predictions of opposites and complements. Unlike the IPC, no pairs of points on the SASB model serve as both opposites and complements. This conceptual clarity has better content validity. An example is that it makes more sense to says that submit complements or goes with control than to say that submit is the opposite of control and then, in another context, to say submit is the complement of control. The better articulation of vertical axes probably is also responsible for the fact that evidence in support of complementarity as defined by the SASB model is strong (Benjamin, 1974; 1994, 2000b; Gurtman, 2001)

The quadrilateral shape of the SASB model is another important difference. It means that points on the SASB model are located most easily by values in a rectangular coordinate system. To illustrate again, the model point <u>114</u> <u>Show empathic understanding</u> is composed of four units of affiliation and five units of autonomy giving. The rectangular coordinates for this point are (4,5), or in general (x,y). A representation on a circular model (circumplex) would base locations of model points on polar instead of rectangular coordinates. In polar coordinates, the values x,y respectively become $r \cos \theta$, and $r \sin \theta$, where θ is the angle between the right-hand side of the x axis and a line drawn from the origin to the point (x,y) on a circle centered at the origin and having the radius r, when $r^2 = x^2 + y^2$. In circumplex literature, r is always set – 1. But in the rectangular version favored by SASB, the value of r would be less than 1 except at the poles of the axes.

Leary's first drawing of the IPC also was a quadrilateral (Laforge, 1985). The switch to a circle likely came from the fact that available statistics are based on operations performed on the squares of differences rather than on absolute values. It is easier to work with squares of difference scores than it is to work with simple difference scores, which require keeping track of signs. The squaring procedure is used in almost all statistics favored by behavioral science, and they relate most directly to models described most simply by polar rather than rectangular coordinates. Even though it is a quadrilateral rather than a circle, for the sake of convenience (e.g., not having to develop factor-analytic methods that work with absolute difference scores rather than squares of differences) and comparability, most tests of SASB structure are based on circumplex methods and logic. At a greater level of precision, lines connecting SASB data points should be linear rather than curvilinear. Nonetheless, the relative orders of magnitudes of relevant parameters (correlations among points; factor loadings; canonical coefficients) are comparable enough whether the model is drawn as a quadrilateral or a circle.

Contemporary IPC research shows considerable concern with establishing perfect circularity in the models (Acton & Revelle, 2002). Even if it is granted that the SASB model should be a circle rather than a quadrilateral, there is no stated logical reason for why the interpersonal model must be a circle (or a square within a circle) rather than an ellipse (or a rectangle within an ellipse). The unexplained reverence for perfect circles seems reminiscent of the Platonic perfect universe and of earlier debates over the shape of the earth's orbit about the sun. Absent compelling theory to the contrary, perhaps data should be allowed to make the decisions regarding optimal shapes of models.

Benjamin (1996c) discusses additional important differences between SASB and the IPC tradition.

Examples of Other Uses of the SASB Model and Technology

A list of identified publications using SASB methods to address a variety of problems is available by writing *Intrex@psych.utah.edu.* Topical areas include validity of SASB; individual, group, and family therapies; psychopathology; personality; prevention; sports psychology; therapist training; behavioral genetics; assessment; and more.

APPLICATION OF SASB AND IRT
TO DSM PERSONALITY DISORDERS

The Wisconsin Personality Inventory

The WISPI (Klein et al., 1983) is based on interpersonally oriented items that reflect Benjamin's (1993, 1996a) descriptions of DSM Axis II personality disorders. Benjamin's view of Axis II was derived from SASB coding DSM-III-R and DSM-IV items (American Psychiatric Association, 1987, 1994) and using the SASB predictive principles, guided by clinical experience, to infer prototypical interpersonal interactive styles as well as their likely historical antecedents. Benjamin's descriptions contributed significantly to the writing of the DSM-IV text about the respective disorders (A. Francis, Editor, and R. Ross, science writer, of DSM-IV, personal communications, 1994).

The WISPI was written to makes sense from the perspective of the rater. For example, consider DSM-IV item 5 for BPD: "Recurrent suicidal threats, gestures, or behavior, or self-mutilating behavior" (p. 654). The corresponding WISPI item is: "I like to be intimate with people, and if I sense any rejection, I deliberately hurt myself by doing something like cutting or burning myself. Then I feel better" (x item #183). The item adds a likely interpersonal stimulus (perceived abandonment) to the behavioral symptom described by DSM (self-attack). The combination of current interpersonal context and history helps "explain" the self-mutilating behavior in terms that are consistent with IRT and that were applied to this disorder by Benjamin (1996a). The contextual detail surrounding the DSM item (self-mutilation) enhances the likelihood it will be endorsed (only) by those self-mutilators who fit the BPD template described by Benjamin (1996a).

*Agreement between the WISPI and Other Methods for
Defining Personality Disorder*

For Axis II diagnoses, agreement among the different methods has been notably poor (Klein, 1983; Fiedler, 1995). Klein et al. (1993) noted that correlations of the WISPI scores for the DSM-III version and counterpart scales of other self-report scales averaged .39 for the MCMI and .69 for the Personality Diagnostic Questionnaire (PDQ); when corrected for attenuation, the coefficients were .43 and .93, respectively (Klein et al., 1993). More recently, Smith et al. (2003) compared diagnoses on the WISPI and the Structured Clinical interview for DSM-IV Axis II Personality Disorder (SCID-II; First, Spitzer, Gibbon, Williams, & Benjamin, 1997) for DSM-IV in a sample of 75 inpatients. They reported poor convergence for categorical diagnoses but quite strong associations between dimensional scores for personality disorders by the two methods. The average *r* between dimensional profiles on DSM-IV versions of the WISPI and the SCID-II for the respective disorders was .61. Correlations between specific scale scores for the respective disorders according to the two methods averaged .48. The average correlation for off-diagonal (i.e., scale scores for a given disorder according to one method correlated with scale scores for a different disorder according to the other method) scores was .14. Results therefore showed good discriminant and convergent validity when diagnosis was by dimensional rather than categorical descriptions.

*Use of the WISPI to test Benjamin's Descriptions of
Personality Disorder*

Klein, Wonderlich, and Crosby (2001) tested Benjamin's (1996a) predictions about differences in self-concept among disorders on a sample of 366 patients who rated both the WISPI (DSM-IV version) and the Intrex introject measure of self-concept.

> There was a high degree of intercorrelation among the WISPI personality disorder scores and also among the adjacent SASB clusters in the introject measure. Therefore, partial correlation analysis was used to control for the variance shared between personality disorder dimensions and the SASB clusters when estimating the association between a given personality disorder scale and a given SASB cluster score. For example, when the correlation between scores on the Paranoid Scale and SASB Cluster 1 was computed, the WISPI scores for the ten other personality disorder scales and the seven other SASB clusters were first partialled out of the analysis so that a partial correlation coefficient represented the unique association between the paranoid score and SASB cluster 1. (p. 153)

They summarized:

> Although there was some overlap between categories, most were associated with fairly distinct patterns of self-concept. The disorders also clustered together in meaningful ways along the major axes of Benjamin's interpersonal model of the self-concept. (p. 150)

There are three data bases available for assessing the interpersonal aspects of personality disorder (in addition to the introject aspect examined by Klein et al., 2001), along with the historical predictions. They are:

1. A sample of 185 psychiatric inpatients collected by Benjamin, using the Morey, Waugh, and Blashfield (1985; see also Morey, 1988) DSM-III definitions of personality disorder based on MMPI-I scores.
2. A sample of 227 outpatients and normals collected by Rothweiler (2003) using the MCMI-III as a measure of personality disorder.
3. A sample of 88 inpatients gathered by Smith (2001) using the WISPI as a measure of personality disorder.

All original analyses in this chapter (e.g., Table 4.1; Figures 4.5–4.8) are based on the data set for sample 1 or other Benjamin data banks, unless Smith or Rothweiler are specifically cited. There are substantial convergences among these three data bases, and there are discrepancies as well. Because her study defined personality disorder (PD) via the WISPI, Smith's tests of Benjamin's DSM-IV-based predictions are discussed here for comparisons of Intrex and WISPI PD scores. Although there are several ways to define PD using the WISPI, and many possible methods of testing associations between Intrex interpersonal scores and PD, the simplest methods are illustrated here. Results are based on WISPI mean dimensional scores correlated with SASB mean cluster scores.

Seventy-five of Smith's inpatients completed the SCID II, the WISPI, and Intrex measures. This provided sufficient n to test selected features of Benjamin's predictions for the following diagnoses: AVD, obsessive–compulsive disorder (OCD), and BPD. Significant r between the dimensional score for a given personality disorder and a SASB cluster score identified interpersonal features associated with that disorder. According to this method, Smith's results showed BPD was characterized by SELF-NEGLECT and SELF-ATTACK, and by a propensity to ATTACK his or her significant other person. Parents of patients with BPD were seen as NEGLECTing and ATTACKing.

The descriptions of relations with self and with others and of the perceived history were generally consistent with Benjamin's interpersonal description of BPD, but they were not complete. Benjamin described BPD as follows:

> There is a morbid fear of abandonment and a wish for protective nurturance, preferably received by constant physical proximity to the rescuer (lover or caregiver). The baseline position is friendly dependency on a nurturer, which becomes hostile control if the caregiver or lover fails to deliver enough (and there never is enough). There is a belief that the provider secretly if not overtly likes dependency and neediness, and a vicious introject attacks the self if there are signs of happiness or success. (p. 119)

The suggested historical antecedents of BPD were growing up with a chaotic, soap-opera lifestyle and traumatic abandonment experiences that fused (confused) pain and love, helplessness and omnipotence, and idealization and devaluation and involved reckless coercion. Self-definition and happiness were attacked, and sickness elicited nurturance.

Unfortunately, the Intrex ratings cannot test for context in which the behaviors occur (e.g., that attack is triggered by perceived abandonment and that self-attack occurs in a context of perceived success). However, the description of individuals with BPD as ATTACKing of self and significant other is confirming of predictions, as is their reckless self-neglect. The finding that parents were seen to IGNORE and ATTACK confirms both copy process theory (parental neglect is internalized to self-neglect; parental attack is imitated), and DSM-based predictions by Benjamin (1996a).

One unanticipated result was a significant association between BPD scale scores and hostile compliance by the mother (SULK). However the additional data sets describing the complementary set—"I focused on mother"—suggest that several of the Cluster B personality disorders were likely to score relatively high on blaming parents. Yet the correlation between BPD scores and "I blamed mother" was not significant in Smith's sample. A trend to orient around that cluster is suggested by circumplex order to the results, centering on BLAME. Successive r become progressively larger as the blame cluster (item 6) is approached. Correlations for the eight clusters in Figure 4.4, starting at the top and proceeding clockwise were .04, .11, .07, .17, .28, .34, .24, .20. Although not significant in Smith's data set, *correlations between the single cluster for I blamed mother and BPD dimensional scores were highly significant in the other two data bases.* Circumplex order was observed there, too.

Smith's results for OCD and AVD were likewise generally supportive of Benjamin's predictions. Many significant r between OCD and SASB clusters had to do with enmeshment involving varying degrees of CONTROL and deference in different contexts. For AVD, significant clusters had to do with interpersonal distance and self-blame. Again, there were features of the predictions that could not be tested, and there also were prediction fail-ures, though some could be interpreted as indirect support. For example, mothers of individuals with AVD did not show the predicted BLAME, but they did show significant deficits in AFFIRM, the opposite of BLAME. This unexpected result was also found in the other two available data bases (Rothweiler, 2003; Benjamin, as described above).

On the Usefulness of Testable Theory and Surprises in Data Bases

The unpredicted result that mothers of individuals with BPD tended to SULK (submit) in relation to them led to inspection of the complementary set of I focused on mother and yielded the suggestion that those with BPD tend to blame their mothers. That trend (BPD correlates with BLAME mother) was highly significant in the other two data bases (Rothweiler, 2003; Benjamin, described above). It makes sense that diagnostic groups that often direct hostile control toward others would have a history of con-trolling their parents.

DSM did not explicitly mark the closely related tendency to control others as a diagnostic indicator for any disorder other than OCD (item 6). Benjamin's predictions (1996a, p. 286), however, marked blame as a base-line feature for the adult behaviors in 8 of the 11 personality disorders and control as a baseline feature for 7 of them. Benjamin was silent on whether these behaviors were shown during childhood. The tendency for several of the PD groups to blame and control is recognized clinically. That, plus the predictions based on Benjamin's SASB codes of DSM items and the correla-tions between blame and control with personality measured three different ways in as many different data bases, suggests that perhaps blame and con-trol should explicitly be included in DSM descriptions of PDs. These results are examples of how SASB can contribute to better descriptions of PD. The addition of predicted links to early learning can help explain how individu-als with personality disorders learned to behave in problematic ways. That, in turn, has both prevents and treatment implications.

Clinical Implications of Using Absolute (Anchored by Content Analysis) or Relative Scores

Mean scores based on raw data describe "level," while scores based on cor-relations or profiles describe "pattern." It can be clinically important to recognize the differences between working with parameters that directly reflect raw scores (e.g., mean of raw scores), transformations that represent relations among raw scores (e.g., profile of means of raw scores), or com-parisons between raw scores and some standard (e.g., normed scores).

For example, consider the significant correlations between BPD dimensional scores and the SASB cluster BLAME when rating "I focused on mother." Let blaming of mother be inspected at an absolute level. This can be done, even in a dimensional set of PD scores, by casting individuals scoring above a criterion (such as having a standard BPD score above 1.64 on any of the three measures of PD in the respective three data bases) into a BPD group and the remainder into an "other" group. In all three data sets, if the ratings for "I focused on my mother/father" for BPD defined this way are compared to the ratings for subjects in the other group, the BPD subjects do *not* have average scores that place them in the region of hostile control of mother. The weighted Affiliation, Autonomy score for BPD places them in the region of friendly autonomy giving when focusing on mother. But for the same subjects, weighted autonomy scores for *normed* SASB scores place BPD clearly in BLAME region of the model.

Thus by one method (scores compared to norms) individuals with BPD blame mother. By the other method (absolute scores), they do not. The reason for the discrepancy is that even though those with BPD have an average absolute position described as friendy autonomy giving to their mothers, *compared to normals*, they are much more blaming. If a clinician or researcher read a profile based on normed scores, he or she might conclude that blaming was characteristic of BPD interactions with mothers. However, the proper interpretation is that individuals with BPD are more likely to give their mothers very moderate amounts of friendly autonomy than they are to blame them. But compared to normals, they do a lot of blaming.

This problem is hard to see unless one is working with a psychometric instrument, such as SASB, that offers parameters with absolute meaning (i.e., objectively established content validity). Recall that for the example under discussion, the SASB items are rated for elements of interdependence or affiliation by naïve judges. This dimensional-ratings method has established that their content is as claimed. Blame is judged to consist of ATTACK and CONTROL. Instruments that lack formal content analyses are difficult to interpret in this same absolute sense. Simple means of ratings for blame do represent a position that involves hostile control. Normed means represent something else that may or may not lead to the same conclusion. A more complete discussion of the SASB-based perspective on this problem and its implications for the measurement of personality appears elsewhere (Benjamin & Critchfield, 2004).

Annie's Axis I and II Profiles

Figure 4.6 shows the changes in Annie's WISPI profile from the time she started treatment with the first IRT trainee to the time of termination with the second IRT trainee (and to whom she much later wrote the note quoted

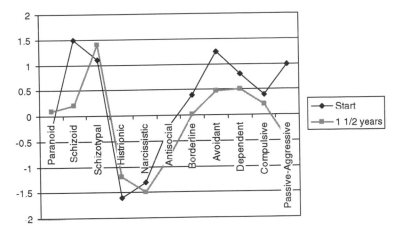

FIGURE 4.6. WISPI profile for Annie.

at the beginning of this chapter). Inspection of the figure shows that Annie was more than 1 standard deviation about the norm on the scales for schizoid, schizotypal, avoidant, and passive–aggressive personality disorders. These disorders share the characteristic of social withdrawal. One and a half years later, all Annie's scores had dropped to less than one-half of a standard deviation above the norm, except for schizotypal, which had increased to 1½ standard deviations above normal. At that time, Annie was very upset about the involuntary termination, and the voices had returned with a vengeance. They were managed medically by the next therapist, a psychiatry resident who consulted with the IRT supervisor. He continued with the plan of helping Annie control the voices by challenging the memory of her uncle, the template for the voices. He also provided kindly supportive therapy for the next 6 months.

Like most nonresponder patients, Annie had high comorbidity between Axis I and II. Figure 4.7 indicates that Annie was above the 80th outpatient percentile on nearly every symptom scale, and above the 90th on many. Every scale but the psychoticism scale showed some decreases by termination time, although she clearly remained highly symptomatic. Despite the severity of Annie's presentation, the fact that she subsequently made no suicidal attempts and needed no additional hospitalization, combined with her later description of dramatic and positive life changes, which she attributed to IRT, provides informal validation of effectiveness of IRT. Like most interpersonal approaches, IRT starts a helpful learning process that, if properly implemented and embraced by the patient, continues long after termination.

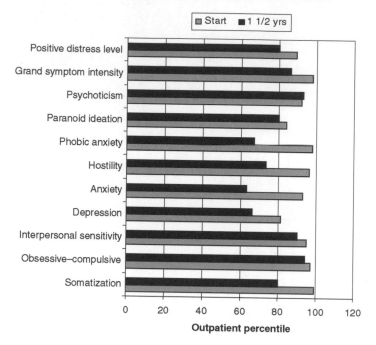

FIGURE 4.7. SCL-90-R for Annie.

Under Current Rules, Effective Treatments for Highly Comorbid Patients Cannot Be Found

Severely disordered patients such as Annie are almost always excluded from research protocols. Effectiveness studies typically focus on a single disorder, with little tolerance for comorbidity. Most of them permit no ongoing suicidality or recurrent psychotic symptoms. Hence, Annie would be unlikely to enter into a federally funded treatment validation study. Any privately or unfunded study that accepted participants such as Annie would be unlikely to be viewed favorably by contemporary standards for editorial review because there is too much comorbidity. Replication studies would be unliklely because most investigators of psychotherapy treatments do not permit highly suicidal or psychotic patients to enter or remain on protocol. *According to contemporary rules and practices for treatment effectiveness studies, like those reviewed and criticized from a clinical perspective by Levant (2003), effective treatments for nonresponders (who by definition already have failed to respond to empirically validated approaches) are unlikely ever to be established.* Nonresponders are excluded from protocol because of their extensive comorbidity ("impurity"), the severity of their disturbance (e.g., psychotic features), and their dangerousness to self or others.

Annie's Intrex Profiles

The Intrex seeks directly to assess and summarize a patient's view of self and important others. This is directly relevant to the main IRT agenda: Identify presenting problems and link them to patterns established in relation to key figures. To illustrate how this can work, Annie's ratings for her relationship with her mother are presented here. They are consistent with the descriptions in her therapy narrative, and they are consistent with the trends identified for mother focused on me (Figure 4.5) for individuals with SZT—Annie's most resistant of her several predominant patterns of personality.

Annie's view of her mother's focus on her is summarized by the cluster score profile for mother from the medium form, shown in Figure 4.8. The center of gravity for the eight clusters representing focus on other (the leftmost set of eight clusters in Figure 4.8) is summarized by the weighted Affiliation (AF), Autonomy (AU) vector of (–29.4, –63.6). This places

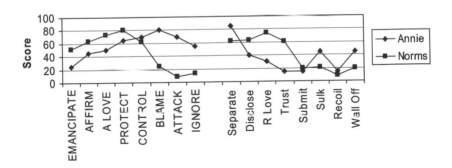

FIGURE 4.8. Annie's view of her mother. The left side shows Intrex ratings of items that describe mother focusing on Annie; the right side shows ratings of mother reacting to her. Annie's mother focused on her with more hostility than do mothers of normal raters, and Annie's mother reacted to her with markedly less friendliness. Various parameters that summarize the trends observed here for Annie's internalized representation of her mother are discussed in the text.

mother's focus on Annie in the lower-left-hand quadrant of the SASB models, the region of hostile control. The method of computing the AF/AU vector was described earlier.

The goodness-of-fit parameter for this set of eight clusters was .82 for the pattern "blaming." The best-fit parameter is the largest of 21 correlations between a given subject's profile of eight clusters, and 21 theoretical profiles that are associated with predetermined sensible names. For example, the pattern for the curve "blaming" peaks on the BLAME cluster and becomes progressively smaller as distance from blaming increases.

The Attack (ATK), Control (CON), and Conflict (CFL) parameters were .816, .770, −.34, respectively. These coefficients come from the set of 21 theoretical coefficients too but are the largest from a small pool of similar curves centered about the poles of the axes. The ATK coefficients represent the best-fit curve from the set of theoretical curves oriented on the horizontal axis. The CON coefficients represent the best-fit curve from the set oriented on the vertical axes. Annie's mother had a large ATK and CON coefficients, in agreement with the AF, AU vector placement of her focus in the quadrant of hostile control. The CFL coefficient represents the largest of the curves describing endorsements of opposites. Positive CFL reflect opposing endorsements on the vertical (interdependence) axis, while negative CFL represent opposing endorsements on the horizontal (attachment) axis. Normally, CFL coefficients tend to be positive. Annie's score of −.34 for mother places her in about the 5th percentile. Annie's mother's love/ hate conflict when focusing on Annie was quite noticeable, compared to that of normal mothers. Unlike the AF, AU vectors, which reflect magnitudes of endorsement, the ATK, CON, and CFL patterns only reflect profiles—relations among clusters without regard for absolute level.

The internal consistency for mother focused on me, which is the correlation between version 1 and version 2 of the medium form, was .48. Internal consistency normally is much higher (mean = .82, SD = .21). This indicates there was instability in Annie's view of her mother's focus. Details about procedures and interpretations of these various parameters and their norms are in the Intrex user's manual (Benjamin, 2000b).

Annie's view of her mother reacting to Annie is shown in eight right-hand clusters of Figure 4.8. The weighted AF, AU vector for this set was (−5.06, 82.31), and places Annie's mother very near the top of the autonomy pole, slightly in the hostile direction. The goodness-of-fit parameter was .73 for the pattern named "Very separate." The ATK, SUB, and CFL patterns were −.44, −.73, and .42. These suggest that Annie's mother reacted to her with some warmth, much autonomy, and some conflict on the vertical axis (submit vs. separate). The internal consistency was .33.

Figure 4.8 objectifies Annie's view of her mother. The summaries provided by the best-fit coefficients are *blaming* and *very detached*. Hostile control and detachment are characteristic of mothers of patients rating high for SZT (Figure 4.5), and they are for Annie too. Copy process theory relates identified caregiver patterns to the patterns of the disorder, and those predictions can be tested for an individual patient or in a diagnostic group of patients using the Intrex ratings.

The Intrex system describes every rated relationship in the manner just explained in association with Figure 4.8. For research users, parameters are output in blocks that are easily read into standard data bases such as the Statistical Package for the Social Sciences. The Intrex questions are very simple, expressed in everyday words written at the sixth-grade level. The output is equally straightforward. SASB is one of the more rater-friendly psychometrics available, if measured by the immediacy, relevance, and validity of the feedback *to the rater*. The concepts are explained without jargon, and the simplicity of explanations based on IRT copy process theory is apparent.

CONCLUDING REMARKS

Most of the goals mentioned in the first edition of this chapter have been addressed in the intervening 8 years. The University of Utah Neuropsychiatric Institute has started a low-cost IRT clinic devoted to the goals of treatment, research, and teaching. Patients admitted are nonresponders, who are highly likely to have personality disorders. Intrex and SASB codes of videotapes of assessment interviews and selected therapy sessions are included in an array of measures used to document change during treatment with IRT. Research, teaching, and service are the goals of the clinic, and each is well underway. Students are learning to develop case formulations, including identifying key figures, and relating them to presenting symptoms. Tests of reliability are being conducted jointly with an IRT team in Wisconsin, led by Kathleen Levenick, MD. A treatment manual has been published (Benjamin, 2003). Unusually specific methods of defining adherence are in place and will be related to outcome. The reasoning is that if adherence measures cover nearly every intervention, and reliably relate in detail to algorithms in the treatment manual, better adherence should lead to better outcome. Further discussion of the advantages of using comprehensive and detailed measures of adherence to relate to outcome to measure effectiveness will appear subsequently.

Much more could be said about IRT and SASB. Ideally, this chapter gives the reader a helpful introduction to the basics of IRT theory and practice and to the structure and selected uses of SASB.

ACKNOWLEDGMENT

I would like to thank Tracey L. Smith for her helpful reading of this chapter, and for many other contributions to the growth and development of IRT and SASB.

NOTE

1. This intellectual property has been gifted to the University of Utah and is available to qualified users through Intrex at the Department of Psychology, University of Utah, Salt Lake City, UT 84112. In 2000, the Intrex manual was updated and expanded; the software was revised to be more user friendly, and is compatible with Windows 2000 and XP. Details can be found by searching for SASB or Intrex on the University website.

REFERENCES

Acton, G. S., & Revelle, W. (2002). Interpersonal personality measures show circumplex structure based on new psychometric criteria. *Journal of Personality Assessment, 79*, 446–471.

Adler, A. (1955). Individual psychology, its assumptions and its results. In C. Thompson, M. Mater, & E. Witenberg (Eds.), *An outline of psychoanalysis* (pp. 283–297). New York: Modern Library.

Ainsworth, A. D. F., Blehar, M. C., Waters, E., & Wall, S. (1978). *Patterns of attachment*. Hillsdale, NJ: Erlbaum.

Allport, G. W. (1937). *Personality. A psychological interpretation*. New York: Henry Holt.

American Psychiatric Association. (1987). *Diagnostic and statistical manual of mental disorders* (3rd ed., rev.). Washington, DC: Author.

American Psychiatric Association. (1994). *Diagnostic and statistical manual of mental disorders* (4th ed.). Washington, DC: Author.

Armelius, K., & Granberg, A. (2000). Self image and perception of mother and father in borderline and psychotic patients. *Psychotherapy Research, 10*, 147–158.

Bateson, G., Jackson, D. D., Haley, J., & Weakland, J. (1956). Toward a theory of schizophrenia. *Behavioral Science, 1*, 251–264.

Benjamin, L. S. (1974). Structural analysis of social behavior. *Psychological Review, 81*, 392–425.

Benjamin, L. S. (1978). Use of Structural Analysis of Social Behavior (SASB) and Markov chains to study dyadic interactions. *Journal of Abnormal Psychology, 88*, 303–319.

Benjamin, L. S. (1979). Structural analysis of differentiation failure. *Psychiatry, 42*, 1–23.

Benjamin, L. S. (1986). Operational definition and measurement of dynamics shown in the stream of free associations. *Psychiatry: Interpersonal and Biological Processes, 49*, 104–129.

Benjamin, L. S. (1987). Use of the SASB dimensional model to develop treatment plans for personality disorders, I: Narcissism. *Journal of Personality Disorders, 1*, 43–70.

Benjamin, L. S. (1988a). *Short form Intrex user's manual*. Salt Lake City: University of Utah.

Benjamin, L. S. (1988b). Is chronicity a function of the relationship between the person and the auditory hallucination. *Schizophrenia Bulletin, 15*, 291–310.

Benjamin, L. S. (1992). An interpersonal view of borderline personality disorder. In J. Clarkin, E. Marzialli, & H. Monroe-Blum (Eds.), *Borderline personality disorder* (pp. 161–196). New York: Guilford Press.

Benjamin, L. S. (1993). Every psychopathology is a gift of love. *Psychotherapy Research, 3*, 1–24.

Benjamin, L. S. (1994). SASB: A bridge between personality theory and clinical psychology. *Psychological Inquiry, 5*, 273–316.

Benjamin, L. S. (1995). Good defenses make good neighbors. In H. R. Conte & R. Plutchik (Eds.), *Ego defenses: Theory and measurement* (pp. 38–78). New York: Wiley.

Benjamin, L. S. (1996a). *Interpersonal diagnosis and treatment of personality disorders* (2nd ed.). New York: Guilford Press.

Benjamin, L. S. (1996b). Introduction to the special section on Structural Analysis of Social Behavior (SASB). *Journal of Consulting and Clinical Psychology, 64*, 1203–1212.

Benjamin, L. S. (1996c). A clinician-friendly version of the interpersonal circumplex: Structural Analysis of Social Behavior (SASB). *Journal of Personality Assessment, 66*, 248–266

Benjamin, L. S. (1997). Human imagination and psychopathology. *Journal of Psychotherapy Integration, 7*, 195–211.

Benjamin, L. S. (2000a). Interpersonal diagnosis and treatment in group therapy. In A. Beck & C. Lewis (Eds.), *The process of group psychotherapy: Systems for analyzing change* (pp. 381–412). Washington, DC: American Psychological Association.

Benjamin, L. S. (2000b). *Intrex user's manual*. Salt Lake City: University of Utah.

Benjamin, L. S. (2003). *Interpersonal reconstructive therapy: Promoting change in nonresponders*. New York: Guilford Press.

Benjamin, L. S. (2004). *Personality guided interpersonal reconstructive therapy for anger, anxiety and depression*. Washington, DC: American Psychological Association.

Benjamin, L. S., & Critchfield, K. L. (2004). *Interpersonal and/or statistical descriptions of personality disorder*. Manuscript in preparation.

Benjamin, L. S., & Cushing, G. (2000). *Manual for coding social interactions in terms of structural analysis of social behavior*. Salt Lake City: University of Utah.

Benjamin, L. S., Cushing, G., Schloredt, K., Callaway, K., & Gelfand, D. (2005). *Transmission of depression through mother–infant interactions*. Manuscript in preparation.

Benjamin, L. S., & Friedrich, F. J. (1991). Contributions of Structural Analysis of

Social Behavior (SASB) to the bridge between cognitive science and a science of object relations. In M. J. Horowitz (Ed.), *Person schemas and maladaptive behavior* (pp. 379–412). Chicago: University of Chicago Press.

Benjamin, L. S., & Pugh, C. (2001). Using interpersonal theory to select effective treatment interventions for personality disorder. In W. J. Livesley (Ed.), *Handbook of personality disorders* (pp. 414–436). New York: Guilford Press.

Benjamin, L. S., & Wonderlich, S. (1994). Social perceptions and borderline personality disorder: The relationship to mood disorders. *Journal of Abnormal Personality, 103,* 610–624.

Blatt, S. J. (1974). Levels of object representation in anaclitic and introjective depression. *Psychoanalytic Study of the Child, 29,* 107–157.

Bluhm, C., Widiger, T. A., & Miele, G. M. (1990). Interpersonal complementarity and individual differences. *Journal of Personality and Social Psychology, 58,* 464–471.

Bowlby, J. (1969). *Attachment and loss: Vol. I. Attachment.* London: Tavistock.

Bowlby, J. (1977). The making and breaking of affectional bonds. *British Journal of Psychiatry, 130,* 201–210; 421–431.

Bretherton, I. (1985). Attachment theory: Retrospect and prospect. *Monographs of the Society for Research in Child Development, 50*(1–2, Serial No. 209), 3–35.

Burkett, L. P. (1991). Parenting behaviors of women who were sexually abused as children in their families of origin. *Family Process, 30,* 421–434.

Cassano, G. B. Miniati, M, Pini, S., Rotondo, A., Banti, S., Borri, C., Camilleri, V., & Mauri, M. (2003). Six-month open trial of haloperidol as an adjunctive treatment for anorexia nervosa: A preliminary report. *International Journal of Eating Disorders, 33,* 172–177.

Cassidy, J., & Shaver, P. R. (Eds.). (1999). *Handbook of attachment: Theory, research, and clinical applications.* New York: Guilford Press

Constantino, M. J. (2000). Interpersonal process in psychotherapy through the lens of the Structural Analysis of Social Behavior. *Applied and Preventive Psychology: Current Scientific Perspectives, 9,* 153–172.

Cushing, G. (2003). *Interpersonal origins of parenting among addicted and non-addicted mothers.* Unpublished PhD dissertation, University of Utah, Salt Lake City.

Cushing, G., & Benjamin, L. S. (1999). *The effect of maternal depression on mother–infant complementarity defined by SASB.* Paper presented at annual meetings of Society for Theory and Research on Personality, Madison, WI.

Derogatis, L. R. (1977). *SCL-90 administration, scoring and procedures manuals for the revised version.* Baltimore: Author.

Erikson, E. H. (1959). Identity and the life cycle. *Psychological Issues, 1,* 1–171.

Fairbairn, W. R. D. (1952). *An object-relations theory of the personality.* New York: Basic Books.

Fenichel, O. (1945). *The psychoanalytic theory of neurosis.* New York: Norton.

Fiedler, P. (1995). *Zum Stellenwert der Komorbiditatsforschung fur die Verhaltenstherapie.* Paper presented to the conference on Personlichkeitsstorungen. Diagnostik and Psychotherapie, sponsored by the University of Heidelberg, Bad Durkheim.

First, M. B., Spitzer, R. L, Gibbon, M., Williams, J. B. W., & Benjamin, L. S.

(1997). *Structured clinical interview for DSM-IV Axis II personality disorders. (SCID-II).* Washington, DC: American Psychiatric Press.

Freedman, M. B., Leary, T. F. , Ossorio, A. G., & Coffey, H. S. (1951). The interpersonal dimensions of personality. *Journal of Personality, 20,* 143–161.

Freud, S. (1959). Heredity and the etiology of the neuroses. In *Sigmund Freud collected papers (Vol. 1)* (J. Riviere, Trans.). New York: Basic Books. (Original work published 1896)

Friedman, M. A., Wilfley D. E., Welch, R. R., & Kunce J. T. (1997). Self-directed hostility and family functioning in normal-weight bulimics and overweight binge eaters. *Addictions Behavior, 22,* 367–375.

Gelfand, D. M., Teti, D. M., & Fox, C. E. R. (1992). Sources of parenting stress for depressed and nondepressed mothers of infants. *Journal of Clinical Child Psychology, 21,* 262–272.

Goedken, J. (2004). *Representations of self and important others in depression. Exploration of unique and qualitative distinctions using Structural Analysis of Social Behavior.* Unpublished PhD dissertation, University of Utah, Salt Lake City.

Greenberg, J. R., & Mitchell, S. A. (1983). *Object relations in psychoanalytic theory.* Cambridge, MA: Harvard University Press.

Greenberg, L. S., & Foerster, F. S. (1996). Task analysis exemplified: The process of resolving unfinished business. *Journal of Consulting and Clinical Psychology, 64,* 439–446.

Gurtman, M. (1996). Interpersonal problems and the psychotherapy context: The construct validity of the Inventory of Interpersonal Problems. *Psychological Assessment, 8,* 241–255.

Gurtman, M. (2001). Interpersonal complementarity: Integrating interpersonal measurement with interpersonal models. *Journal of Counseling Psychology, 48,* 97–110.

Guttman, L. (1966). Order analysis of correlation matrixes. In R.B. Cattell (Ed.), *Handbook of multivariate experimental psychology* (pp. 439–458). Chicago: Rand McNally.

Harlow, H. (1958). The nature of love. *American Psychologist, 13,* 673–685.

Harlow, H. F., & Harlow, M. K. (1962). Social deprivation in monkeys. *Scientific American, 203,* 136–146.

Hartkamp, N., & Schmitz, N. (1999). Structures of introject and therapist patient interaction in a single case study of inpatient psychotherapy. *Psychotherapy Research, 9,* 199–215.

Henry, W. P., Schacht, T. E., & Strupp, H. H. (1986). Structural analysis of social behavior: Application to a study of interpersonal process in differential psychotherapeutic outcome. *Journal of Consulting and Clinical Psychology, 54,* 27–31.

Hilliard, R. B., Henry, W. P., & Strupp, H. H. (2000). An interpersonal model of psychotherapy: Linking patient and therapist developmental history, therapeutic process and types of outcome. *Journal of Consulting and Clinical Psychology, 68,* 125–133.

Holmqvist, R., & Armelius, K. (2000). Countertransference feelings and the psychiatric staff's self-image. *Journal of Clinical Psychology, 56*(4), 475–490.

Horowitz, L. M. (1996). The study of interpersonal problems: A Leary legacy. *Journal of Personality Assessment, 66,* 283–300.

Humes, D. L., & Humphrey, L. L. (1994). A multimethod analysis of families with a polydrug-dependent or normal adolescent daughter. *Journal of Abnormal Psychology, 103,* 676–685.

Humphrey, L. L., & Benjamin, L. S. (1986). Using Structural Analysis of Social Behavior to assess critical but elusive family processes: A new solution to an old problem. *American Psychologist, 41,* 979–989.

Jay, P. (1965). The common langur of North India. In I. DeVore (Ed.), *Primate behavior: Field studies of monkeys and apes* (pp. 197–249). New York: Holt, Rinehart & Winston.

Jorgensen, C.R. (2000). The dynamic assessment interview (DAI), interpersonal process measured by Structural Analysis of Social Behavior (SASB) and therapeutic outcome. *Psychotherapy Research, 10,* 181–195.

Karpiak, C. P., & Benjamin, L. S. (2004). Therapist affirmation and the process and outcome of psychotherapy: Two sequential analytic studies. *Journal of Personality, 60,* 1–18.

Klein, M. (1975). On the theory of anxiety and guilt. *Envy and gratidue and other works, 1946–1963.* New York: Delacorte Press. (Original work published 1948)

Klein, M. H. (1983, Spring). Issues in the assessment of personality disorders. *Journal of Personality Disorders* (Suppl.), 18–33.

Klein, M. H., Benjamin, L. S., Rosenfeld, R., Treece, C., Husted, J., & Greist, J. (1993). The Wisconsin Personality Disorders Inventory: I. Development, reliability, and validity. *Journal of Personality Disorders, 7,* 285–303.

Klein, M. H., Wonderlich, S. A., & Crosby, R. (2001). Self-concept correlates of the personality disorders. *Journal of Personality Disorders, 15,* 150–156.

Kupfer, D. J., First, M., & Regier, D. (2002). *A research agenda for DSM-V.* Washington, DC: American Psychiatric Press.

LaForge, R. (1985). Early development of the Freedman–Leary–Coffey interpersonal system. *Journal of Personality Assessment, 49,* 611–621.

Leary, T. (1957). *Interpersonal diagnosis of personality: A functional theory and methodology for personality evaluation.* New York: Ronald Press.

Levant, R. F. (2003). The empirically validated treatments movement: A practitioner perspective. *Psychotherapy Bulletin, 38,* 36–39.

Lorr, M. (1991). A redefinition of dominance. *Personality and Individual Differences, 12,* 877–979.

Lorr, M., & Strack, S. (1999). A study of Benjamin's eight facet Structural Analysis of Social Behavior (SASB) Model. *Journal of Clinical Psychology, 55,* 207–215.

MacKenzie, K. R. (1990). Time limited group psychotherapy. Washington, DC: American Psychiatric Press.

Mahler, M. (1968). *On human symbiosis and the vicissitudes of individuation.* New York: International Universities Press.

Meltzoff, A. N., & Moore, M. K. (1977). Imitation of facial and manual gestures by human neonates. *Science, 198,* 75–78.

Moore, A. M. (1998). *Why people drink: An interpersonal analysis.* Unpublished PhD dissertation, University of Utah, Salt Lake City.

Morey, L. C. (1988). *The MMPI Personality Disorder Scales: A manual and guide to interpretation.* Unpublished manuscript, Vanderbilt University, Nashville, TN.

Morey, L. C., Waugh, M. H., & Blashfield, R. K. (1985). MMPI scales for DSM-IIII personality disorders: Their derivation and correlates. *Journal of Personality Assessment, 49,* 245–251.

Murray, H. A. (1938). *Explorations in personality.* New York: Oxford University Press.

Mussen, P. H., Conger, J. J., & Kagan, J. (1971). *Child development and personality* (3rd ed.). New York: Harper & Row.

O'Connor, B. P., & Dyce, J. A. (1998). A test of models of personality disorder configuration. *Journal of Abnormal Psychology, 107,* 3–16.

Orford, J. (1986). The rules of interpersonal complementarity: Does hostility beget hostility and dominance, submission? *Psychological Review, 93,* 365–377.

Pavio, S. C., & Bahr, L. M. (1998). Interpersonal problems, working alliance, and outcome in short-term experiential therapy. *Psychotherapy Research, 8,* 392–407.

Pincus, A. L. (1998). Structural Analysis of Social Behavior (SASB) circumplex analyses and structural relations with the interpersonal circle and the five-factor model of personality. *Journal of Personality and Social Psychology, 74,* 1629–1645.

Pincus, A. L., Dickinson, K. A., Schut, A. J., Castonguay, L. G., & Bedics, J. (1999). *European Journal of Psychological Assessment, 15,* 206–220.

Pincus, A. L., Newes, S. L., Dickinson, K. A., & Ruiz, M. A. (1998). A comparison of three indexes to assess the dimensions of Structural Analysis of Social Behavior. *Journal of Personality Assessment, 70,* 145–170.

Prochaska, J. O., DiClemente, C. C., & Norcross, J. C. (1992). In search of how people change: Applications to addictive behaviors. *American Psychologist, 47,* 1102–1114.

Ratti, L. A., Humphrey, L. L., & Lyons, J. S. (1996). Structural analysis of families with a polydrug-dependent, bulimic, or normal adolescent daughter. *Journal of Consulting and Clinical Psychology, 64,* 1255–1262.

Rothweiler, J. (2003). *An evaluation of the internal and external validity of the Intrex and Interpersonal Adjective Scales.* Unpublished PhD dissertation, University of Utah, Salt Lake City.

Rudy, J. P., McLemore, C. W., & Gorsuch, R. L. (1985). Interpersonal behavior and therapeutic progress: Therapists and clients rate themselves and each other. *Psychiatry, 48,* 264–281.

Rueck, C., Andreewitch, S., Flyckt, K., Edman, G., Nyman, H., Meyerson, B. A., Lippitz, B. E., Hindmarsh, T., Svanborg, P., Mindus, P., & Asberg, M. (2003). Capsulotomy for refractory anxiety disorders: Long-term follow-up of 26 patients. *American Journal of Psychiatry, 160,* 513–521.

Safran, J. D., & Muran, J. C. (1996). The resolution of ruptures in the therapeutic alliance. *Journal of Consulting and Clinical Psychology, 64,* 447–458.

Sandor, C. M. (1996). *An interpersonal approach to substance abuse.* Unpublished PhD dissertation, University of Utah, Salt Lake City.

Schaefer, E. S. (1965). Configurational analysis of children's reports of parent behavior. *Journal of Consulting Psychology, 29,* 552–557.

Sim, J. P., & Romney, D. M. (1990). The relatinoship between a circumplex model of interpersonal behaviors and personal disorders. *Journal of Personality Disorders, 4,* 329–341.

Skinner, B. F. (1990). Can psychology be a science of mind? *American Psychologist, 45,* 1206–1210.

Smith, T. L. (2001). *Psychosocial perceptions and symptoms of personality and other disorders.* Unpublished PhD dissertation, University of Utah, Salt Lake City.

Smith, T. L., Klein, M. H., & Benjamin, L. S. (2003). Validation of the Wisconsin Personality Disorders Inventory—IV with the SCID-II. *Journal of Personality Disorders, 17,* 173– 187.

Solomon, R. L., & Wynne, L. C. (1953). Traumatic avoidance learning: acquisition in normal dogs. *Psychological Monographs, 67*(4, Whole no. 354).

Sullivan, H. S. (1953). *The interpersonal theory of psychiatry.* New York: Norton.

Thase, M. E., Friedman, E. S., & Howland, R. H. (2001). Management of treatment-resistant depression: Psychotherapeutic perspectives. *Journal of Clinical Psychiatry (Supplement 18), 62,*18–24.

Widiger, T. A., & Costa, P. T. (1994). Personality and personality disorders. *Journal of Abnormal Psychology, 103,* 78–91.

Wiggins, J. S. (1978). A psychological taxonomy of trait-descriptive terms: The interpersonal domain. *Journal of Personality and Social Psychology, 37,*395–412.

Wiggins, J. S. (1982). Circumplex models of interpersonal behavior in clinical psychology. In P. C. Kendall & J. N. Butcher (Eds.), *Handbook of research methods in clinical psychology* (pp. 183–221). New York: Wiley.

Wiggins, J. S. (1995). *Interpersonal Adjective Scales. Professional manual.* Odessa, FL: Psychological Assessment Resources.

Wiggins, J. S., & Broughton, R. (1985). The interpersonal circle: a structural model for integrating personality research. In R. Hogan & W. H. Jones (Eds.), *Perspectives in Personality* (Vol., pp. 1–47). Greenwich, CT: JAI Press.

Wonderlich, S., Klein, M. H., & Council, J. R. (1996). Relationship of social perceptions and self-concept in bulimia nervosa. *Journal of Consulting and Clinical Psychology, 64,* 1231–1237.

Wynne, L. C., & Singer, M. T. (1963). Thought disorder and family relations of schizophrenics II: A classification of forms of thinking. *Archives of General Psychiatry, 9,* 199–206.

Zinbarg, R. E., Barlow, D. H., Brown, T. A., & Hertz, R. M. (1992). Cognitive behavioral approaches to the nature and treatment of anxiety disorders. *Annual Review of Psychology, 43,* 235–268.

CHAPTER 5

■ ■ ■

An Attachment Model
of Personality Disorders

BJÖRN MEYER
PAUL A. PILKONIS

Attachment theory has enjoyed increasing popularity among developmental, social, personality, and clinical researchers (cf. Cassidy & Shaver, 1999; Simpson & Rholes, 1998) since the publication of Bowlby's (1969, 1973, 1980) seminal works. The question of how personality disorders might be understood from the perspective of attachment theory, however, is only beginning to receive systematic attention (e.g., Bartholomew, Kwong, & Hart, 2001; Brennan & Shaver, 1998; Fossati et al., 2003; Lyddon & Sherry, 2001). Attachment theory has the potential to inform etiological models of personality disorders because it seeks to explain how early interpersonal experiences influence personality and psychosocial functioning later in life. Because it also tries to explain how ineffective emotion regulation, unstable relationships, and problematic mental representations are maintained once formed, attachment theory can inform models concerned with the tenacity of personality maladjustment.

We begin by reviewing basic elements of attachment theory and then describe the role attachment processes might play in DSM-IV personality disorders. The focus is primarily theoretical, although we summarize empirical data where relevant and report briefly on the results of a pilot study. Our introductory review of attachment touches on basic elements of the theory, its history, measurement issues, and relevant recent research and controversies. More comprehensive descriptions have appeared elsewhere (e.g., Bowlby, 1969, 1973, 1980; Cassidy & Shaver, 1999).

231

BACKGROUND AND BASIC PRINCIPLES

The origins of the theory date from the mid-20th century when Bowlby, just graduated from Cambridge University, began to study how disruptions in the mother–child relationship influenced emotional distress in children and the later emergence of psychopathology. Among Bowlby's early discoveries was that a predictable sequence—angry protest followed by despair—occurred when children were separated from their mothers, indicating the existence of a special emotional bond between mother and child. It became clear that this bond was not well explained by psychoanalytical and social learning theories, both of which held that infants became attached to adults who fed them or provided other forms of gratification or reinforcement. Animal studies (cf. Harlow, 1958; Lorenz, 1935), however, demonstrated that attachments unrelated to feeding were common, and later studies with human infants confirmed this idea (e.g., Ainsworth, 1967). Not only did human infants attach to mothers regardless of feeding practices, but they attached even to abusive caregivers.

Based on such insights, and drawing on ethology, evolutionary biology, cognitive science, and control systems theory, Bowlby formulated attachment theory in the following decades (Bowlby, 1958, 1969, 1973, 1980). His theory stressed the importance of actual life events, rather than the child's internal experience, as causal factors in the development of psychopathology and personality disturbance—an emphasis that reflected a major departure from traditional psychoanalytic conceptions and, not surprisingly, alienated many of his psychoanalytically oriented colleagues (cf. Kobak, 1999).

Attachment theory proposes that young children are equipped with an innate, biologically based motivational system—the *attachment behavioral system*—whose function is to promote proximity between child and caregiver, especially in situations signaling threat or danger. Attachment motivation is proposed to be distinct from other motivations, such as feeding or sex. The attachment system is thought to have evolved because it conferred an adaptive advantage in the ancestral environment—children who were motivated to seek proximity and protection in threatening situations were more likely to survive. Becoming attached to others, then, is not as an indication of weakness or immaturity but a functional adaptation that leads to increased safety and ultimately to enhanced exploration and mastery of the environment, once safety has been established.

According to the theory, the attachment system can be activated by external or internal cues. External cues include the presence of a threatening stimulus or excessive distance from the caregiver, whereas internal cues refer to fear, injury, illness, or fatigue, all of which signal to the child that resources for independent mastery of the environment are compromised.

Once the system is activated, children are thought to respond by emitting characteristic attachment behavior. The function of this behavior—the goal of regulating the child's actions—is to attain a sense of *felt security* that results from the caregiver's comforting and protective presence. The means by which this goal can be attained depend on the situational context as well as the child's behavioral repertoire. For example, some attachment behaviors indicate an interest in interaction to the caregiver (e.g., smiling and vocalizing), others are aversive behaviors that indicate the child's distress (e.g., crying) to the caregiver, and yet others are direct efforts (e.g., approaching and following) to increase proximity to the caregiver. When the caregiver is successful in promoting the child's sense of security, attachment behavior is terminated. Thus, the attachment figure functions as a *safe haven* to which the child turns (and returns) in times of difficulty. Attachment theory also proposes that the attachment figure functions as a *secure base* from which children set out to explore their environment. Children's perception that others will be available and willing to provide support when needed encourages exploration, play, and other social behaviors.

The discovery of three distinct patterns of children's attachment—secure, ambivalent, and avoidant—by Mary Ainsworth and her colleagues was a landmark event in attachment research (Ainsworth, Blehar, Waters, & Wall, 1978). In Ainsworth's experimental procedure—the *Strange Situation*—the exploratory and proximity-seeking behavior of infants was observed under conditions of varying stress (e.g., departure of the attachment figure, introduction of a stranger, and reunion with the caregiver). This research showed that infants with a secure attachment pattern typically engage in confident exploration of the environment when the caregiver is present. In conditions of threat, securely attached infants respond with distress and seek proximity with the caregiver, and they are relatively easily consoled when the caregiver returns.

Infants with insecure forms of attachment, by contrast, do not use the attachment figure in this manner. Those with *anxious–resistant* or *ambivalent* attachment respond with intense distress when separated from the caregiver and are not easily consoled upon reunion, displaying instead a mixture of continued distress and contact seeking. Infants with this attachment pattern tend to remain preoccupied with monitoring the proximity of caregivers; instead of engaging in play or exploration, their attention tends to remain focused on the caregiver, seemingly in an effort to ensure the caregiver's uncertain presence. Infants showing *avoidant* attachment do not appear overtly distressed by the caregivers' departure, and they tend to ignore or actively avoid the caregiver upon reunion.

In addition to these three patterns, other forms of insecure attachment have been described. The avoidant/ambivalent pattern (Crittenden, 1988), for example, refers to children who display a mixture of avoidant and ambivalent behaviors, and Main and Solomon's (1990) disorganized–disoriented pattern refers to infants who exhibit contradictory or disoriented behaviors. Such children appear unable to maintain a consistent strategy for dealing with the stress in the Strange Situation. Recent discussions of disorganized attachment have focused on the dilemma created for the child by "frightened or frightening parental behavior" and the "fright without solution" that it evokes (Lyons-Ruth & Jacobvitz, 1999, p. 520). A meta-analysis of attachment studies suggested that 55% of all infants can be classified as secure, 23% as avoidant, 8% as ambivalent, and 15% as disorganized (van IJzendoorn, 1995).

The origins of these infant attachment patterns have been examined in many studies, and a preliminary conclusion is that caregiver sensitivity and responsiveness exert a reliable but moderate influence on the emergence of secure and insecure attachment (DeWolff & van IJzendoorn, 1997; Goldsmith & Alansky, 1987). A typical finding is that mothers of infants with secure attachment tend to be consistently responsive, whereas mothers of infants with ambivalent attachment are inconsistent and inept in their responsiveness, and mothers of infants with avoidant attachment tend to be cold and rejecting or, in some cases, intrusive and overcontrolling (cf. Belsky, 1999). Infant temperament may also play a role in the genesis of attachment patterns, but research does not support the idea of a simple linear path from temperament to attachment (Vaughn & Bost, 1999).

FROM CHILDHOOD ATTACHMENT
TO ADULT PERSONALITY DISORDERS

Secure and insecure patterns of infant attachment have clear and documented consequences for children's subsequent psychosocial adjustment. For example, Weinfield, Sroufe, Egeland, and Carlson (1999) concluded in their review that those with anxious–ambivalent attachment are at risk for the development of anxiety-related problems, presumably as a consequence of having learned that caregivers cannot be relied on and must be monitored vigilantly. Those with avoidant as well as disorganized/disoriented attachment, by contrast, may be prone to develop anger- and aggression-related problems, possibly because of the early rejection and insensitivity they experienced from caregivers. Children with secure attachment, however, typically experience more optimal trajectories; they tend to be adept at responding sensitively to emotional cues, to engage in empathic behavior, to form loyal friendships, and to be regarded as competent leaders by others (cf. Weinfield et al., 1999), all of which may protect them from later personality maladjustment.

These psychosocial consequences begin to suggest pathways through which early attachment patterns might influence the later development of personality disorder. Children with anxious-ambivalent attachment, for example, tend to be anxiety prone and easily frustrated (Weinfield et al., 1999), which might increase their risk for avoidant, obsessive–compulsive, dependent, borderline, or histrionic personality disorders. Those with avoidant attachment tend to feel alienated from others and lack empathy and are prone to experience hostile anger (Weinfield et al., 1999), suggesting that they may be at risk to develop antisocial, narcissistic, or paranoid personalities. Finally, disorganized attachment tends to be linked with incoherent behavioral strategies and trance-like states (Weinfield et al., 1999), suggesting risk for borderline and possibly schizotypal personality disorders.

Early insecure forms of attachment may also indirectly affect risk for personality disorders by interfering with the ability to establish stable, supportive relationships. The ensuing social isolation or interpersonal turmoil may then constitute pathogenic stressors in themselves (Hawkley & Cacioppo, 2003) or limit the availability of social support as a buffer of stress (Coyne & Downey, 1991). Such social isolation or detachment may follow not only as a consequence of early insecure attachment, but also when attachment needs themselves are underdeveloped or impoverished—which may be a rare event, given that the "need to belong" is often regarded as a fundamental human motivation (Baumeister & Leary, 1995). Among people with a lack of attachment motivation, the failure to seek out and enjoy contact with others may increase the risk for personality disorders such as the schizoid and perhaps schizotypal patterns. Empirical evidence supporting the links between early attachment histories and later psychopathology is beginning to emerge, although most studies in this area tend to focus on symptoms such as anxiety, depression, or conduct problems rather than personality disorder features per se (e.g., Carlson, 1998; Warren, Huston, Egeland, & Sroufe, 1997).

There are additional routes by which early attachment experiences might plausibly contribute to later personality problems. For example, early attachment relationships might affect brain development and thus influence the neurological basis of personality (Schore, 1997, 2000; Young, 2002). Early attachment relationships might also determine the child's learning of and later capacity for effective emotion regulation (Cassidy, 1994; Zimmerman, 1999). That is, learning early that distress can be externally regulated by involving caregivers in affect regulation might facilitate the later emergence of effective internal emotion regulation. Yet another plausible pathway is that early attachment relationships contribute to children's learning of effective interpersonal skills (Anders & Tucker, 2000; Mallinckrodt, 2000). By interacting with caregivers in a manner that leads to need fulfillment and goal attainment, children learn how to interact in a reciprocal and skilled way, which then yields dividends in adult relatedness.

Perhaps the most theoretically compelling way in which early attachment experiences might influence later personality development is through their effects on "internal working models." Bowlby (1969, 1973, 1980) proposed that child–caregiver interaction patterns become encoded in the form of such models—sets of beliefs and expectations about the likelihood of other people providing help and nurturance when needed and about the degree to which the self is viewed by others as worthy of care and nurturance (for a recent review, see Bretherton & Munholland, 1999). Children whose caregivers are consistently responsive tend to develop positive schemas about the self, others, and relationships more generally, which enhance the likelihood that they approach later relationships with comfort and confidence. Children whose parents are not responsive but rather are neglectful, intrusive, or abusive are thought to develop negatively toned mental representations, enhancing the likelihood that they enter adult relationships with less comfort and confidence and with poorer prospects for relationship stability.

Regardless of the relative importance of the mechanisms mediating between early parenting and adult psychopathology, early interpersonal experiences probably do not affect adult personality in an absolute, deterministic sense. Significant interpersonal experiences later in life, such as loss of a parent, improvements in parenting, therapy, or marital success versus conflict might all alter the direction of a person's path toward, or away from, optimal adjustment. In this regard, Bowlby (1988) stressed the necessity

> to think of each personality as moving through life along some developmental pathway, with the particular pathway followed always being determined by the interaction of the personality as it has so far developed and the environment in which it is then finding itself. . . . So long as family conditions are favorable the pathway will start and continue within the bounds of healthy and resilient development; but should conditions become sufficiently unfavorable at any time, it may deviate . . . towards some form of disturbed and vulnerable development. . . . [My] hypothesis is that the pathway followed by each developing individual and the extent to which he or she becomes resilient to stressful life events is determined to a very significant extent by the pattern of attachment he or she develops during the early years. (pp. 171–172)

Empirical evidence supports Bowlby's hypothesis. For example, Fraley (2002) reanalyzed longitudinal data from 25 studies to examine the malleability of attachment from infancy to adulthood. The data were found to fit better with a "prototype" model, which assumes that early representations remain unchanged over the course of development and influence adult functioning directly. The "revisionist" model, according to which adult attachment representations are entirely predicted by concurrent interpersonal experience, was not supported in these analyses. Fraley (2002) concluded that "the estimated prototype model indicates that the true degree of attachment stability between age 1 and subsequent ages is roughly equivalent to a correlation of .39" (p. 136).

ADVANCES IN RESEARCH ON ADULT ATTACHMENT

Through the 1970s, attachment research focused primarily on children, but two events in the mid-1980s initiated an increasing emphasis on adults. One was the development of the Adult Attachment Interview (AAI; George, Kaplan, & Main, 1985; Main, Kaplan, & Cassidy, 1985), a method that revealed associations between parents' attachment-related thoughts and their children's attachment patterns, and the other was the publication of Hazan and Shaver's (e.g., 1987, 1990, 1994) work on adult romantic relationships from an attachment perspective.

Hazan and Shaver (1987) pioneered the use of questionnaires to assess attachment styles in adults. Their original measure required adults to read a prototypical description of secure, anxious–ambivalent, and avoidant features and then rate which description matched their own style the best. This measure has been revised and expanded numerous times, and several multi-item adult attachment measures have also appeared in the literature (cf. Brennan, Clark, & Shaver, 1998). According to Hazan and Shaver (e.g., 1994), it is sensible to study attachment in adulthood because adult peer and romantic relationships fulfill many of the same functions that characterize the infant–caregiver dyad earlier in life. For instance, adult intimate partners tend to serve as safe haven and secure base for one another (whereas, in infancy, the relationship is asymmetrical—the caregiver serves as secure base and safe haven for the infant, but not the other way around).

Adult romantic attachment styles, as measured by the various self-report questionnaires, have been linked with a host of theoretically predicted outcomes (for reviews, see Feeney, 1999; Simpson & Rholes, 1998; Shaver & Mikulciner, 2002). For example, those with a secure attachment style tend to form more stable, longer-lasting, conflict-free relationships than do others; they tend to respond to interpersonal stress by seeking proximity; they are more flexible in their cognitive styles; and they are more resilient in the face of stress. Those with anxious–ambivalent (preoccupied) styles, by contrast, tend to have stormy, conflict-ridden relationships, and those with avoidant attachment tend to have brief, superficial relationships.

A major development in the adult attachment literature was the model described by Bartholomew and Horowitz (1991) according to which four adult attachment patterns can be distinguished based on the possible combinations of positive and negative internal working models of self and others (see Figure 5.1). The valence of the self-model can also be interpreted as degree of attachment anxiety: People with positive self-representations experience low levels of attachment anxiety; their sense of self-worth is not easily compromised by inadequate external validation. Those with negative self-representations, by contrast, tend to feel highly anxious about potential rejection, and they rely and depend on others' approval to maintain a sense of self-worth. Mental representations of others, in this model, relate to people's approach-versus-avoidance tendencies in response to attachment needs. Holding positive views of others motivates people to approach others, to rely on them in difficult times, and to value and pursue intimacy in relationships. Construing others in a negative light, by contrast, motivates people to avoid closeness, to prefer a safe distance from others, and to value solitary pursuits over those involving intimacy (cf. Brennan et al., 1998).

The anxiety and avoidance dimensions, as shown in Figure 5.1, can be assessed with a variety of adult attachment measures. One example is the Experiences in Close Relationships questionnaire, which was recently revised using models based on item response theory (Brennan et al., 1998; Fraley, Waller, & Brennan, 2000). Such self-reports of romantic attach-

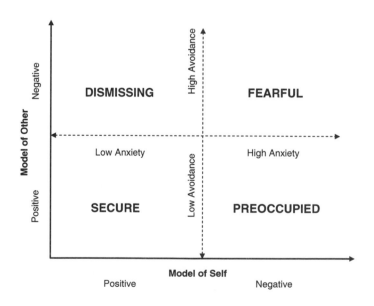

FIGURE 5.1. Two-dimensional attachment model.

ment, however, are not the only method for assessing attachment-relevant constructs. Studies in the AAI tradition rely on a narrative approach to assess the cognitive structures underlying individual differences in adult attachment. AAI coders evaluate *how* adults speak in response to a semistructured interview about significant attachment-related experiences. By rating the style and coherence with which such childhood memories are conveyed, AAI coders gain insight into adults' "states of mind" with regard to attachment. The content and valence of their memories—whether attachment relationships are remembered as pleasant or problematic—are less important in this approach than the ability of adults to present attachment-related recollections in an emotionally balanced, genuine, and coherent manner (cf. Hesse, 1999).

Research with the AAI has confirmed that, as predicted, securely attached infants tend to have parents who speak with coherence and emotional balance about their own childhood experiences, whereas infants with avoidant attachment tend to have parents who speak in a dismissing, minimizing manner about attachment-related childhood events (cf. Hesse, 1999). Infants classified with anxious–resistant attachment, in turn, typically have parents who are preoccupied with their childhood experiences; their narratives suggest that they often feel emotionally overwhelmed by attachment-related memories (cf. Hesse, 1999; Main et al., 1985; van IJzendoorn, 1995).

In addition to the AAI and romantic attachment self-reports, other methods for the assessment of adult attachment have been developed (cf. Stein, Jacobs, Ferguson, Allen, & Fonagy, 1998). One such method is Pilkonis's (1988) *adult attachment prototype rating method*, which was developed in the context of research on depressive symptoms. Pilkonis (1988) sought to examine whether more fine-grained differentiations could be made among depressed patients who present with either excessively dependent or excessively autonomous personality styles—two dimensions that had been described by a number of authors as theoretically important personality configurations among depressives (e.g., Beck, 1983; Blatt, Quinlan, Chevron, McDonald, & Zuroff, 1982). These dimensions can be interpreted as conceptually similar to the two main axes of adult attachment space, with excessive dependency corresponding to the attachment anxiety axis and excessive autonomy corresponding to the attachment avoidance axis.

In Pilkonis's (1988) study, 88 descriptors of excessively avoidant or excessively dependent individuals were extracted from the clinical literature, and cluster analyses were performed on clinicians' ratings of these descriptors to yield a number of "attachment prototypes." Three facets of excessive autonomy emerged and were labeled (1) defensive separation (similar in content to other measures of avoidant attachment); (2) lack of interpersonal sensitivity and antisocial features (similar in content and empirically related to antisocial personality disorder; cf. Meyer, Pilkonis, Prioetti, Heape, & Egan, 2001); and (3) obsessive–compulsive features (similar in content to obsessive–compulsive personality disorder; cf. Meyer et al., 2001). For excessive dependency, two facets were observed and were labeled (1) excessive dependency (similar in content to other measures of preoccupied attachment, and empirically and semantically related to dependent personality disorder; cf. Meyer et al., 2001) and (2) borderline features (similar in content and empirically related to borderline personality disorder; cf. Meyer et al., 2001).

In later work with this method, a prototype labeled compulsive caregiving was added as another facet of excessive dependency and preoccupied attachment. In addition, a prototype for secure attachment was added when it became clear that low ratings on the insecure prototypes did not necessarily capture security of attachment (Strauss, Lobo-Drost, & Pilkonis, 1999). The convergent validity of the attachment prototype rating method vis-à-vis other established measures of attachment is not yet clear, but initial evidence appears promising (Buchheim et al., 2003).

PERSONALITY DISORDERS AS AUTOMATIZED COGNITIVE–AFFECTIVE–MOTIVATIONAL PATTERNS

Up to this point, we have briefly summarized basic principles of attachment theory, potential pathways from early attachment to later personality disturbance, and different approaches to the measurement of attachment in childhood and adulthood. A piece that is still missing, however, is an explicit conceptualization of the terms "personality" and "personality disorder"—terms that are as central to our chapter as they are infamous for resisting unambiguous definition.

A number of theorists have recently defined personality in terms of networks of "cognitive and affective units" that create patterns of behavior consistent over time but also dependent on situational context (e.g., Cervone & Shoda, 1999; Mischel & Shoda, 1995; Zayas, Shoda, & Ayduk, 2002). This dynamic view emphasizes that personality is more than "traits" in the traditional sense of behavioral stability across situations. What is stable, in this view, are the underlying cognitive and affective units, but not necessarily the overt behavior across different situations. Only certain cognitive–affective units are activated at any given time and in any given context, and, depending on the particular pattern of activation or inhibition, complex patterns can emerge. These complex patterns may form unique (and relatively consistent) behavioral "signatures," but such profiles are difficult to capture within a traditional trait perspective.

In Mischel and Shoda's (1995) cognitive–affective personality systems (CAPS) model, key personality units include mental representations of self and others, goals and the strategies used to pursue them, expectancies about future outcomes, and affects experienced in response to specific situations. This construal of personality is compatible with attachment theory, given that attachment behaviors arise as a joint function of particular situations (e.g., threats to personal security) and the activation of cognitive and affective representations (e.g., internal working models). Mischel and Shoda (1995) described the process by which these units become activated in certain situations and lead to behavior:

> When certain configurations of situation features are experienced by an individual, a characteristic subset of cognitions and affects becomes activated through this distinctive network of connections in the encoding process. . . . Within any individual a rich system of relationships among the cognitive and affective units guides and constrains further activation of other units throughout the network, ultimately activating plans, strategies, and potential behaviors in the behavior generation process. . . . Units that become activated in the personality system activate other units through their distinctive organization in a network of relations, ultimately generating observable behaviors (pp. 254–255)

Interestingly, evidence suggests that many of these processes can occur *automatically*, beyond conscious awareness and without volitional intent (e.g., Bargh, 1997; Bargh & Ferguson, 2000). To document this type of automaticity, research subjects are sometimes exposed unobtrusively to information that activates target mental representations, and the effects on tangible behavior are later assessed. When people are primed with words activating the concept of "rudeness," for example, they are more likely to behave impolitely by disrupting a conversation, even though they may not recognize any connection between the priming and their own behavior (Bargh, Chen, & Burrows, 1996). Presumably, attachment-related mental representations, goals, and strategies can become activated automatically in a similar manner in day-to-day situations.

The possibility that attachment-related goals and strategies are automatically pursued in this manner was also noted recently by Carver and Scheier (1998), theorists who have traditionally emphasized the purposive, goal-directed, and conscious control of behavior and personality:

> The idea that people have goals that influence their actions outside awareness means they can be actively trying to do things they don't realize they're doing. These attempts at goal conformity simply blend into the backdrop of the personalized sense of normalcy. . . . Pursuit of [some] goals may be automatic because the goals were particularly important early in life. Thus efforts to

attain them were overlearned, and became automatized to the point where they're no longer noticed. . . . Presumably a particular manner of attaining relationship-relevant goals was overlearned during early attachment, and has now become automatic. . . . This portrayal . . . implies that determining the goals that constitute any person's self-structure will involve a lot of guesswork. . . . Somewhat to our surprise, we find ourselves in the position of saying that it can be hard to know what motives underlie behavior, including one's own behavior. This is a point of contact between self-regulatory and psychodynamic models that we wouldn't have expected 20 years ago. (pp. 219–220)

To illustrate how this model of automatized cognitive–affective personality units might be relevant to attachment and personality disorders, Figure 5.2 provides a conceptual application to a patient with borderline personality disorder and a preoccupied attachment style. In this example, the salient interpersonal situation is one in which a therapist announces to her patient that she is about to rotate to a new clinic and will have to transfer the case to another clinician. Instead of encoding all aspects of this situation, though, the patient hears primarily that "someone valued will abandon me"—a selective encoding facilitated by already activated models of others as rejecting and of the self as unlovable. These activated self- and other-models, and the salient expectation of impending abandonment, all trigger affective reactions and appraisals, such as intense self-hatred; anxiety and anger about the impending abandonment; and ambivalent feelings at the prospect of losing a valued other. These affective experiences, in turn, facilitate the formulation and activation of interpersonal goals, intentions, and ultimately actions.

In this case, the preoccupied borderline personality feels ambivalent—angry at the prospect of being abandoned but simultaneously desiring and valuing the guidance and nurturance associated with the therapist. This ambivalent motivation is translated into the intention to escalate the situation into a crisis and demand a greater level of care—an intention that combines both hostile (alienating demandingness) and proximity-enhancing (needy care-seeking) elements. Ultimately, the intentions facilitate action; the action affects the environment (i.e., the therapist reacts in some way to the patient's behavior), and thus the behavior feeds back to the patient in the form of a new and revised interpersonal situation.

To summarize, we propose that symptoms of personality disorder can be understood as the manifestations and consequences of complex interactions among cognitive–affective units that are triggered by specific situational contingencies and, through synergistic and recursive activation, lead to characteristic patterns of action, thoughts, and feelings. From this perspective, personality disorder symptoms can be understood as motivated, goal directed, or strategic, even though neither the goals

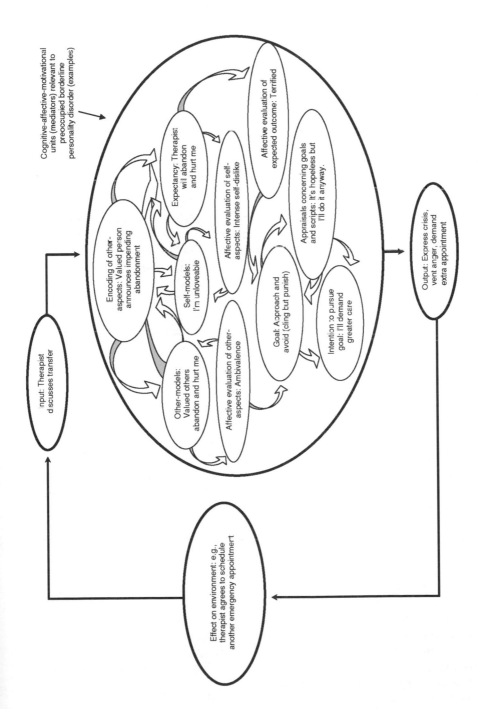

FIGURE 5.2. Conceptual analysis of potential CAPS processes in preoccupied borderline personality.

nor the strategies to pursue the goals may be consciously accessible or under easy volitional control. We propose that differences among personality disorders reflect systematic variations in the content and in the reciprocal activation and inhibition among these cognitive–affective units. Attachment theory, in our view, is fully compatible with this conceptualization of personality disorders, and—more important—the theory suggests an organizing structure for the bewildering complexity of the cognitive—affective units by emphasizing the conceptual primacy of models of self and others and of the interpersonal goals and strategies that flow from these models.

This conceptualization of personality disorders as automatized cognitive–affective–motivational patterns overlaps with other models, especially cognitive models. According to Beck, Freeman, and Associates (1990), for example, personality disorders can be understood as cognitive–affective–motivational strategies that are triggered by cognitive appraisals. Similar to our interpretation, Beck et al. (1990) do not regard these strategies as conscious—even though they are oriented toward goal attainment.

We should also note that there are alternative conceptualizations of personality and personality disorders, and attachment theory has much to say about such approaches as well. One popular alternative is the "Big Five" model of universal personality traits (e.g., Costa & Widiger, 2002). The relations between adult attachment and the Big Five traits are not entirely clear, although preliminary suggestions have been offered. For example, Bartholomew et al. (2001) speculated that introverted individuals might have more weakly developed attachment needs than extraverts, which could increase their risk for schizoid, schizotypal, paranoid, or antisocial personality disorder. High neuroticism, in turn, might be linked with attachment anxiety and rejection sensitivity, which could increase risk for borderline, histrionic, avoidant, and dependent personality disorders. These plausible associations, however, still await empirical confirmation. Furthermore, even if the empirical links between the Big Five traits and attachment styles were identified definitively, the even more important question (in our view) of which cognitive, affective, and motivational processes account for such associations would still not be answered.

Taking DSM-IV as a descriptive framework, our goal in the remainder of the chapter is to elaborate on the attachment-related structures and processes we regard as important in each of the personality disorders. These processes include positive and negative representations of the self and of others and the strategies used habitually to structure the interpersonal environment. To orient the reader to the relations among attachment dimensions and specific personality disorders, however, we first present the results of a pilot study in which the structural associations among attachment styles and personality disorders were explored.

EMPIRICAL LINKS BETWEEN ATTACHMENT STYLES
AND PERSONALITY DISORDERS: A PILOT STUDY

In a pilot study, we administered brief personality disorder and attachment style questionnaires to 176 undergraduate students at a large university in the southeastern United States (mean age = 20.21; *SD* = 2.36; 84% female; see Meyer, Pilkonis, & Beevers, 2004, for a detailed description of this study). To measure personality disorder features, the Structured Clinical Interview for DSM-IV, Axis II (SCID-II) questionnaire (First, Spitzer, Gibbon, & Williams, 1997) was administered, and to measure attachment styles, Brennan et al.'s (1998) Experiences in Close Relationships (ECR) questionnaire (ECR) was given. The SCID-II questionnaire alone—without the usual follow-up interview—is an imperfect measure of personality disorders but was used here for its brevity and convenience and because of its close ties with specific DSM-IV symptoms. The SCID-II questionnaire includes items that inquire about the presence of each personality disorder symptom using everyday language. For example, a question about the presence of unstable relationships (a borderline personality disorder diagnostic criterion) inquires, "Do your relationships with people you really care about have lots of extreme ups and downs?" Each question was rated here on a 4-point scale, including the following anchors: 1 ("Never or not at all"), 2 ("Sometimes or a little"), 3 ("Often or moderately"), and 4 ("Very often or extremely"). The version of the SCID-II used in our pilot study included items for all of the 10 DSM-IV personality disorders except antisocial personality.

The ECR (Brennan et al., 1998) is a 36-item questionnaire of adult attachment styles, with items culled from other attachment questionnaires. The ECR yields scores on two attachment dimensions—anxiety and avoidance. Sample items for anxiety include "I worry about being abandoned" and "I often wish that my partner's feelings for me were as strong as my feelings for him/her." Sample items for avoidance include "I get very uncomfortable when a romantic partner wants to be very close" and "I try to avoid getting too close to my partner." Responses are made on a 7-point scale, ranging from "Disagree Strongly" (1) to "Agree Strongly" (7).

We first inspected correlations between the anxiety and avoidance attachment dimensions and the nine personality disorder scales. As shown in Table 5.1, all personality disorders except schizoid correlated with attachment anxiety, with the strongest links for dependent and borderline personality. Even milder features of personality disorders, then, tend to be associated with heightened attachment anxiety, except for the case of schizoid personality. These analyses also showed that relatively few personality disorder scales were linked with attachment avoidance; significant correlations emerged only for the avoidant, paranoid, and schizoid scales.

TABLE 5.1. Correlations among Attachment and Personality Disorders Self-Reports

Personality Disorder Features: SCID-II Scales	Attachment dimensions: Experiences in Close Relationships (ECR) Scales	
	Avoidance	Anxiety
Avoidant	.22**	.37**
Dependent	.06	.47**
Obsessive–Compulsive	.09	.25**
Paranoid	.19*	.42**
Schizotypal	.07	.37**
Schizoid	.16*	−.01
Histrionic	−.02	.26**
Narcissistic	.07	.32**
Borderline	.13	.45**

Note. $n = 176$.
*$p < .05$; **$p < .01$.

Our second approach to analyzing this data set was to select approximately the top 15% (n's ranged from 22 to 28 per group) of participants on each of the personality disorder scales and to estimate where those with the strongest relative disturbance would fall within the two-dimensional attachment space defined by anxiety and avoidance (Figure 5.3). Thus, we computed and plotted the mean anxiety and avoidance scores for each of the nine personality disorder groups. For comparison, we also selected 28 "normal control" participants who scored low (below a mean of 1.3) on all SCID-II scales.

Note, however, that these groups were not mutually exclusive. For example, of the 27 in the avoidant personality group, 9 were also in the borderline group, 8 were in the schizotypal group, and some others were in additional groups. Similarly, of the 25 in the narcissistic group, 12 were also in the paranoid group, 11 were in the obsessive–compulsive group, and so forth. Thus, each of the groups reflects dominant features of the respective personality disorder but also includes considerable heterogeneity, which is similar to the mixed diagnoses observed in typical clinical settings.

As expected, Figure 5.3 shows that normal control participants—those without self-reported personality disorder features—were most likely to be securely attached. Three personality disorders—histrionic, borderline, and dependent—were located fairly clearly in the preoccupied quadrant. Four other ones—paranoid, obsessive–compulsive, narcissistic, and schizotypal—were located at the border between preoccupied and fearful attachment. Avoidant personality was somewhat more clearly in the fearful quadrant, and only schizoid personality was in the dismissing quadrant.

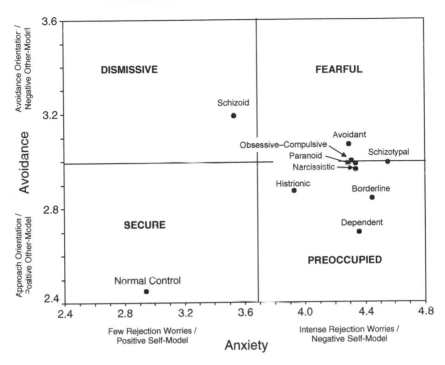

FIGURE 5.3. DSM-IV personality disorder features in attachment space (undergraduate self-reports).

COMPARISON WITH A CLINICAL SAMPLE

To compare these nonclinical findings with those from a clinical group, we constructed a similar plot based on a sample described in a previous report (see Meyer et al., 2001). In that study, 152 diagnostically heterogeneous adult patients at a psychiatric hospital were studied (80% outpatients; 57% female; mean age = 34.5, SD = 9.3). Trained clinicians conducted semi-structured interviews with each patient and, in a majority of cases, with significant others. Pilkonis's (1988) attachment prototype rating method was employed to estimate attachment styles of each patient, and clinical consensus ratings were used to determine the severity of each personality disorder symptom for each patient. To construct the plot shown in Figure 5.4, we selected only those 10–15% of patients with the highest relative severity scores on each personality disorder scale. Thus, between 19 and 28 individuals per group were selected, and their mean scores on the preoccupied ("excessive dependency") and avoidant ("defensive separation") attachment prototype scales were plotted.

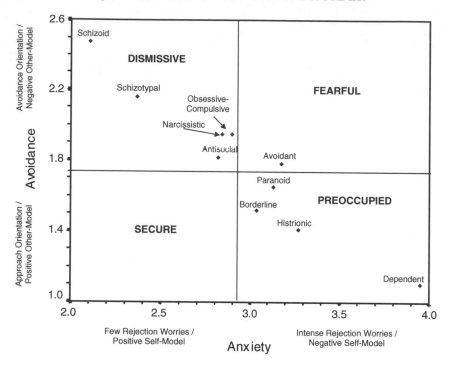

FIGURE 5.4. Personality disorder features in attachment space (clinical ratings of psychiatric patients).

Figures 5.3 and 5.4 reveal notable similarities but also several differences between the clinical and nonclinical groups. In the clinical as well as the student sample, schizoid personality fell in the dismissive quadrant; avoidant in the fearful; and borderline, histrionic, and dependent in the preoccupied quadrant. Locations of the other personality disorders, though, varied slightly; for example, schizotypal personalities appeared more dismissive in the clinical group but at the interface between preoccupied and fearful attachment in the student group. Differences in measurement and sample type may account for some of these observed differences, but regardless of their precision and generalizability, the purpose of presenting these pilot findings here is to provide a heuristic orientation to how DSM-IV personality disorders might relate to the four adult attachment patterns. Our interpretation of how these links can be understood follows in the next section.

Our review of the 10 DSM-IV Axis II disorders focuses on elements that we consider to be critical cognitive–affective–motivational determinants of personality. They include the content and valence of models of the self and others as well as the dominant goals and strategies each personality habitually uses in relating to the interpersonal environment. In most personality disorders, mental representations of self and others combine various negative qualities, although the specific content and connotations of the negativity differ among disorders. It is not enough, of course, to know that mental models are "bad"; to understand their implications for personality disorders, one also needs to describe what information these models contain beyond mere valence. In this section, we speculate on the content of these representations across the DSM-IV personality disorders, and we discuss briefly possible developmental antecedents and relevant empirical findings on the links between attachment and personality disorders.

PREOCCUPIED PERSONALITIES: DEPENDENT, BORDERLINE, AND HISTRIONIC

Dependent Personality

Dependent personalities are described as having "a pervasive and excessive need to be taken care of that leads to submissive and clinging behavior and fears of separation" (American Psychiatric Association, 1994, p. 665). They are said to have low self-confidence, to feel uncomfortable or helpless when alone, and to yearn for nurturance, support, guidance, advice, and reassurance from others (American Psychiatric Association, 1994). Most classical descriptions concur that the combination of an inadequate self-image and clinging submission to others constitute core features of the dependent personality (see Millon & Davis, 1996).

The etiology of dependent personality remains speculative owing to a lack of longitudinal data. Much of the clinical literature, though, suggests that submission-inducing parenting styles can promote adult dependency. This might include, for example, a combination of dominant–authoritarian, overindulgent, and overprotective parenting, where the child learns that submission to others is a necessary and efficient way to attain gratification (cf. Millon & Davis, 1996). Overprotection may also convey the message that the child is incapable of independent mastery of the environment, which encourages a passive–submissive style along with representations of the self as incompetent. Studies with retrospective designs tend to confirm that adults with dependent personality recall their parents as authoritarian or overprotective (e.g., McCranie & Bass, 1984; Parker & Lipscombe, 1980).

The self-model in prototypical dependent personality, then, may be construed as negative in the sense that the self is viewed as inept, incompetent, or incapable of autonomous mastery of the environment. However, self-representations may also have positive aspects, given that dependent personalities believe that others are, in principle, willing to engage with them in relationships and to provide nurturance and support. The self is viewed as inept but nevertheless as worthy of other people's attention, guidance, and nurturance.

The dependent personality's prototypical model of others, in contrast, appears to be mostly positive—others are viewed as indispensable sources of nurturance and direction. In the dependent personality's world view, "only others possess the requisite talents and experience to attain the rewards of life" (Millon & Davis, 1996, p. 332). Viewing others as inherently superior and the self as inept and inferior, the dependent personality seeks to loyally submit to the nurturing authority expected from others. However, other-models may also have secondary negative aspects. Dependent personalities are acutely aware that others might leave or abandon them—the possibility of rejection is chronically salient and further strengthens their submission tendencies, motivated by the desire to avoid potential rejection.

Thus, active submission in dependent personality can be construed as flowing primarily from approach motivation (desiring proximity to obtain guidance and nurturance) but also, secondarily, from avoidance motivation (pleasing and appeasing others to avoid feared rejection). In terms of the balance between appealing versus threatening aspects of other-representations, positive aspects can be viewed as dominant, given that dependent personalities readily approach and enter into relationships. The pattern of mostly negative self-views and mostly positive other-views in dependent personality corresponds to preoccupied adult attachment. When negative other-models outweigh positive ones, though, a shift toward fearful attachment and avoidant personality features would seem likely.

The potentially confusing mix of active versus passive strategies in dependent personality is resolved by recognizing that the underlying goal motivating the dependent personality's actions is the maintenance of close, nurturing relationships (i.e., proximity to attachment figures). This goal, however, can sometimes be achieved by behaving passively and submissively and sometimes by pursuing more active routes. This point was also expressed by Bornstein (1992) in his review of the motivational dynamics underlying dependency:

> How can we reconcile the seemingly inconsistent findings that dependent people are passive and acquiescent in certain contexts and relatively active and assertive in others? By examining the motivations that underlie the dependent person's behavior in different situations. . . . [One] central goal underlies much of the dependent person's behavior: obtaining and maintaining nurturant, supportive relationships. This core motivation of the dependent person is reflected in a wide variety of situations and settings, albeit in different ways. (p. 18)

Not surprisingly, empirical evidence confirms that features of dependent personality relate to measures of preoccupied attachment. Among 149 psychiatric patients, for example, an interview-based measure of preoccupied attachment correlated highly ($r = .73$, $p < .001$) with DSM-III-R features of dependent personality disorder (Meyer et al., 2001). The magnitude of this association suggests strong overlap between the constructs or, alternatively, a degree of redundancy between measures. Indeed, Pilkonis's (1988) preoccupied attachment prototype has previously been labeled "excessive dependency" and includes items such as "tends to be anxious and insecure because of the fear that s/he may lose an important relationship or person" and "tends to depend too much on other people; becomes 'clingy' in relationships." Such content overlap between attachment and dependent personality features is also evident in other measures, such as Hazan and Shaver's (1987) anxious–ambivalent attachment item (e.g., "I often worry that my partner doesn't really love me or won't want to stay with me. I want to get very close to my partner, and this sometimes scares people away"). These parallels suggest, perhaps, that dependent personality and anxious–ambivalent/preoccupied attachment truly overlap on both theoretical and empirical levels of analysis. Several studies have also confirmed close associations between dependent personality and anxious–preoccupied forms of attachment (e.g., Brennan & Shaver, 1998; West, Rose, & Sheldon-Keller, 1994).

In summary, dependent personality indicates the presence of high levels of attachment anxiety, coupled primarily with interpersonal approach strategies. This pattern reflects the presence of mostly (but not entirely) negative self-representations, coupled with mostly (but not entirely) positive other-representations. This prototypical constellation of preoccupied attachment in dependent personality may be summarized by phrases such as "The inept, helpless but still loveable self submits to revered others in order to receive guidance and nurturance" (see Figure 5.5). We do not think that such phrases are consciously salient to these personalities, but their symptoms suggest that they structure and strategically organize their interpersonal environment based on such implicit principles.

Although the prototypical attachment pattern in dependent personality is preoccupied, in our view, it is also possible that other attachment variants of dependency exist. For example, dependency might arise when securely attached persons construe the self as worthy and lovable but nevertheless as oriented primarily toward the provision of support and nurturance for others (i.e., a caregiving orientation). Such positive self-views may be coupled with positive other-models; when others are revered as providers of guidance (and as appreciative receivers of nurturance), and the self is appraised positively (but as a caregiver rather than care receiver), dependent personality features would seem a logical consequence. Empirically,

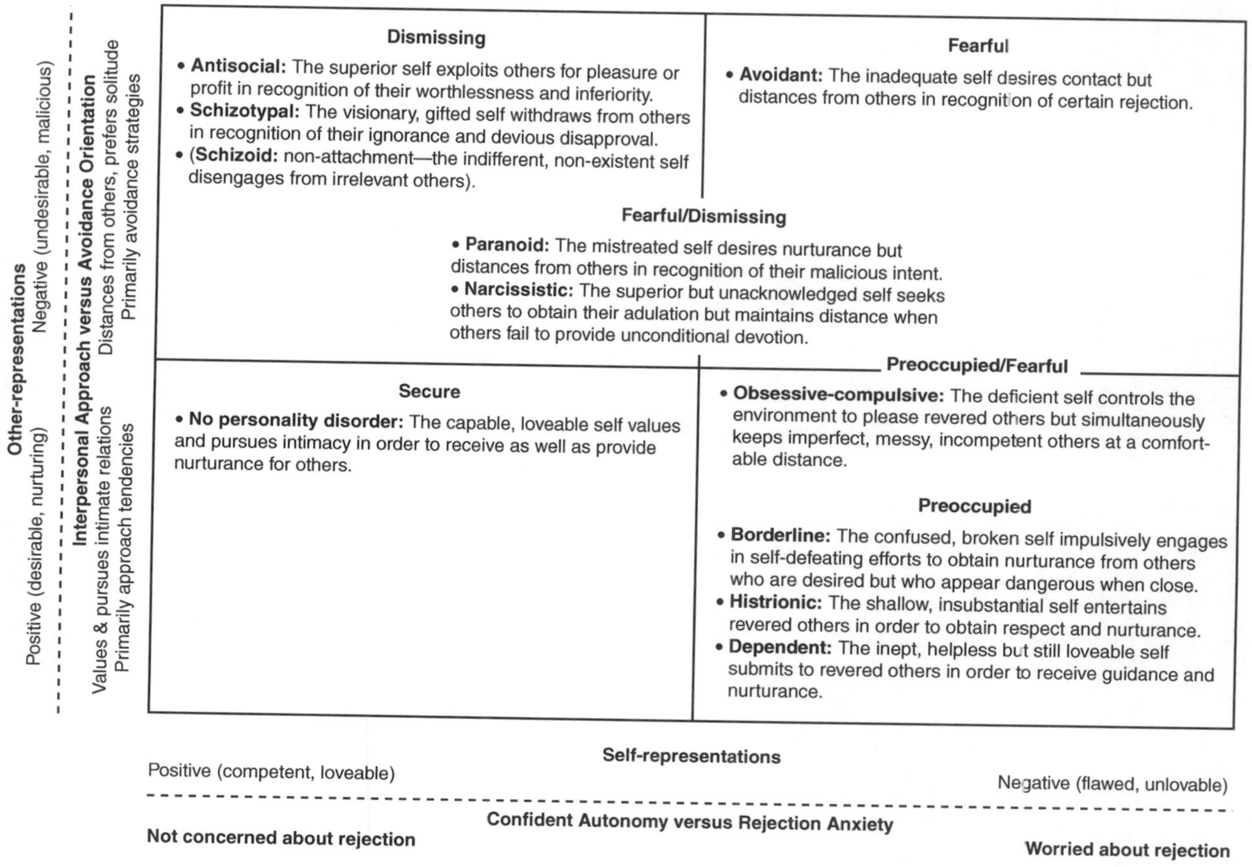

Dismissing

- **Antisocial:** The superior self exploits others for pleasure or profit in recognition of their worthlessness and inferiority.
- **Schizotypal:** The visionary, gifted self withdraws from others in recognition of their ignorance and devious disapproval.
- **(Schizoid:** non-attachment—the indifferent, non-existent self disengages from irrelevant others).

Fearful

- **Avoidant:** The inadequate self desires contact but distances from others in recognition of certain rejection.

Fearful/Dismissing

- **Paranoid:** The mistreated self desires nurturance but distances from others in recognition of their malicious intent.
- **Narcissistic:** The superior but unacknowledged self seeks others to obtain their adulation but maintains distance when others fail to provide unconditional devotion.

Preoccupied/Fearful

- **Obsessive-compulsive:** The deficient self controls the environment to please revered others but simultaneously keeps imperfect, messy, incompetent others at a comfortable distance.

Preoccupied

- **Borderline:** The confused, broken self impulsively engages in self-defeating efforts to obtain nurturance from others who are desired but who appear dangerous when close.
- **Histrionic:** The shallow, insubstantial self entertains revered others in order to obtain respect and nurturance.
- **Dependent:** The inept, helpless but still loveable self submits to revered others in order to receive guidance and nurturance.

Secure

- **No personality disorder:** The capable, loveable self values and pursues intimacy in order to receive as well as provide nurturance for others.

Self-representations

Positive (competent, loveable) — — — — — — — — — — — — — — Negative (flawed, unlovable)

Confident Autonomy versus Rejection Anxiety

Not concerned about rejection — — — — — — — — — — — — — Worried about rejection

Interpersonal Approach versus Avoidance Orientation

Distances from others, prefers solitude — Values & pursues intimate relations
Primarily avoidance strategies — Primarily approach tendencies

Other-representations

Negative (undesirable, malicious) — — — — Positive (desirable, nurturing)

252

FIGURE 5.5. Attachment variants of personality disorders (implicitly held mental representations and interpersonal strategies).

though, such a securely attached variant of dependent personality disorder remains speculative.

Borderline Personality

Of the nine DSM-IV criteria for borderline personality disorder, one describes both a high level of attachment anxiety and a particular style of coping with this anxiety: "Frantic efforts to avoid real or imagined abandonment" (American Psychiatric Association, 1994, p. 654). If this were the only borderline criterion, an attachment interpretation would be straightforward, but the symptoms also include unstable relationships with alternating idealization and devaluation; unstable self-representations; impulsive, potentially self-damaging behavior; recurrent suicidality or self-mutilation; unstable and highly reactive mood; feelings of emptiness; anger-related problems; and transient psychotic symptoms.

From an attachment perspective, some of these symptoms can be interpreted in terms of the content and coherence of internal working models (e.g., fluctuating self and other-representations). Other symptoms can be interpreted as responses to underlying attachment anxiety or as interpersonal strategies that are habitually employed to manage omnipresent threats of rejection. What is perplexing about borderline personalities is the intensity, violence, and unpredictability of their "efforts to avoid abandonment." The unpredictably shifting, erratic, and intense nature of these borderline symptoms suggests that underlying mental models and interpersonal strategies are also internally conflicted, incoherent, or unstable. In borderline personality disorder (BPD), it seems that not *one* dominant attachment goal is pursued persistently (e.g., greater intimacy) but that the goals and strategies themselves fluctuate dramatically, with previously desirable targets suddenly switching into strongly valenced opposites, creating an intense, confusing, and dissatisfying roller-coaster of vacillating approach and avoidance efforts. Approach strategies may dramatically switch into avoidance when intimacy itself is recognized as dangerous, which would seem plausible in light of the typical developmental antecedent reported by these personalities (i.e., abuse histories).

In terms of underlying mental representations, the presence of intense attachment anxiety suggests a fundamentally negative self-model, whereas unstable approach–avoidance fluctuations indicate conflicted models of others, entailing positive and negative aspects that cannot easily be reconciled. The content of the negative self-model in an individual with BPD may differ profoundly from those in other disorders. For example, whereas dependent personalities view themselves as inept but potentially lovable, the borderline's self-image has more fatalistic connotations. Borderline personalities may experience themselves as utterly damaged or "broken" on a deep, fundamental level (cf. Beck et al., 1990). Once such self-representations are activated, self-loathing can become so intense that it motivates self-harm, reflected in suicidal and self-injurious behavior. Studies have confirmed that individuals with BPD endorse strongly negative self-beliefs, viewing the self as weak, needy, helpless, and incapable (e.g., Butler, Brown, Beck, & Grisham, 2002).

Similarly, in individuals with BPD, mental representations of others appear to take on unique connotations, characteristically different from those in individuals with other disorders. Generally positive other-representations (reflected in a desire for intimacy and concern over potential rejection) may be linked with strongly negative aspects that ironically become activated primarily when intimacy is approached. This dynamic change in the valence of the other-model might account for the overt fluctuations between other-idealization and devaluation, and perhaps contributes to symptoms such as sudden anger outbursts, relationship instability, and dangerous impulsivity. As the individual with BPD approaches the goal of intimacy, the intimacy goal itself switches and becomes a danger signal (i.e., an avoidance rather than approach goal; cf. Carver & Scheier, 1998), from which only the most dramatic actions promise escape. Such dynamic changes in other-representations have yet to be examined, but consistent with this idea, evidence confirms that other-models in borderline personality tend to be ambivalent, such that others are strongly desired but simultaneously feared and mistrusted (e.g., Butler et al., 2002).

In terms of its location in contemporary attachment space, BPD fits primarily into the preoccupied quadrant, marked by high attachment anxiety and primarily approach rather than avoidance tendencies. Because a key feature of BPD is instability, though, we would not expect such personalities to remain fixed within the preoccupied quadrant. Instead, as noted previously, negative aspects of other-representations may suddenly overwhelm the salience of positive ones, leading to temporary shifts toward fearful attachment, where both self- and other-models are strongly negative.

Empirical studies of attachment in BPD are more numerous than for other personality disorders. Patrick, Hobson, Castle, Howard, and Maughn (1994), for example, compared attachment-related mental representations, as assessed with the AAI, among 12 dysthymic and 12 borderline women who were matched for age, education, and socioeconomic status. Most of the participants with BPD were rated as confused, fearful, and overwhelmed with regard to early attachment experiences. Furthermore, 10 of the 12 (88%) borderline patients were rated as fearfully preoccupied by trauma or loss, pointing to the importance of this etiological pathway. In a larger sample of psychiatric inpatients, Fonagy et al. (1996) confirmed this finding, although the proportion of participants with BPD rated as preoccupied with trauma or loss was somewhat lower than Patrick et al.'s (1994) study. Similar findings were reported by Stalker and Davies (1995) and by Rosenstein and Horowitz (1996), who found that 9 of 14 adolescents with DSM-III-R (American Psychiatric Association, 1987) borderline features fit the AAI-based preoccupied attachment classification.

In a study in which Pilkonis's (1988) prototype-rating method of attachment was used (Meyer et al., 2001), borderline features were also linked with several indexes of insecure attachment. Specifically, among 149 psychiatric patients, DSM-III-R borderline features were moderately and inversely linked with a prototype measuring security of attachment, and there was a weak, positive association between borderline pathology and a measure of preoccupied attachment. In our pilot study described earlier, borderline features were relatively strongly linked with attachment anxiety but not avoidance.

Several other studies have also examined relations between self-reports of attachment and borderline symptoms. Brennan and Shaver (1998), for example, found that both preoccupied and fearful attachment were linked with BPD. Dutton, Saunders, Starzomski, and Bartholomew (1994) found that a borderline self-report measure was linked with preoccupied as well as fearful attachment. Further support for the notion of broad attachment disturbance in BPD was provided by Sack, Sperling, Fagen, and Foelsch (1996), who found that patients with BPD scored high on a number of measures of insecure attachment.

In summary, substantial evidence concurs that attachment disturbances play an important role in the etiology and maintenance of borderline personality pathology. Extreme violations within the early parent–child bond—such as chronic abuse, parental neglect, or emotional invalidation—may all interfere with the formation of positive, stable, and coherent mental representations of self and others, thereby placing the abuse victim on an early trajectory toward greater borderline risk (e.g., Yen et al., 2002; Zanarini et al., 1997). The maltreatment experienced by these children may impair their ability to reflect on other people's mental states (e.g., Fonagy, Gergely, Jurist, & Target, 2002) or may lead to tendencies to construe others' motives as malicious (e.g., Arntz & Veen, 2001). Their risk appears to be magnified when other vulnerabilities, such as temperamental emotionality, interact with the adverse effect of early attachment disturbance (cf. Linehan, 1993; Siever & Davis, 1991). In borderline personality, negative, contradictory, and unstable mental representations appear to be carried forward into adulthood, where they manifest in preoccupied strategies, with temporal shifts toward fearful and even dismissing strategies. The instability, incoherence, and extreme negative features of the working models, along with the failure to have evolved effective interpersonal strategies, can then contribute to the emergence and maintenance of numerous variations of adult borderline pathology.

Histrionic Personality

Compared with the intensity and destructiveness of the borderline personality, the histrionic pattern represents a milder expression of preoccupied
attachment. Histrionic personality is defined by symptoms such as excessive emotionality and attention seeking; discomfort upon being ignored;
sexually seductive behavior; shallow, shifting, and theatrical expression of
emotions; impressionistic speech; suggestibility; and tendencies to overem-
phasize or misinterpret intimacy in relationships (American Psychiatric
Association, 1994). At a glance, several of these symptoms seem to indicate
significant concern about potential rejection combined with active efforts
to attract others and thereby prevent rejection. Many early characterizations of histrionic personalities confirm that rejection sensitivity along with
active self-dramatization form the core of this disorder (cf. Millon & Davis,
1996).

Symptoms such as "discomfort when not the center of attention" suggest the presence of high attachment anxiety (and thus a primarily negative
self-model). Histrionic behaviors such as exaggerated displays of emotion
and active seeking of approval from others, by contrast, can be construed
as approach strategies triggered by attachment anxiety and motivated by
the goal to get attachment needs met. Such approach efforts reveal a desire
for intimacy and, thus, a positive other-model. Similar to dependent personality, then, the motivational dynamics underlying the histrionic pattern
fit the preoccupied attachment pattern. However, whereas dependent personalities tend to be aware of their preoccupied intimacy craving, such
attachment needs may be more implicit, unacknowledged, or unconscious
in individuals with histrionic personalities (Bornstein, 1998).

Preoccupied attachment appears to be at the core of the histrionic
personality, but dismissing attachment might also play a role. In dismissing attachment, other-models are negative and self-models are positive,
which often seems evident in those with histrionic personalities who are
charmed and entertained by their own dramatic performances. In such
cases, others are demoted to the role of mere spectators, and thus their
other-models are superficially positive but, at a deeper level, dismissive
and shallow and, in that sense, negative. Bartholomew et al. (2001)
described a histrionic personality for whom this pattern seemed to fit:
"She was highly sexually active (describing getting men as 'a hobby'),
though these liaisons never satisfied her craving for love and attention"
(p. 216). These tendencies could be interpreted as "secondary dismissing
elements—a tendency to objectify others, and a tendency to cut off
threatening feelings of vulnerability by derogating others and focusing on
sexuality at the exclusion of intimacy within relationships" (Bartholomew
et al., 2001, p. 216).

Based on these speculations, we propose that the prototypical other-model in histrionic personality combines several qualities: The positive, ide-alized image of others as potentially nurturing and loving; the positive but shallow, simplistic image of others as providers of recognition and admiration; and the negative, impoverished image of others as mere objects, who are not of interest except for their potential to provide applause. Similarly, we propose that the prototypical histrionic self-model combines positive and negative qualities: the dominant negative self-image of a person who is likely to be rejected and must therefore continuously appear entertaining and seductive and the more brittle positive self-image of the effective entertainer who dazzles and bewitches others. The implicit principle guiding the actions of an individual with a histrionic personality could thus be summarized as "the shallow, insubstantial self entertains revered others in order to obtain respect and nurturance" (see Figure 5.5). Such beliefs and scripts might perpetuate histrionic symptoms as they guide how others are approached and interpreted, how the self is defined in relation to others, and what kinds of actions tend to be pursued to get attachment needs met.

The developmental pathways leading to adult histrionic personality remain speculative. Lyddon and Sherry (2001), like others before them, suggested that minimal or inconsistent parenting might facilitate histrionic trajectories, as children in such environments must resort to extreme, dramatic measures to receive attention. In situations in which parental attention is made contingent upon theatrical displays, histrionic behaviors are shaped and reinforced. Bornstein (1999) also noted this (yet untested) pathway: "Like the infant whose caregivers do not respond until she screams at the top of her lungs, the histrionic child eventually learns that the way to get what she wants from others is to draw attention to herself through every means available—the more intrusive the better" (p. 547).

Empirical studies investigating the role of attachment in histrionic personality, unfortunately, are rare. We reported previously that histrionic personality features correlated weakly with a measure of preoccupied attachment and weakly and inversely with measures of avoidant and secure attachment (Meyer et al., 2001). In our pilot study (see Table 5.1), histrionic features were linked weakly but specifically with attachment anxiety. These associations are consistent with our interpretation that histrionic personality reflects working models that combine positive and negative qualities, but that the negative self-model and positive other-model predominate, justifying the view of histrionic personality as primarily a manifestation of preoccupied attachment. In Brennan and Shaver's (1998) study, the majority of histrionic participants were classified as secure, consistent with the view that this disorder reflects a milder variant of attachment disturbance, compared to the more harmful preoccupied pattern in borderline personality.

PRIMARILY FEARFUL ATTACHMENT: AVOIDANT PERSONALITY

Avoidant personalities desire close relationships but simultaneously fear humiliation, are convinced of their personal inadequacy, and therefore tend to avoid social situations that entail the potential for embarrassment (American Psychiatric Association, 1994; Millon & Davis, 1996). DSM-IV emphasis is on inhibition, restraint, and shame in interpersonal situations and inadequate self-image; craving for intimacy, however, is relatively deemphasized (Pilkonis, 1995). The pattern of high attachment anxiety (intense worries about rejection and humiliation) coupled with active avoidance strategies to prevent the threat of rejection suggests the presence of generalized fearful attachment, such that others in general—not just one specific attachment figure—are regarded as potentially rejecting and are therefore avoided.

Several studies have confirmed the construal of avoidant personality as a disorder of fearful attachment. Sheldon and West (1990), for example, reported that strong desires for attachment coupled with fears of rejection were common among 47 adults diagnosed with avoidant personality disorder. In Brennan and Shaver's (1998) study, most avoidant participants could also be classified as fearfully attached. In our pilot study, avoidant personality features correlated with both avoidant and anxious attachment (see Table 5.1), and in both a clinical and nonclinical sample, avoidant features tended to fall within the fearful attachment quadrant (see Figures 5.3 and 5.4).

The fearful attachment in avoidant personality may originate from childhood adversity, and many theorists have noted the plausibility of such a pathway (e.g., Beck et al., 1990; Millon & Davis, 1996). Beck et al. (Beck & Freeman, 1990), for example, proposed that "as children, [individuals with APD] may have had a significant person (parent, sibling, peer) who was highly critical and rejecting of them" (p. 261). Similarly, Stravynski, Elie, and Franche (1989) reported that patients diagnosed with avoidant personality disorder (APD) remembered their parents as more rejecting, guilt-inducing, and less affectionate than did a control group. In another study, narratives of childhood memories were rated more negatively among college students who endorsed more avoidant personality features (Meyer & Carver, 2000).

From an attachment perspective, it is unfortunate that the definition in DSM-III-R and DSM-IV shifted toward general social discomfort and away from the attachment-consistent view that desire for, but fear of, dyadic intimacy constitutes the core features of avoidant personality. DSM-IV emphasis on shame and embarrassment may also magnify the often noted overlap with generalized social phobia (Feske, Perry, Chambless, Renneberg, &

Goldstein, 1996; Herbert, Hope, & Bellack, 1992). If avoidant personality is defined primarily as a disorder of general social discomfort, the overlap with fearful attachment is obscured—many people are timid and fearful of embarrassment in social situations, but they nevertheless manage to have close, mutually nurturing relationships. Those personalities whose core motivation revolves around the desire for intimacy, fear of rejection, and avoidance of others as strategy to prevent potential rejection would fit the prototype of fearful attachment more closely. We agree in this respect with Bartholomew et al. (2001), who proposed that "the critical features of this disorder are a desire for close relationships, coupled with an extreme fear of disapproval and rejection, leading to avoidance of becoming intimately involved with others" (p. 219).

Attachment theory also clarifies the overlap among avoidant, schizoid, and dependent personalities (cf. Trull, Widiger, & Frances, 1987). Individuals with both avoidant and dependent personalities share a high degree of attachment anxiety, marked by fear of rejection or abandonment. A difference, however, is that an individual with APD fears *entering* into relationships, whereas the individual with a dependent personality fears being left or rejected *once in a relationship*. Similarly, whereas those with APD rely on interpersonal strategies that establish a social environment marked by safe distance from others and relative solitude, those with dependent personality disorder use strategies that bring at least one person into continuous proximity. Thus, individuals with APD pursue avoidance-oriented strategies in response to attachment anxiety, whereas individuals with dependent personalities employ approach-oriented strategies. Despite their dominant social avoidance, it has been noted clinically that individuals with APD occasionally manage to enter into close relationships, in which case they often may shift toward a more dependent stance with that person (cf. Bartholomew et al., 2001; Lyddon & Sherry, 2001).

BETWEEN FEARFUL AND DISMISSING ATTACHMENT: PARANOID AND NARCISSISTIC PERSONALITIES

Paranoid Personality

Paranoid personalities mistrust and are suspicious of other people's motives; they inappropriately infer from innocuous cues that others intend to exploit, deceive, or harm them; and they often angrily "counterattack" against perceived threats that are not apparent to others (American Psychiatric Assocation, 1994). Unlike the other two disorders in which paranoia features prominently—paranoid schizophrenia and delusional disorder—individuals with paranoid personalities tend to be suspicious but not psychotic in the sense of experiencing frequent delusions or hallucinations.

The consistent mistrust that individuals with paranoid personalities harbor against others suggests the presence of predominantly negative other-models, whereas views of the self as the innocent, persecuted victim suggest at least somewhat positive self-models—a constellation that would seem to indicate dismissing attachment. In datasets we analyzed (see Figures 5.3 and 5.4), however, paranoid features corresponded to a mixture of preoccupied and fearful attachment, suggesting negative self- and ambivalent other-models. In Brennan and Shaver's (1998) study, most paranoid personalities were classified as fearful (34%), an almost equally large percentage as secure (29%), and smaller percentages as dismissing or preoccupied (18% each). Rosenstein and Horowitz (1996) found that dismissing attachment was significantly more common than preoccupied attachment among adolescents with paranoid features. These mixed findings suggest that it may be difficult to assign paranoid personality to a single, prototypical attachment pattern.

Despite this ambiguity, some authors have speculated that paranoid personality is a syndrome of predominantly fearful attachment (e.g., Lyddon & Sherry, 2001). In this view, paranoia emerges when parents persistently monitor, harass, and disapprove of their children. Such parenting is thought to facilitate both a negative self-model (because the self comes to be viewed as incompetent or worthless) and a negative other-model (because others are experienced as malevolent and persistently critical). Once such early experiences have led to the pattern of pervasive suspicion, paranoid styles may become self-perpetuating because "the view that others have malevolent motives often leads to increased social isolation and alienation, further confirming to the person that others cannot be trusted and should be blamed for things that go wrong" (Lyddon & Sherry, 2001, p. 409).

In his review of paranoid conditions, Blaney (1999) highlighted that many etiological models hold that paranoia emerges as a compensation for underlying negative self-models, including views of the self as helpless, meaningless, lonely, or powerless. Individuals with paranoid personalities are thought to be reluctant, however, to fully recognize their own negative self-views and instead defensively blame others for negative outcomes. There is experimental evidence suggesting that paranoid individuals hold implicit negative self-representations that play a part in their tendency to blame others for adverse events (Kinderman & Bentall, 1996, 1997). On the surface, though, individuals with paranoid personalities often experience themselves as important, righteous, justified, and entitled (Blaney, 1999).

Our preliminary attachment interpretation, then, is that prototypical paranoid personality combines implicit negative self-views with a façade of positive self-representations. The self is experienced as the innocent victim of others' harassment, persecution, and malevolence. At the same time, however, there may be a limited recognition that something is not quite right with the self—that the self is questionable, potentially flawed, or somehow compromised in worth or competence. Given the hallmark symptom of suspiciousness, we further propose that prototypical individuals with paranoid personalities hold negative other-representations, viewing others as untrustworthy and malevolent in their intentions. This constellation of mental representations leads individuals with paranoid personalities to adopt primarily avoidant interpersonal strategies (i.e., interpersonal distance is maintained in order to avoid the expected harassment and persecution). As such, we interpret paranoid personality as a cognitive–affective–motivational pattern combining elements of fearful and dismissing attachment (see Figure 5.5).

Narcissistic Personality

Another personality disorder in which both dismissive and fearful attachment may play a role is the narcissistic pattern. Individuals with narcissistic personality disorder are described as grandiose, requiring excessive admiration, and lacking in the capacity for empathy; they present as arrogant and interpersonally exploitative, and they feel superior and entitled to special treatment from others (American Psychiatric Assocation, 1994). An obvious attachment interpretation suggests the presence of extremely positive, inflated self-representations coupled with impoverished, disparaging other-representations. Prototypical narcissists construe others as inferior, have little recognition of others' autonomy and dignity, and are interested in others primarily as subservient providers of nurturance and gratification.

The characterization of narcissists as self-loving, other-despising egotists is straightforward but resembles a caricature more than it reflects the complexities of clinical reality—an assertion already made by Cooper and Sacks (1991, cited in Millon and Davis, 1996) against the DSM conception of narcissistic personality. Indeed, clinical observation suggests that narcissism is often associated with some implicit or explicit recognition of personal inadequacy and envy for the positive qualities of others. Consistent with this idea, theorists have suggested that narcissistic personalities harbor intense self-doubt, feelings of personal inferiority, and sensitivity to interpersonal rejection (cf. Millon & Davis, 1996). These self-doubts are thought to originate either from disparaging, belittling parenting, against which the narcissism emerges as a self-protective but often brittle defense, or from the recognition that parental admiration is not shared by others. In either case, a discrepancy emerges between views of the self as exceptional versus ordinary or even incompetent. Instead of being able to reconcile this conflict, the narcissist is thought to adhere inflexibly to superior self-views.

Empirically, the associations between narcissistic personality and attachment are complex if not confusing. In Brennan and Shaver's (1998) analyses, the conceptualization of narcissistic personalities as predominantly dismissive was not supported; instead, narcissists exhibited a wide range of attachment configurations. Only 16% of narcissistic adults were classified as dismissive, whereas nearly one-third exhibited either dominant secure or fearful attachment, with another 20% in the preoccupied group (Brennan & Shaver, 1998). In a study using Pilkonis's attachment prototype ratings (Meyer et al., 2001), narcissistic DSM-III-R features were inversely related to secure attachment but did not correlate with features of either the preoccupied or avoidant attachment prototype. In our pilot study (see Table 5.1 and Figure 5.4), narcissism correlated with attachment anxiety but not avoidance, suggesting the presence of preoccupied attachment, with some trends toward fearful elements. In Rosenstein and Horowitz's (1996) study, narcissistic adolescents were more likely to be dismissing than preoccupied in their attachment pattern.

In our interpretation, prototypical narcissism is characterized by easily and frequently activated grandiose self-views. Others are typically viewed in instrumental terms as providers of support and admiration rather than as valuable and autonomous persons in their own right. The dominant constellation of superior self-views combined with inferior other-views suggests that narcissistic personality can be construed as a pathology of dismissing attachment. To the degree that negative self-evaluations are also present beyond the more obvious façades of grandiosity, however, fearful attachment may also play a role. One possibility is that subtypes of narcissistic personality can be distinguished along this dimension: At one end would be the "uncomplicated grandiose" type, in which grandiosity is rooted in consistently positive self-representations. At the other end would be the "defensively grandiose" type, in which overt grandiosity masks underlying negative self-views. Similar variants of narcissism have been described by many others (Gabbard, 1989; Wink, 1991) These variations may also be associated with different developmental histories.

One interpersonal influence that promotes narcissism may be overindulgent and acquiescent parenting in which children learn that "the family world revolves around them" and that they are special and entitled to favorable treatment (Millon & Davis, 1996, pp. 419–420). The pathway from parental overindulgence to narcissism has a long history in psychiatric theory and dates from Freud and Horney, among others (cf. Millon & Davis, 1996). At the other extreme is the idea that early parental rejection, coldness, and disapproval create representations of the self as despicable, against which the budding narcissist defends by forming an unrealistically inflated self-image. Such views have also been advanced by psychoanalytically oriented theorists, among them Kernberg and Kohut (cf. Millon &

Davis, 1996). There is little empirical evidence, however, to clarify the degree to which overindulgent versus cold and rejecting parenting can create variations of narcissism.

PREDOMINANTLY (BUT NOT EXCLUSIVELY) DISMISSING ATTACHMENT: ANTISOCIAL AND SCHIZOTYPAL PERSONALITIES

Antisocial Personality

Individuals with antisocial personalities are callous and reckless in their pursuit of personal benefit; they disregard and violate social norms and the rights of others; they lie and deceive others for pleasure or profit; they are impulsive and fail to plan ahead; they are irritable and aggressive; they are irresponsible with work and finances; and they lack remorse (American Psychiatric Association, 1994). Other features include an inability to maintain long-term relationships; a limited capacity to feel empathy and guilt or to learn from punishing experiences; a tendency to infer malicious motives in others and to exploit them; a glib and superficial charm; and an arrogant, self-assured style (American Psychiatric Association, 1994; Millon & Davis, 1996). This pattern of self-centeredness and contemptuous disregard for others suggests that dismissing attachment plays a key role in many cases of antisocial personality.

In a study of men who were in treatment for assaulting their partners and were diagnosed primarily with antisocial personality, dismissing attachment was particularly important (cf. Bartholomew et al., 2001). Bartholomew et al. (2001) noted: "Interestingly, the small subgroup of men whose personality problems appeared limited to antisocial (and perhaps sadistic) characteristics were most likely to be predominantly dismissing" (p. 221). One such case described by Bartholomew included a characteristic developmental history that was described, moreover, in prototypically dismissive style:

> He had a superficial understanding of his childhood, downplayed or was unaware of any effects his upbringing had on him. . . .His mother . . . provided only minimal care and supervision . . . she was unresponsive to [the children's] attempts to gain attention and support . . . He dropped out of school at a young age. . . . His childhood was also permeated with models of threats and violence. . . . His mother was unnecessarily harsh in her sporadic attempts at discipline. (p. 221)

Connections between antisocial personality and dismissing attachment were also observed in a study by Rosenstein and Horowitz (1996). In a sample of psychiatrically hospitalized adolescents, dismissing attachment, assessed by the AAI, was found to relate to both interview-based and self-report measures of conduct disorder and antisocial symptoms (Rosenstein & Horowitz, 1996). Of 13 adolescents with predominant antisocial features, 11 were classified as dismissing. Other studies, however, have failed to uncover this specific association. In a study by Mickelson, Kessler, and Shaver (1997), both anxious–ambivalent and avoidant attachment were linked with antisocial features in a large, nationally representative sample. In analyses we previously reported, neither an anxious–ambivalent/preoccupied nor an avoidant attachment measure related to antisocial tendencies, although a secure attachment prototype was inversely linked with antisocial personality (Meyer et al., 2001). Based on this heterogeneity in findings, we concur with the conclusion reached by Bartholomew et al. (2001): "It appears that insecurity of attachment is related to antisocial tendencies, though perhaps extremity of insecurity . . . is more predictive than a specific attachment orientation" (p. 221). However, it also appears that dismissive attachment is particularly characteristic of psychopathic antisocial personalities who present with lack of empathy, callous disregard for the rights of others, and exploitative tendencies.

Lyddon and Sherry (2001) located the antisocial personality at the interface between fearful and dismissive attachment. In their view, abuse and neglect during childhood are typical antecedents of later antisocial tendencies. Such experiences convey to children that they must not be lovable, promoting negative self-images. However, they speculate that, "alternatively, a positive view of self often develops, possibly as a defense in reaction to this negative view, and may lead to a sense of entitlement" (p. 410). The self-view of the antisocial personality, according to this analysis, is negative at the core but is often masked or replaced by a positive, inflated conception of the self. Other-representations, by contrast, are thought to be more consistently negative, permeated by beliefs that others—like the abusive, vindictive attachment figures earlier in life—will not be willing to provide love and nurturance. These negative models of others, then, justify and motivate the antisocial personality's hostile interpersonal exploitation.

Lyddon and Sherry's (2001) position that the aggrandized self-view in antisocial personality is typically a defense against underlying negative self-views has been shared by some other theorists. For example, Eissler (1949, cited in Millon & Davis, 1996) "portrayed their behaviors as designed to restore feelings of omnipotence that had been severely injured in childhood. Having suffered these injustices or deprivations, these youngsters felt deeply betrayed and, hence, became mistrustful, narcissistic, self-inflating, material-seeking, and addicted to risk and excitement" (p. 438).

Others disagree, however, with the position of antisocial grandiosity as a defense. Millon and Davis (1996) emphasized that "much of the antisocials' habits of social indifference and personal exploitation are driven not by a hateful revenge . . . but by their having neither a basic awareness of others' feelings, nor a disposition to care for their welfare" (p. 461). In this view, the usual developmental precursors involve harsh adversity, but the child, instead of developing negative self-representations, simply learns that he (typically males) must fend for himself because no one else will. The message perceived by the child may not be so much "I must be unlovable because my parents do not behave as if they love me" (Lyddon & Sherry, 2001) but, instead, "It's a dog-eat-dog world: Every man for himself!" The question whether love might be available but is being withheld (and the sense of shame and inadequacy that this recognition could trigger) may never arise in the environments of abuse and neglect that are associated with antisocial behavior—giving and receiving love may truly be "unheard of." In our view, then, the positive self-views of the antisocial personality may more typically arise from the early recognition that callous abuse and exploitation herald success and result in powerful feelings of competence and mastery (see Figure 5.5).

In sum, there appears to be a reasonable consensus that extreme adversity in early child–caregiver relations can promote insecure attachment that increases the risk for later antisocial tendencies (Hill, 2003; Luntz & Widom, 1994; Rothbaum & Weisz, 1994). This prototypical developmental history may encourage the dismissive antisocial pattern, but variations around this theme appear to be common. Other risk factors, however, such as a biologically mediated incapacity to experience fear or be able to learn from punishment (e.g., Newman & Kosson, 1986; Patrick, 1994), may interact with insecure attachment in the development of later antisocial behavior. Despite the intuitively plausible pathway from early abuse or neglect to later insecure–dismissive attachment and antisocial personality, however, more longitudinal research is needed to test such models and determine the degree to which early psychopathic tendencies might cause, rather than result from, early attachment disturbances (cf. Hare, Cooke, & Hart, 1999).

Schizotypal Personality

Individuals with schizotypal personalities are acutely uncomfortable with, and have a reduced capacity for, close relationships (American Psychiatric Association, 1994). They tend to mistrust others; their appearance and behavior are eccentric or odd; they hold unusual beliefs; and they exhibit abnormalities in thinking, speech, and affect (American Psychiatric Association, 1994). Individuals with schizotypal personalities share with those having avoidant and schizoid personalities "an impoverished social life [and] a distancing from close interpersonal relationships" (Millon & Davis,

1996, p. 613). However, compared to those with avoidant and schizoid personalities, "because of their more advanced state of pathology, schizotypals frequently lead a meaningless, idle, and ineffectual existence, drifting from one aimless activity to another, remaining on the periphery of societal life, and rarely developing intimate attachments or accepting enduring responsibilities" (Millon & Davis, 1996, p. 613).

Lyddon and Sherry (2001) proposed that schizotypal personalities fit within the fearful and dismissing attachment patterns. In their view, schizotypal mistrust and suspicion suggest the presence of negative other-representations, whereas self-representations appear to vacillate "between a positive, negative, and almost nonexistent view" (Lyddon & Sherry, 2001, p. 410). These authors speculated that such mental representations flow from a cold and derogatory parenting style, where caregivers convey messages such as "You're a strange bird." Empirical evidence suggests that schizotypal personality features correlate with early adversity, such as a history of childhood sexual abuse (Norden, Klein, Donaldson, Pepper, & Klein, 1995). However, such assocations are not specific; in Norden et al.'s study, borderline, self-defeating, narcissistic, histrionic, and sadistic personality disorders were all correlated with childhood sexual abuse.

In a sample of psychiatric patients, schizotypal features correlated inversely with a secure attachment prototype, confirming that schizotypals are unlikely to feel comfortable in close relationships and have little trust that others will provide support when needed (Meyer et al., 2001). Indeed, the correlation between schizotypal features and secure attachment ($r = -.41$, $p < .01$) was relatively strong in magnitude, exceeded only by that between borderline features and secure attachment ($r = -.45$, $p < .01$). In that study, schizotypal features were also inversely related to a preoccupied attachment prototype and were positively related to an avoidant attachment prototype (Meyer et al., 2001). This pattern of correlations is consistent with the idea that insecure attachments—especially the fearful and dismissing patterns—play a significant role in this disorder. Further support was reported by Brennan and Shaver (1998), who found that the largest proportion (39%) of those with schizotypal personality fit within the fearfully attached group, whereas the smallest proportion (16%) was classified as secure.

In our view, schizotypal personality symptoms are theoretically most closely associated with dismissing attachment configurations (see Figure 5.4). Other-representations are dominantly negative, consistent with the defining feature of chronic suspiciousness and mistrustful anxiety among schizotypals. Mental representations of the self, however, may contain both positive and negative qualities, although the positive tend to be more salient than the negative qualities. In the dismissing schizotypal, the self might be experienced as exceptional or gifted, whose special talents are unfortunately misunderstood, ignored, or rejected by others (see Figure 5.5). Fearfully attached schizotypals, by contrast, might recognize to some degree that aspects of the self are somehow odd or peculiar and will likely be met with disapproval or rejection from other people. Beyond attachment processes, of course, it is important to recognize that biological processes might play a critical role in the pathogenesis of the schizotypal pattern (e.g., Dickey, McCarley, & Shenton, 2002).

ATTACHMENT VARIANTS OF OBSESSIVE–COMPULSIVE PERSONALITY

Individuals with obsessive–compulsive personality disorder (OCPD) are preoccupied "with orderliness, perfectionism, and mental and interpersonal control, at the expense of flexibility, openness, and efficiency" (American Psychiatric Association, 1994). They tend to be excessively devoted to work; their perfectionism tends to interfere with task completion; and they present as overly conscientious, rigid, and stubborn (American Psychiatric Assocation, 1994).

Millon and Davis (1996), like others before them, proposed that such symptomatology relates to internal conflicts between strongly opposing motives (akin to classic Freudian conceptions of struggles between id and superego): On the one hand, the individual with OCPD is thought to harbor hostile, oppositional, even antisocial urges (thought to be largely unconscious), and on the other, more conscious desires to submit and conform. In Millon and Davis's (1996) words:

> Inwardly, [obsessive–compulsive personalities] churn with defiance like the antisocial personality; consciously and behaviorally, they submit and comply like the dependent. To bind their rebellious and oppositional urges, and to ensure that these do not break through their controls, compulsives become overly conforming and overly submissive. (p. 506)

From an attachment perspective, this conceptualization suggests the presence of negative other-representations that motivate aggressive or oppositional urges that are, however, kept in check by compensatory conformity. Directly contrasting with this view, however, other theorists have proposed that individuals with OCPD hold positive other-models. In Lyddon and Sherry's (2001) interpretation, for example, individuals with OCPD fit into the preoccupied cluster, where negative self-models are combined with positive other-models. They speculated that OCPD styles can be traced to rigid, achievement-oriented parenting, in which nurturance was made contingent upon the child's achievement. In terms of self-models, however, "these children . . . ultimately develop a view of themselves that is inherently negative because, although they see themselves as reliable and competent, they continually fall short in the eyes of the parental figure" (pp. 408–409). The emergence of compulsive workaholism and perfectionism can be interpreted, in this view, as a continued effort to gain acceptance from attachment figures.

The conceptualization of the obsessive–compulsive personality as insecure or self-doubting is mirrored in many classical descriptions of compulsive, perfectionistic, or anankastic personalities (cf. Millon & Davis, 1996). For example, Schneider (1923, cited in Millon & Davis, 1996) held that "[this personality] is always trying to hide a nagging inner uncertainty under various forms of compensatory or overcompensatory activity. . . . Outer correctness covers an imprisoning inner insecurity" (p. 507). Such characterizations indicate negative models of the self as flawed.

To complicate matters, theorists have also proposed that the self-representations of obsessive-compulsive personalities contain certain positive elements, or may even be dominantly positive. Lyddon and Sherry (2001) noted that, despite their negative conception of consistently falling short of internalized parental standards, those with OCPD also come to view the self as reliable, competent, and righteous. Similarly, Millon and Davis (1996) noted that "these personalities see themselves as devoted to work, as industrious, reliable, meticulous, and efficient individuals" (p. 516). Leary (1957, cited in Millon & Davis, 1996) also wrote that "they present themselves as reasonable, successful, sympathetic, mature. . . . They do not complain of timidity, isolation, distrust, etc. . . . Why then, do they come to the clinic? The overwhelming majority of these patients are not self-referred" (p. 511).

Even a cursory overview, then, suggests that a conceptualization of obsessive–compulsive personality informed by attachment theory is not straightforward. In Brennan and Shaver's (1998) analyses, college students identified as obsessive–compulsive could be grouped across all four attachment types, with approximately one-third falling into the secure and fearful categories, respectively. In analyses from a psychiatric sample, DSM-III-R obsessive–compulsive features correlated slightly and inversely with secure attachment but did not correlate with preoccupied or avoidant attachment prototypes (Meyer et al., 2001). Our preliminary interpretation of these complex theoretical and empirical findings is that the obsessive–compulsive personality does not seem to correspond with great clarity to any one attachment pattern. Instead, varieties of obsessive–compulsive personalities may be distinguished across all four attachment patterns.

We propose that the obsessive–compulsive personality, in its most interpersonally responsive form, corresponds most closely to the preoccupied attachment pattern, indicating a combination of attachment anxiety and an approach orientation. According to this conceptualization, those with OCPD harbor negative self-views (the self as inferior or flawed) and desire approval from others. To prevent the feared rejection and disapproval, they compensate for perceived flaws by minimizing errors and striving for control in all domains of life. In this sense, their perfectionism can be viewed as a motivated (but not necessarily conscious) strategy to cope with rejection anxiety and to fulfill attachment needs.

Other variants of obsessive–compulsive personality, however, also appear plausible and may be common clinically. For example, some fearful individuals with OCPD seem to experience the self as deeply inadequate and feel certain that rejection would follow if others were allowed to penetrate the "defensive armor" of pedantic perfectionism. In this case, obsessive–compulsive symptoms function defensively to create interpersonal distance in order to prevent otherwise certain rejection. In dismissing individuals with OCPD, a positive view of the self as righteous and responsible is coupled with negative views of others as messy and undependable. Symptoms such as the characteristic orderliness can be understood as motivated (but not necessarily conscious) efforts to maintain positive self-representations and create distance from inferior others. The empirical merit of these speculations, of course, remains to be evaluated. The fact that such variants seem plausible clinically highlights the importance of determining the motives underlying attachment behavior rather than relying on the form of the behavior alone, an observation that applies not only for obsessive-compulsive personality disorder but for all others as well.

DIMINISHED ATTACHMENT MOTIVATION: SCHIZOID PERSONALITY

Current definitions of schizoid personality characterize this disorder as stemming from "a fundamental defect in the ability to form social relationships and an underreponsiveness to all forms of stimulation" (Millon & Davis, 1996, p. 217). Individuals with schizoid features are disinterested in sexual and other close relationships; they prefer solitary activities; and they present as aloof, detached, emotionally bland, passive, and lacking in empathy (American Psychiatric Organization, 1994; Millon & Davis, 1996). In contrast to avoidant personality, where the solitary style is explained by a fear of humiliation coupled with a desire for close relationships, the solitary nature of schizoid personality is not regarded as self-protective or defensive. Instead, schizoid personalities are viewed as truly—and simply—incapable of and disinterested in forming attachments.

Theorists have offered contrasting interpretations regarding the processes accounting for the schizoid's social indifference and detachment.

One view is that constitutional risk factors (e.g., passive temperament and neurological deficits) operate to create the lack of sociability of the schizoid personality. Once this social incapacity is in place, regardless of its specific origin, the detachment is viewed as self-perpetuating. A contrasting view highlights the influence of early family transactions, which might interact with preexisting vulnerabilities. Millon and Davis (1996) speculated on this pathway:

> Constitutionally unresponsive infants . . . who evoke few reactions from the environment, may experience a compounding of their initial activation and sensory deficits. Such children receive little attention, cuddling, and affection from their parents and, as a consequence, are deprived of the social and emotional cues requisite to learning human attachment behaviors. (p. 246)

From an attachment perspective, the indifferent distancing in schizoid personality disorder appears to indicate a fundamental incapacity to form attachments—literally a detachment. Not all attachment theorists agree, though, with this interpretation. For example, Brennan and Shaver (1998), West, Rose, and Sheldon-Keller (1994), and Lyddon and Sherry (2001) argued that schizoid personality might indicate dismissing attachment rather than below-average attachment motivation. Clinically, however, people with dismissing attachment tend to be at least somewhat interested in, and have some capacity for, forming attachments, even though they typically prefer interpersonal distance (Bartholomew et al., 2001). Indeed, those with dismissing attachments often do have sexual relationships (unlike schizoid personalities), and they often use casual sexual relationships as an alternative to more psychologically risky, committed partnerships (Brennan & Shaver, 1995).

Unfortunately, there is a lack of data to clarify whether dismissing attachment or an inherent attachment incapacity might better explain the prototypical schizoid personality. In a diagnostically heterogeneous sample, the severity of schizoid symptoms correlated inversely with a measure of preoccupied attachment and positively with a measure of avoidant attachment, suggesting that dismissive avoidance might well play a role in this disorder (Meyer et al., 2001). Similarly, in our pilot study (see Table 5.1), schizoid features among undergraduates correlated slightly with avoidance but not with attachment anxiety, and those with relatively pronounced schizoid features could be located within the dismissing attachment quadrant (see Figure 5.4). Nevertheless, such cross-sectional associations do not reveal whether the strength of attachment motivation itself is also compromised and is perhaps a better indicator of schizoid features. In our view, clinical and theoretical descriptions suggest that a failure to develop attachments rather than classic dismissing attachment is a core feature in schizoid personality. As a disorder of detachment, we would expect the self- and other-models of schizoid personalities to be underdeveloped and impoverished. Representations of others by prototypical schizoids may be simple, sterile, and lacking in affect. This characterization should apply equally to self-models in schizoid personality, which are confined primarily to descriptions of outward characteristics and social roles, without significant development of psychological attributes (e.g., hopes, wishes, fears, goals, intentions, or values) or the use of attachment terms. In this respect, there might be some resemblance between schizoid personality and certain forms of autistic spectrum disorders (Millon & Davis, 1996). Nevertheless, schizoid personality and autism are clearly distinct. Individuals with schizoid personalities, for example, often appear outwardly "normal," have no obvious disturbances in language, and fit in society despite inner detachment (cf. Millon & Davis, 1996).

SUMMARY AND CONCLUSIONS

We argued in this chapter that attachment theory can add to our understanding of the etiology and motivational dynamics creating and maintaining personality disorders. Nevertheless, it would be unrealistic to expect that Bowlby's theory could or should replace models that examine personality disorders from other conceptual perspectives. In our interpretation, adult attachment patterns and personality disorders are "made of the same stuff"—both can be construed as cognitive–affective–motivational patterns that are triggered in response to situational contingencies and have a partial "agentic" character. That is, they are motivated and goal directed but nevertheless are triggered automatically and executed without full volitional control. Among the many cognitive–affective units that mediate both attachment patterns and personality disorder symptoms, we highlighted the importance of mental representations of self and others and the interpersonal strategies facilitated by such models. Many of the personality disorders described in the current diagnostic nomenclature can be construed as prototypical patterns of mental representations, of characteristic early experiences that give rise to these representations, and of distinctive interpersonal goals and strategies that are linked to these models and that provide the mechanisms by which these personalities create the particular social environments that perpetuate their maladjustment.

We agree with other theorists who view some, but not all, DSM-IV personality disorders as conceptually amenable to an attachment perspective (e.g., Bartholomew et al., 2001). Specifically, dependent, borderline, and histrionic personalities can be construed as variants of preoccupied attachment and avoidant personality as a variant of fearful attachment.

Attachment interpretations of other personality disorders are somewhat more difficult and tentative, however. In schizoid personality, a dismissing pattern in which others are devalued and ignored appears common, although schizoid detachment might be even better construed as stemming from impoverished, underdeveloped attachment needs. In some cases of narcissistic, schizotypal, paranoid, antisocial, and obsessive–compulsive personality, negative other-models may also be present and motivate a preference for distancing, avoidant strategies. Thus, these disorders may combine aspects of fearful and dismissing attachment. Finally, obsessive–compulsive strategies may flow from any of the attachment patterns, although psychosocial consequences and phenomenology may differ depending on which motivational currents direct the pedantic and perfectionistic obsessive–compulsive strategies.

One general conclusion, then, is that models assuming a one-to-one correspondence between each personality disorder and a particular attachment pattern are not reasonable. The cognitive–affective–motivational patterns defining personality disorders can reflect, and be motivated by, various combinations of attachment-related mental models and interpersonal strategies. For example, as outlined previously, pedantic perfectionism among obsessive–compulsive personalities may be motivated by the desire to gain approval from others in order to maintain positive self-views, or—in another variant—by the desire to avoid rejection and negate negative self-views. Such differences between approach versus avoidance motivation are not trivial and have clear implications for symptomatic experience and well-being (Emmons, 1996; Higgins, 1996).

A related conclusion is that insecure forms of attachment are probably best viewed as risk factors but not absolute determinants of specific forms of later personality pathology (cf. Pilkonis, 2001). That is, most people with insecure attachment do not go on to develop such pathology, even though a high proportion of those with significant personality disturbance may exhibit early as well as concurrent attachment disturbances.

There are additional questions we hope to have raised in this chapter. Our review suggests, for instance, that many personality disorders may combine "core" negative self-representations with "defensive" positive self-models. Thus, narcissistic grandiosity may sometimes emerge in response to intense self-doubts, obsessive–compulsive perfectionism in response to inadequate self-views, and paranoid righteousness as a compensation for views of the self as injured and mistreated. But how and why do such compensatory processes occur? And to what degree are they central to the etiology and maintenance of personality disorder symptoms?

One answer to these questions relates to people's ubiquitous desire to maintain positive self-regard. The need for self-worth is often considered central in human motivation (e.g., Baumeister, 1991), and social psychologists have described many ways in which even those without personality disorders habitually distort reality or strategically defend against threats to their positive self-images. When events are encountered that have clear negative implications for the self (such as being repeatedly rejected), people often engage in strategic action to minimize or defuse the threat. They may avoid thinking in detail about the events; they may reinterpret the meaning of the events or reframe them in a positive light; they may mentally relegate the events to the past, thereby defusing their negative implications for self-worth; and they may avoid situations entailing the risk for additional humiliation or defeat (cf. Baumeister, 1996).

We suspect that, in a similar fashion, the positive façades in some of the personality disorders may come to exist through repeated and motivated efforts to maintain self-regard amidst adversity and humiliation. Attachment theory suggests that some of the most profound forms of adversity are early interpersonal experiences of loss, separation, rejection, and neglect that skew internal models of self and others. Facing and accepting undesirable self-aspects may be too threatening, in many cases, and the escape into unrealistically positive fictions about the self—which later become self-perpetuating—may be a preferred and less painful alternative. In that sense, the grandiose, righteous, or perfect views of the narcissistic, paranoid, and obsessive–compulsive personalities, respectively, may be understood as stemming from avoidance maneuvers. The painful confrontation with an unpleasant reality about the self is avoided, but at the cost of sustaining false self-images. It is increasingly recognized that such forms of experiential avoidance may be at the core of many forms of psychopathology, not just personality disorders (Hayes, Wilson, Gifford, Follette, & Strosahl, 1997). Even in anxiety disorders, alcohol problems, or eating disorders, pathology may arise or be intensified by consistent efforts to avoid dealing with unpleasant aspects of physical or mental reality.

IMPLICATIONS FOR INTERVENTION

From the perspective of attachment theory, one of the most important messages for parents is that, contrary to still common but misleading assumptions, "consistently providing infants' needs does not condemn them to perpetual dependency, but in fact serves as the springboard for self-reliance because it instills a sense of efficacy concerning the environment" (Weinfield et al., 1999, p. 78). In addition, there are other, more direct implications of attachment theory for therapeutic practice, and a literature is emerging in recent years that documents empirically how attachment styles are associated with aspects of the therapeutic alliance and outcome (Meyer & Pilkonis, 2002).

One of the crucial tasks for therapists working from an attachment perspective with patients with personality disorders may be to insist on an attachment "diagnosis," that is, to incorporate into their work an assessment of specific models of self and others and the relations between the two as well as dominant interpersonal strategies. For that purpose, the recently developed attachment questionnaires may be good starting point, but a reliance only on questionnaires would be insufficient. Therapists must also cultivate their listening skills in order to infer what patients' conversational styles reveal about their internal models. In short, they must become implicit and accurate AAI raters, constantly attending to parameters such as the coherence, emotional balance, and genuineness of patients' interpersonal accounts. Slade (1999), for example, refuses to advocate for a specific form of "attachment therapy" but argues instead that "an understanding of the nature and dynamics of attachment *informs* rather than *defines* intervention and clinical thinking" (p. 577).

Therapists and therapy researchers also are called on to study how to establish optimal alliances with patients with different attachment patterns. Skillfully building a therapeutic alliance also requires therapists to develop an awareness of the complexities with which cognitive–affective units interact in creating personality disturbance. Therapists can, and must, learn how to recognize which situational triggers "turn on" the dominant, problematic interpersonal strategies, but also which contingencies "turn off" or deactivate such patterns. Despite Slade's reservations about "attachment therapy" per se, patients are likely to benefit from psychoeducation about attachment themes as they influence the development of personality, adaptation, and coping. Patients are often quick to recognize themselves in the typologies and dimensions proposed for attachment behavior, precisely because struggles regarding attachment are universal developmental issues. Finally, patients may be willing to collaborate in changing attachment styles as a goal of therapy, and we hope that our observations here may encourage such work.

REFERENCES

Ainsworth, M. D. S. (1967). *Infancy in Uganda: Infant care and the growth of attachment.* Baltimore: Johns Hopkins University Press.
Ainsworth, M. D., S., Blehar, M. C., Waters, E., & Wall, S. (1978). *Pattern of attachment: Psychological study of the Strange Situation.* Hillsdale, NJ: Erlbaum.
American Psychiatric Association. (1987). *Diagnostic and statistical manual of mental disorders* (3rd ed., rev.). Washington, DC: Author.
American Psychiatric Association. (1994). *Diagnostic and statistical manual of mental disorders* (4th ed.). Washington, DC: Author.

Anders, S. L., & Tucker, J. S. (2000). Adult attachment style, interpersonal communication competence, and social support. *Personal Relationships, 7*, 379–389.

Arntz, A., & Veen, G. (2001). Evaluations of others by borderline patients. *Journal of Nervous and Mental Disease, 189*, 513–521.

Bargh, J. A. (1997). The automaticity of everyday life. In R. S. Wyer, Jr. (Ed.), *Advances in social cognition* (Vol. 10, pp. 1–61). Mahwah, NJ: Erlbaum.

Bargh, J. A., Chen, M., & Burrows, L. (1996). Automaticity of social behavior: Direct effects of trait construct and stereotype activation on action. *Journal of Personality and Social Psychology, 71*, 230–244.

Bargh, J. A., & Ferguson, M. J. (2000). Beyond behaviorism: On the automaticity of higher mental processes. *Psychological Bulletin, 126*, 925–945.

Bartholomew, K., & Horowitz, L. (1991). Attachment styles among young adults: A test of a model. *Journal of Social and Personality Psychology, 61*, 226–244.

Bartholomew, K., Kwong, M. J., & Hart, S. D. (2001). Attachment. In J. W. Livesley (Ed.), *Handbook of personality disorders: Theory, research, and treatment* (pp. 196–230). New York: Guilford Press.

Baumeister, R. F. (1991). *Meanings of life.* New York: Guilford Press.

Baumeister, R. F. (1996). Self-regulation and ego threat: Motivated cognition, self deception, and destructive goal setting. In P. M. Gollwitzer & J. A. Bargh (Eds.), *The psychology of action: Linking cognition and motivation to behavior* (pp. 27–47). New York: Guilford Press.

Baumeister, R. F., & Leary, M. R. (1995). The need to belong: Desire for interpersonal attachments as a fundamental human motivation. *Psychological Bulletin, 117*, 497–529.

Beck, A. T. (1983). Cognitive therapy of depression: New approaches. In P. Clayton & J. Barrett (Eds.), *Treatment of depression: Old and new approaches* (pp. 265–290). New York: Raven Press.

Beck, A. T., & Freeman, A., & Associates. (1990). *Cognitive therapy of personality disorders.* New York: Guilford Press.

Blaney, P. H. (1999). Paranoid conditions. In T. Millon, P. H. Blaney, & R. D. Davis (Eds.), *Oxford textbook of psychopathology* (pp. 339–361). New York: Oxford University Press.

Blatt, S. J., Quinlan, D. M., Chevron, E. S., McDonald, C., & Zuroff, D. (1982). Dependency and self-criticism: Psychological dimensions of depression. *Journal of Consulting and Clinical Psychology, 50*, 113–124.

Bornstein, R. F. (1992). The dependent personality: Developmental, social, and clinical perspectives. *Psychological Bulletin, 112*, 3–23.

Bornstein, R. F. (1998). Implicit and self-attributed dependency needs in dependent and histrionic personality disorders. *Journal of Personality Assessment, 71*, 1–14.

Bornstein, R. F. (1999). Dependent and histrionic personality disorders. In T. Millon, P. H. Blaney, & R. D. Davis (Eds.), *Oxford textbook of psychopathology* (pp. 535–554). New York: Oxford University Press.

Bowlby, J. (1958). The nature of the child's tie to his mother. *International Journal of Psycho-Analysis, 39*, 350–373.

Bowlby, J. (1969). *Attachment and loss: Vol. 1. Attachment.* New York: Basic Books.

Bowlby, J. (1973). *Attachment and loss: Vol. 2. Separation.* New York: Basic Books.

Bowlby, J. (1980). *Attachment and loss: Vol. 3. Loss.* New York: Basic Books.

Bowlby, J. (1988). *A secure base: Clinical applications of attachment theory.* London: Routledge.

Brennan, K. A., Clark, C. L., & Shaver, P. R. (1998). Self-report measurement of adult attachment: An integrative overview. In J. A. Simpson & W. S. Rholes (Eds.), *Attachment theory and close relationships* (pp. 46–76). New York: Guilford Press.

Brennan, K. A., & Shaver, P. R. (1995). Dimensions of adult attachment, affect regulation, and romantic relationships functioning. *Personality and Social Psychology Bulletin, 21,* 267–283.

Brennan, K. A., & Shaver, P. R. (1998). Attachment styles and personality disorders: Their connections to each other and to parental divorce, parental death, and perceptions of parental caregiving. *Journal of Personality, 66,* 835–878.

Bretherton, I., & Munholland, K. A. (1999). Internal working models in attachment relationships: A construct revisited: A. In J. Cassidy & P. R. Shaver (Eds.), *Handbook of attachment: Theory, research, and clinical applications* (pp. 89–111). New York: Guilford Press.

Buchheim, A., Kächele, H., Pokorny, D., Strauss, M., Simons, C., Hölzer, M, & Strauss, B. (2003, June). *Convergent validity of different attachment measures in patients with anxiety disorders: A pilot study.* Paper presented at the annual convention of the Society for Psychotherapy Research, Weimar, Germany.

Butler, A. C., Brown, G. K., Beck, A. T., & Grisham, J. R. (2002). Assessment of dysfunctional beliefs in borderline personality disorder. *Behaviour Research and Therapy, 40,* 1231–1240.

Carlson, E. (1998). A prospective longitudinal study of attachment disorganization/disorientation. *Child Development, 69,* 1107–1128.

Carver, C. S., & Scheier, M. F. (1998). *On the self-regulation of behavior.* New York: Cambridge University Press.

Cassidy, J. (1994). Emotion regulation: Influences of attachment relationships. *Monographs of the Society for Research in Child Development, 59,* 228–283.

Cassidy, J., & Shaver, P. R. (1999). *Handbook of attachment: Theory, research, and clinical applications.* New York: Guilford Press.

Cervone, D., & Shoda, Y. (1999). *The coherence of personality.* New York: Guilford Press.

Costa, P. T. Jr., & Widiger, T. A. (2002). *Personality disorders and the five-factor model of personality* (2nd ed.). Washington, DC: American Psychological Association.

Coyne, J. C., & Downey, G. (1991). Social factors and psychopathology: Stress, social support, and coping processes. *Annual Review of Psychology, 42,* 401–425.

Crittenden, P. M. (1988). Relationships at risk. In J. Belsky & T. Neyworski (Eds.), *Clinical implications of attachment* (pp. 136–174). Hillsdale, NJ: Erlbaum.

DeWolff, M., & van IJzendoorn, M. (1997). Sensitivity and attachment: A meta-analysis on parental antecedents of infant attachment. *Child Development, 68,* 571–591.

Dickey, C. C., McCarley, R. W., & Shenton, M. E. (2002). The brain in schizotypal personality disorder: A review of structural MRI and CT findings. *Harvard Review of Psychiatry, 10*, 1–15.

Dutton, D. G., Saunders, K., Starzomski, A., & Bartholomew, K. (1994). Intimacy-anger and insecure attachment as precursors of abuse in intimate relationships. *Journal of Applied Social Psychology, 24*, 1367–1386.

Emmons, R. A. (1996). Striving and feeling: Personal goals and subjective well-being. In P. M. Gollwitzer & J. M. Bargh (Eds.), *The psychology of action: Linking cognition and motivation to behavior* (pp. 313–337). New York: Guilford Press.

Feeney, J. A. (1999). Adult romantic attachment and couple relationships. In J. Cassidy & P. R. Shaver (Eds.), *Handbook of attachment: Theory, research, and clinical applications* (pp. 355–377). New York: Guilford Press.

Feske, U., Perry, K. J., Chambless, D. L., Renneberg, B., & Goldstein, A. J. (1996). Avoidant personality disorder as a predictor for treatment outcome among generalized social phobics. *Journal of Personality Disorders, 10*, 174–184.

First, M. B., Spitzer, R. L., Gibbon, M., & Williams, J. B. W. (1997). *User's guide for the Structured Clinical Interview for DSM-IV Axis II disorders.* Washington, DC: American Psychiatric Press.

Fonagy, P., Gergely, G., Jurist, E. L., & Target, M. (2002). *Affect regulation, mentalization, and the development of self.* New York: Other Press.

Fonagy, P., Leigh, T., Steele, M., Steele, H., Kennedy, R., Mattoon, G., Target, M., & Gerber, A. (1996). The relation of attachment status, psychiatric classification, and response to psychotherapy. *Journal of Consulting and Clinical Psychology, 64*, 22–31.

Fossati, A., Feeney, J. A., Donati, D., Donini, M., Novella, L., Bagnato, M., Carretta, I., Leonardi, B., Mirabelli, S., & Maffei, C. (2003). Personality disorders and adult attachment dimensions in a mixed psychiatric sample: A multivariate study. *Journal of Nervous and Mental Disease, 191*, 30–37.

Fraley, R. C. (2002). Attachment stability from infancy to adulthood: Meta-analysis and dynamic modeling of developmental mechanisms. *Personality and Social Psychology Bulletin, 6*, 123–151.

Fraley, R. C., Waller, N. G., & Brennan, K. A. (2000). An item response theory analysis of self-report measures of adult attachment. *Journal of Personality and Social Psychology, 78*, 350–365.

Gabbard, G. (1989). Two subtypes of narcissistic personality disorder. *Bulletin of the Menninger Clinic, 53*, 527–532.

George, C., Kaplan, N., & Main, M. (1985). *The adult attachment interview.* Unpublished manuscript, University of California at Berkeley, Department of Psychology.

Goldsmith, H. H., & Alansky, J. A. (1987). Maternal and infant temperamental predictors of attachment: A meta-analytic review. *Journal of Consulting and Clinical Psychology, 55*, 805–816.

Hare, R. D., Cooke, D. J., & Hart, S. D. (1999). Psychopathy and sadistic personality disorder. In T. Millon, P. H. Blaney, & R. D. Davis (Eds.), *Oxford textbook of psychopathology* (pp. 555–584). New York: Oxford University Press.

Harlow, H. F. (1958). The nature of love. *American Psychologist, 13*, 673.

Hawkley, L. C., & Cacioppo, J. T. (2003). Loneliness and pathways to disease. *Brain, Behavior and Immunity, 17,* 98–105.

Hayes, S. C., Wilson, K. G., Gifford, E. V.. Follette, V. M., & Strosahl, K. (1996). Emotional avoidance and behavioral disorders: A functional dimensional approach to diagnosis and treatment. *Journal of Consulting and Clinical Psychology, 64,* 1152–1168.

Hazan, C., & Shaver, P. R. (1987). Romantic love conceptualized as an attachment process. *Journal of Personality and Social Psychology, 52,* 511–524.

Hazan, C., & Shaver, P. R. (1990). Love and work: An attachment theoretical perspective. *Journal of Personality and Social Psychology, 59,* 270–280.

Hazan, C., & Shaver, P. R. (1994). Attachment as an organizational framework for research on close relationships. *Psychological Inquiry, 5,* 1–22.

Herbert, J. D., Hope, D. A., & Bellack, A. S. (1992). Validity of the distinction between generalized social phobia and avoidant personality disorder. *Journal of Abnormal Psychology, 101,* 332–339.

Hesse, E. (1999). The Adult Attachment Interview: Historical and current perspectives. In J. Cassidy & P. R. Shaver (Eds.), *Handbook of attachment: Theory, research, and clinical applications* (pp. 395–433). New York: Guilford Press.

Higgins, E. T. (1996). Ideals, oughts, and regulatory focus: Affect and motivation from distinct pains and pleasures. In P. M. Gollwitzer & J. A. Bargh (Eds.), *The psychology of action: Linking cognition and motivation to behavior* (pp. 91–114). New York: Guilford Press.

Hill, J. (2003). Early identification of individuals at risk for antisocial personality disorder. *British Journal of Psychiatry, 182*(Suppl. 44), 11–14.

Kinderman, P., & Bentall, R. P. (1996) Self-discrepancies and persecutory delusions: Evidence for a defensive model of paranoid ideation. *Journal of Abnormal Psychology, 105,* 106–114.

Kinderman, P., & Bentall, R. P. (1997). Causal attributions in paranoia and depression: Internal, personal, and situational attributions for negative events. *Journal of Abnormal Psychology, 106,* 341–345.

Kobak, R. (1999). The emotional dynamics of disruptions in attachment relationships: Implications for theory, research, and clinical intervention. In J. Cassidy & P. R. Shaver (Eds.), *Handbook of attachment: Theory, research, and clinical applications* (pp. 21–43). New York: Guilford Press.

Linehan, M. (1993). *Cognitive-behavioral treatment of borderline personality disorder.* New York: Guilford Press.

Lorenz, K. (1935). Der Kumpan in der Umwelt des Vogels. *Journal of Ornithology, 83,* 137–413.

Luntz, B. K., & Widom, C. S. (1994). Antisocial personality disorder in abused and neglected children grown up. *American Journal of Psychiatry, 151,* 670–674.

Lyddon, W. J., & Sherry, A. (2001). Developmental personality styles: An attachment theoretical conceptualization of personality disorders. *Journal of Counseling and Developing, 70,* 405–414.

Lyons-Ruth, K., & Jacobvitz, D. (1999). Attachment disorganization: Unresolved loss, relational violence, and lapses in behavioural and attentional strategies. In J. Cassidy & P. R. Shaver (Eds.), *Handbook of attachment: Theory, research, and clinical applications* (pp. 520–554). New York: Guilford Press.

Main, M., Kaplan, N., & Cassidy, J. (1985). Security in infancy, childhood, and adulthood: A move to the level of representation. In I. Bretherton & E. Waters (Eds.), *Growing points in attachment theory and research* (pp. 66–104). *Monographs of the Society for Research in Child Development, 50*, Serial No. 209.

Main, M., & Solomon, J. (1990). Procedures for identifying insecure-disorganized/disoriented infants: Procedures, findings, and implications for the classification of behavior. In M. Greenberg, D. Cicchetti, & M. Cummings (Eds.), *Attachment in preschool years: Theory, research, and intervention* (pp. 121–160). Chicago: University of Chicago Press.

Mallinckrodt, B. (2000). Attachment, social competencies, social support, and interpersonal process in psychotherapy. *Psychotherapy Research, 10*, 239–266.

McCranie, E. W., & Bass, J. D. (1984). Childhood family antecedents of dependency and self-criticism. *Journal of Abnormal Psychology, 93*, 3–8.

Meyer, B., & Carver, C. S. (2000). Negative childhood accounts, sensitivity, and pessimism: A study of avoidant personality disorder features in college students. *Journal of Personality Disorders, 14*, 233–248.

Meyer, B., & Pilkonis, P. A. (2002). Attachment style. In J. A. Norcross (Ed.), *Psychotherapy relationships that work: Therapists' relational contributions to effective psychotherapy* (pp. 367–382). London: Oxford University Press.

Meyer, B., Pilkonis, P. A., & Beevers, C. G. (2004). What's in a (neutral) face?: Personality disorders, attachment styles, and the appraisal of ambiguous social cues. *Journal of Personality Disorders, 18*, 320–336.

Meyer, B., Pilkonis, P. A., Proietti, J., Heape, C., & Egan, M. (2001). Attachment styles and personality disorders as predictors of treatment response. *Journal of Personality Disorders, 15*, 371–389.

Mickelson, K. D., Kessler, R. C., & Shaver, P. R. (1997). Adult attachment in a nationally representative sample. *Journal of Personality and Social Psychology, 73*, 1092–1106.

Millon T., & Davis, R. D. (1996). *Disorders of personality: DSM-IV and beyond.* New York: Wiley.

Mischel, W., & Shoda, Y. (1995). A cognitive-affective system theory of personality: Reconceptualizing situations, dispositions, dynamics, and invariance in personality structure. *Psychological Review, 102*, 246–268.

Newman, J. P., & Kosson, D. S. (1986). Passive avoidance learning in psychopathic and nonpsychopathic offenders. *Journal of Abnormal Psychology, 95*, 252–256.

Norden, K. A., Klein, D. N., Donaldson, S. K, Pepper, C. M., & Klein, L. M. (1995). Reports of the early home environment in DSM-III-R personality disorders. *Journal of Personality Disorders, 9*, 213–223.

Parker, G., & Lipscombe, P. (1980). The relevance of early parental experiences to adult dependency, hypochondriasis and utilization of primary physicians. *British Journal of Medical Psychology, 53*, 355–363.

Patrick, C. J. (1994). Emotion and psychopathology: Startling new insights. *Psychophysiology, 31*, 319–330.

Patrick, M., Hobson, R. P., Castle, D., Howard, R., & Maughn, B. (1994). Personality disorder and the mental representation of early social experience. *Development and Psychopathology, 6,* 375–388.

Pilkonis, P. A. (1988). Personality prototypes among depressives: Themes of dependency and autonomy. *Journal of Personality Disorders, 2,* 144–152.

Pilkonis, P. A. (1995). Commentary on avoidant personality disorder: Temperament, shame, or both? In W. J. Livesley (Ed.), *The DSM-IV personality disorders* (pp. 234–238). New York: Guilford Press.

Pilkonis, P. A. (2001). Treatment of personality disorders in association with symptom disorders. In J. W. Livesley (Ed.), *Handbook of personality disorders: Theory, research, and treatment* (pp. 541–554). New York: Guilford Press.

Rosenstein, D. S., & Horowitz, H. A. (1996). Adolescent attachment and psychopathology. *Journal of Consulting and Clinical Psychology, 64,* 244–253.

Rothbaum, F., & Weisz, J. (1994). Parental caregiving and child externalizing behavior in nonclinical samples: A meta-analysis. *Psychological Bulletin, 116,* 55–74.

Sack, A., Sperling, M. B., Fagen, G., & Foelsch, P. (1996). Attachment style, history, and behavioral contrasts for a borderline and nomal sample. *Journal of Personality Disorders, 10,* 88–102.

Schore, A. N. (1997). Early organization of the nonlinear right brain and development of a predisposition to psychiatric disorders. *Development and Psychopathology, 9,* 595–631.

Schore, A. N. (2000). Attachment and the regulation of the right brain. Attachment and *Human Development, 2,* 23–47.

Shaver, P. R., & Mikulciner, M. (2002). Attachment-related psychodynamics. *Attachment and Human Development, 4,* 133–161.

Sheldon, A. E. R., & West, M. (1990). Attachment pathology and low social skills in avoidant personality disorder: An exploratory study. *Canadian Journal of Psychiatry, 35,* 596–599.

Siever, L. J., & Davis, K. L. (1991). A psychobiological perspective on the personality disorders. *American Journal of Psychiatry, 148,* 1647–1658.

Simpson, J. A., & Rholes, W. S. (Eds.). (1998). *Attachment theory and close relationships.* New York: Guilford Press.

Slade, A. (1999). Attachment theory and research: Implications for the theory and practice of individual psychotherapy with adults. In J. Cassidy & P. R. Shaver (Eds.), *Handbook of attachment: Theory, research, and clinical applications* (pp. 575–594). New York: Guilford Press.

Stalker, C., & Davies, F. (1995). Attachment organization and adaptation in sexually abused women. *Canadian Journal of Psychiatry, 40,* 234–240.

Stein, H., Jacobs, N. J., Ferguson, K. S., Allen, J. G., & Fonagy, P. (1998). What do adult attachment scales measure? *Bulletin of the Menninger Clinic, 62,* 33–82.

Strauss, B. M., Lobo-Drost, A. J., & Pilkonis, P. A. (1999). Einschätzung von bindungsstilen bei erwachsenen: Erste erfahrungen mit der deutschen version einer prototypenbeurteilung (Evaluation of attachment styles among adults: First experiences with the German version of a prototype rating system). *Zeitschrift für Klinische Psychologie, Psychiatrie, und Psychotherapie, 47,* 347–422.

Stravynski, A., Elie, R., & Franche, R. L. (1989). Perceptions of early parenting by patients diagnosed with avoidant personality disorder: A test of the overprotection hypothesis. *Acta Psychiatrica Scandinavica, 80,* 415–420.

Trull, T. J., Widiger, T. A., & Frances, A. (1987). Covariation of criteria sets for avoidant, schizoid, and dependent personality disorders. *American Journal of Psychiatry, 144,* 767–771.

van IJzendoorn, M. H. (1995). Adult attachment representations, parental responsiveness, and infant attachment: A meta-analysis on the predictive validity of the Adult Attachment Interview. *Psychological Bulletin, 117,* 387–403.

Vaughn, B. E., & Bost, K. K. (1999). Attachment and temperament: Redundant, independent, or interacting influences on interpersonal adaptation and personality development? In J. Cassidy & P. R. Shaver (Eds.), *Handbook of attachment: Theory, research, and clinical applications* (pp. 198–225). New York: Guilford Press.

Warren, S. L., Huston, L., Egeland, B., & Sroufe, L. A. (1997). Child and adolescent anxiety disorders and early attachment. *Journal of the American Academy of Child and Adolescent Psychiatry, 36,* 637–644.

Weinfield, N. S., Sroufe, A. L., Egeland, B., & Carlson, E. A. (1999). The nature of individual differences in infant-caregiver attachment. In J. Cassidy & P. R. Shaver (Eds.), *Handbook of attachment: Theory, research, and clinical applications* (pp. 68–88). New York: Guilford Press.

West, M., Rose, S., & Sheldon-Keller, A. (1994). Assessment of patterns of insecure attachment in adults and application to dependent and schizoid personality disorders. *Journal of Personality Disorders, 8,* 249–256.

Wink, P. (1991). Two faces of narcissism. *Journal of Personality and Social Psychology, 61,* 590–597.

Yen, S., Sr., Shea, M. T., Battle, C. L., Johnson, D. M., Zlotnick, C., Dolan-Sewell, R., Skodol, A. E., Grilo, C. M., Gunderson, J. G., Sanislow, C. A., Zanarini, M. C., Bender, D. S., Rettew, J. B., & McGlashan, T. H. (2002). Traumatic exposure and posttraumatic stress disorder in borderline, schizotypal, avoidant and obsessive–compulsive personality disorders: Findings from the Collaborative Longitudinal Personality Disorders Study. *Journal of Nervous and Mental Disease, 190,* 510–518.

Young, L. J. (2002). The neurobiology of social recognition: Approach, and avoidance. *Biological Psychiatry, 51,* 18–26.

Zanarini, M. C., Williams, A. A., Lewis, R. E., Reich, R. B., Vera, S. C., Marino, M. F., Levin, A., Yong, L., & Frankenburg, F. R. (1997). Reported pathological childhood experiences associated with the development of borderline personality disorders. *American Journal of Psychiatry, 154,* 1101–1106.

Zayas, V., Shoda, Y., & Ayduk, O. N. (2002). Personality in context: An interpersonal systems perspective. *Journal of Personality, 70,* 851–900.

Zimmerman, P. (1999). Structure and functions of internal working models of attachment and their role for emotion regulation. *Attachment and Human Development, 1,* 291–306.

CHAPTER 6

■ ■ ■

A Contemporary Integrative Interpersonal Theory of Personality Disorders

AARON L. PINCUS

In this chapter, I continue to develop an approach to the definition and description of personality disorders based on a contemporary integrative interpersonal theory (CIIT) of personality (Pincus & Ansell, 2003). I begin with a discussion of some current issues in the classification and diagnosis of personality disorders in order to contextualize this effort and highlight salient concerns that the application of CIIT attempts to address. This is followed by an outline of the theoretical foundations of CIIT and sections that apply the theory to both definition of personality disorder and description of individual differences in the expression of personality pathology (see also Pincus, in press).

A NEW ERA IN THE STUDY
OF PERSONALITY DISORDERS

Since the earliest clinical nosologies of the 20th century (e.g., Abraham, 1921/1927; Kraepelin, 1907; Reich, 1933/1949; Schneider, 1923/1950), psychopathologists, personologists, and practitioners have recognized the existence of abnormal personalities and the therapeutic benefits of conceptualizing and classifying them as pathological phenomena that are relatively distinct from symptom syndromes. In many ways, these efforts culminated in the publication of the third edition of the *Diagnostic and Statistical Manual of Mental Disorders* (DSM-III; American Psychiatric Association, 1980), which was clearly a landmark event for the clinical science of personality disorder. DSM-III provided a separate diagnostic axis (Axis II) on which personality disorders were to be evaluated and also introduced the contemporary categories of avoidant, borderline, dependent, and narcissistic personality disorder to the official nomenclature. For twenty years, DSM-III Axis II and its subsequent revisions (DSM-III-R [American Psychiatric Association, 1987], DSM-IV [American Psychiatric Association, 1994], and DSM-IV-TR [American Psychiatric Association, 2000]) provided a stimulus and an organizing framework for a remarkably rich period of theoretical development and empirical investigation into the nature, classification, and treatment of personality disorders. The advances stimulated by the DSM Axis II categories of personality disorder have been invaluable to clinical science and practice; however, it appears that the by the end of 20th century the benefits of the approach were exhausted. There has clearly been a shift in the *zeitgeist* of clinical science of personality disorders and efforts to define, classify, diagnose, and treat personality disorders in the 21st century are emerging in the post DSM-III/DSM-IV era (Livesley, 2001).

This shift has accelerated in recent years as a number of leading personality disorder investigators have published increasingly explicit and critical assessments of the DSM system of classifying and diagnosing personality disorders based on psychometric, theoretical, and clinical grounds (Bornstein, 1997, 2003; Clark, Livesley, & Morey, 1997; Cloninger, 2000; Endler & Kocovski, 2002; Hartung & Widiger, 1998; Livesley, 2001; Millon, 2000; Parker et al., 2002; Westen & Arkowitz-Westen, 1998; Westen & Shedler, 2000; Widiger, 2000; Widiger & Sankis, 2000). For example, Livesley (2001) stated:

> Despite the progress of the last 20 years, problems with the DSM model are all too obvious. The approach has limited clinical utility. Diagnostic overlap is a major problem, and there is limited evidence that current categories predict response to treatment. In sum, the construct validity of the system has yet to be established. Problems are equally apparent from a research perspective. DSM diagnoses are too broad and heterogeneous to use in investigations of biological and psychological mechanisms, forcing investigators to use alternative constructs and measures. (pp. 6–7)

Similarly, Cloninger (2000) declared:

> Our current official classification of personality disorders is fundamentally flawed by its assumption that personality disorder is composed of multiple discrete categorical disorders. The current list of clusters and categories are highly

redundant and overlapping. Systematic diagnosis of so many categories is not feasible in clinical practice and unjustifiable in psychometric research. Predictive power of categorical diagnoses is weak and inconsistent. (pp. 106–107)

Finally and perhaps most directly, Westen and Shedler (2000) asserted, "The increasing consensus among personality disorder researchers is that Axis II does not rest on a firm enough foundation. We may do well to rebuild it from the basement up rather than trying to plug the leaks or replace the roof" (p. 110).

The shift in *zeitgeist* has also become apparent from "behind the scenes." For those of us who regularly review empirical and theoretical manuscripts on personality disorders that are submitted for publication, the receptiveness to approaches that are anchored strictly to DSM Axis II categories has diminished. Submitted articles often note the increasing criticism of the DSM categories yet limit operationalization of personality disorders to measures of DSM constructs or offer only translations of the extant categories. For example, there have now been more than 56 published studies that examined the description, classification, or understanding of DSM personality disorders in terms of the five-factor model of personality (Widiger & Costa, 2002). While early efforts in this regard were highly relevant and provided the basic scientific evidence for considering alternative approaches from the science of individual differences (e.g., Costa & McCrae, 1990; Soldz, Budman, Demby, & Merry, 1993; Wiggins & Pincus, 1989), recent work has been met with less enthusiasm by many in the field. To paraphrase a consistent point from a recent set of reviews and the editorial decision for such a submission to a top-tier psychology journal, "The fundamental conceptual problem, in a nutshell, is why bother to predict a criterion that is neither clinically nor conceptually valid? The 'necessary evil' argument isn't a very convincing one." Such a critique was much less likely in the 1980s and 1990s.

This does not mean the DSM nosology is a complete failure by any means. It clearly continues to elaborate on a century clinical observation of abnormal personalities, albeit imperfectly. It has also highlighted the types of issues and concepts that we must empirically and theoretically consider in conceptualizing personality disorder (e.g., categorical vs. dimensional vs. prototypal classification, continuous vs. discontinuous conceptions of the relation between abnormal personality and normal personality, the nature and purpose of classification itself, and many more; see Lenzenweger & Clarkin, 1996). It has taken us into this new era. As we see later, all expressions of personality pathology characterized and labeled in the DSM need not be discarded. It would be foolish to ignore its accumulation of observations and the efforts of many to work these into a reliable diagnostic system. I believe personality concepts such as narcissism and dependency remain clinically relevant beyond DSM Axis II. The shift in attitude about the DSM nosology does, however, have implications for evolving theories of personality disorder. My opinion is that theories of personality disorder in the new era need not, and perhaps should not, anchor themselves to the DSM categories. In the current case, I make explicit that CIIT of personality disorders does not seek to account for or describe DSM categories of personality disorder.

Classification of Personality Disorders: Two Trends in the New Era

Pincus (in press) reviewed the recent literature on classification of personality disorders and noted two trends that were identified as "causal–theoretical approaches" and "practical–empirical approaches" (see Table 6.1). The approaches are not mutually exclusive in terms of their superordinate concerns or even group membership, but they do have several contrasting emphases. Causal–theoretical approaches view classification in the context of explanation and tend to emphasize theory, open concepts, the nature of pathology, and definition of personality disorder. In contrast, practical–empirical approaches view classification in the context of the practical task of diagnosis and tend to emphasize methods, operational definitions, phenomenology, and description of individual differences in personality disorder.

Theory and Open Concepts versus Method and Operational Definitions

Theoretical models of personality disorder usually propose and prioritize fundamental principles that underlie the integrated functioning of the whole person, which is assumed to then organize the contents and functional relationships among domains of personality. All such theories have

TABLE 6.1. Emphases of Two Trends in Personality Disorder Classification

Causal–theoretical approaches	Practical–empirical approaches
Theory	Method
Open concepts	Operational definitions
Pathology	Phenomenology
Definition	Diagnosis
Explanation	Description
Based on theory	Based on empirical data
Based on empirical data	Based on theory
Accept, ignore, or revise DSM system	Revise DSM system

normative and pathological implications. Clarkin and Lenzenweger (1996) and Millon, Meagher, and Grossman (2001) identified the major theoretical approaches to personality disorder as cognitive theories, interpersonal theories, intrapsychic (psychodynamic) theories, evolutionary theories, and neurobiological theories.

While approaches emphasizing theory do not eschew operational definitions completely, they often are reliant on open concepts. These two emphases mark the end points of an epistemological continuum of conceptual breadth versus conceptual specificity (Millon, 1987). Open concepts are more abstract and hypothetical, reflecting the nature of personality constructs as less rigidly organized than many constructs in the hard sciences. That is, in the fields of personology, psychopathology, and psychotherapy, we have few one-to-one relationships between personality, behavior, experience, and development, and we have many more feedback, feedforward, stochastic, and transactional processes involving indeterminate or inferential intervening concepts.

In contrast, practical–empirical approaches emphasize methodologically driven models of personality disorder that do not necessarily make a priori theoretical commitments and thus are free to address any domain (or even several domains) of personality. In such approaches, investigators make few a priori assumptions about what dimensions/domains might emerge. Such approaches rely on operational definitions and attempt to anchor personality disorder directly in the empirical world of observation, linking each pathological attribute to an indicator in a one-to-one fashion. The goal is to reduce inference and maximize the relationship between attribute and method of measurement.

The emphases of both approaches have inherent vulnerabilities. Millon et al. (2001) cautioned that a limitation of many theoretical approaches to personality disorder is their typical allegiance to one domain of personality (e.g., cognition) as central, while casting all other domains as peripheral or derivative. They further cautioned that conceptualizing personality disorder strictly in terms of open concepts runs the risk of growing so circuitous in references as to become tautological and imply no links to anything observable. This undermines the scientific contribution of theory by rendering it both untestable and inapplicable to clinical diagnosis (Millon, 1991). On the other hand, purely methods-based approaches to personality disorder may provide only retrospective rationales for findings and "structure and sufficiency are thus offered in compensation for lack of a compelling theory" (Millon et al., 2001, p. 47). A related concern is that while operational definitions allow for diagnostic indicators to be directly translatable into clinical assessment guidelines that maximize precision (reliability), such approaches can be deficient in scope (validity) if they are based on any single methodological procedure (e.g., factor analysis).

Pathology, Definition, and Explanation versus Phenomenology, Diagnosis, and Description

These concepts are all related to whether one views classification of psychopathology as mainly in the service of understanding the nature of normality and abnormality or mainly in the service of the practical task of clinical identification. A set of diagnostic criteria can be interpreted as defining what the disorder is, or as providing a set of fallible indicators for determining when the disorder is present (Widiger & Trull, 1991). The 10 specific DSM-IV personality disorder criteria sets really serve the latter function as the manual provides a definition of personality disorder distinct from them, but the definition is not systematically and specifically used in making DSM diagnoses. Widiger (1991) suggested that DSM criteria sets tend to describe the phenomenology of individual differences in personality disorder rather than fundamentally defining the pathology of personality disorders in relation to normal personality functioning. Similarly, Parker et al. (2002) suggested that DSM-IV criteria sets mix and confuse indicators of personality dysfunction (which could serve to define and explain personality disorder) with descriptors of personality style (which serve to distinguish and portray individual differences in personality disorder phenomenology). My view is that the clinical science of personality disorders will benefit from clearly recognizing this distinction. Quite simply, the questions of what is personality (disorder) and how to describe it are related but distinct. Classification of personality disorders in the post DSM-III/DSM-IV era will require greater coordination of definitional theories and systems for describing variation in expression of personality pathology (Pincus, in press).

Theoretical versus Empirical Basis for Classification

In reality, I do not believe there is a true distinction here, as few in the field view either source of information as truly distinct and sufficient. For example, of the nine requirements for an empirically based classification provided by Livesley (2001), the fourth was "The classification should be based on empirical evidence" and the fifth was "The classification should be theory based." He noted that current classification is at odds with empirical data, yet he also suggested that no currently existing theory of personality disorder is yet adequate to provide the necessary basis for classification. Similarly, many of their critical issues for *theories* of personality disorder summarized by Lenzenweger and Clarkin (1996) are strongly tied to, and some even derived from, practical–empirical issues (the types of populations used in personality disorder research, the structure of the DSM multiaxial system, etc.). I do think that more integration of theory and method is clearly necessary. When one reviews critiques of personality disorder research (e.g., Bornstein, 2003), there is often little to inform theory development. When one reviews theory, there is often insufficient connection to the issues debated within the practical–empirical approaches.

The DSM System Revisited

Current major theories of personality disorder vary in terms of their assessment of DSM Axis II. Benjamin's (1996b, 1996c) interpersonal theory based on Structural Analysis of Social Behavior (SASB) and Beck's cognitive theory (Beck, Davis, & Associates, 2004; Pretzer & Beck, 1996) both generally accept the DSM classification. Contemporary psychodynamic theories (e.g., Kernberg, 1984, 1996; McWilliams, 1994) and neurobiological theories (e.g., Depue, 1996; Paris, 2000) tend to ignore DSM classification in favor of current or future alternatives. Millon's (1990) evolutionary theory tends to parallel DSM (Millon & Davis, 1996), although he is clear about DSM's limitations (Millon, 2000). Almost all of the recent practical–empirical literature concludes that the DSM system needs revision, although suggestions differ in terms of whether to focus revisions on the structure of the DSM (e.g., Axis I vs. Axis II distinctions, categorical vs. dimensional vs. prototypal classification) or to focus revisions on the nature and scope of diagnostic criteria, or both. CIIT of personality disorder does not attempt to account for all 10 DSM Axis II categories.

Two-Step Diagnostic Approaches

There have been several recent proposals for revising the classification and diagnosis of personality disorders, including prototype matching procedures (Westen & Shedler, 2000), use of a purely dimensional model with empirically derived cutoff scores (Widiger, 2000), developing a classification system anchored in biology/neurobiology (Depue, 1996; Paris, 2000; Silk, 1997), increasing the scope and uniformity of coverage of DSM criteria sets (Millon, 2000), and revising DSM criteria via behaviorally referenced criterion validation based on experimental manipulation of personality disorder processes that produce measurable behavioral change (Bornstein, 2003). All these proposals have merits that will contribute to the study of personality disorders in the new era. Pincus (in press) noted that several substantively divergent alternatives actually converge in proposing a two-step diagnostic process that distinguishes *definition* of personality disorder pathology (Step 1) from *description* of individual differences in personality disorder phenomenology (Step 2). I believe that explicitly decoupling definition of personality disorder and description of individual differences in phenomenological expression is the most promising approach to optimizing classification for psychopathologists, personologists, practitioners, and patients. It appears that the strengths of causal–theoretical approaches may best inform Step 1 and the strengths of practical–empirical approaches may best inform Step 2. Some examples of two-step diagnostic approaches are noted next.

DSM-IV actually took a step in this direction by providing general criteria for personality disorder (Step 1) in a similar format to criteria sets for specific Axis II categories (Step 2). DSM-IV, in a sense, defines personality disorder as clinically significant distress or impairment due to an enduring, inflexible, and pervasive pattern of inner experience and behavior that deviates markedly from cultural expectations as manifested in two or more areas: cognition, affectivity, interpersonal functioning, and impulse control. Such dysfunction may then be expressed in 10 different ways corresponding to the specific Axis II categories, or any unusual pattern of expression, can be labeled "personality disorder not otherwise specified." However, theoretical linkages among the general criteria are not provided, no empirical research has evaluated them, and they are not systematically incorporated into clinical diagnostic practice.

Investigators as diverse as Otto Kernberg and Robert Cloninger have also proposed two steps in personality disorder diagnosis. In Kernberg's (1984, 1996) structural diagnosis of personality, maturational level of object relations defines three levels of personality organization (neurotic, borderline, psychotic) each increasing in level of pathological severity, while character type describes constellations of defenses, needs, and expectancies that give rise to individual differences in the expression of normal and pathological personality organization. Cloninger (2000) proposed that the defining features of personality disorder (Step 1) be based on low levels of the character dimensions of the Temperament Character Inventory (TCI; Cloninger, Przybeck, Svrakic, & Wetzel, 1994): low Self-directedness, low Cooperativeness, low Affective Stability, and low Self-transcendence. Individual differences in personality disorder phenomenology (Step 2) are then described based on variation in combinations and levels of the TCI temperament dimensions of Reward Dependence, Novelty Seeking, and Harm Avoidance.

Parker et al. (2002) provided the longest list of defining features I could identify in the literature, including disagreeableness, inability to care for others, lack of cooperation, causes discomfort to others, ineffectiveness, lack of empathy, failure to form and maintain interpersonal relationships, failure to learn from experience, impulsivity, inflexibility, maladaptability, immorality, extremes of optimism, self-defeating behaviors, low self-directedness, lack of humor, and tenuous stability under stress. There is no doubt that these features are commonly observed in psychotherapy with personality disordered patients. However, it is likely that the larger the set of defining features, the more difficult it will be to decouple definition of personality pathology from description of its phenomenological expression. For example, it is unclear how to distinguish many of the aforementioned features as distinct from the assessment of lower-order traits of personality disorder such as those reflected in Clark's Schedule for Nonadaptive and Adaptive Personality (SNAP; Clark, 1993) and Livesley's Dimensional Assessment of Personality Pathology (DAPP, Livesley & Jackson, in press), both of which would be most suited to describing individual differences in personality disorder phenomenology (Step 2).

In contrast, Livesley (1998, 2001) proposed only two core criteria for defining personality disorder. He concluded that review of the clinical literature on personality disorders reveals two major features of dysfunction that can be used to elegantly and parsimoniously define personality disorder (Step 1). He suggested personality disorder could be clinically defined by *chronic interpersonal dysfunction* and *problems with self or identity*. The former is characterized by pervasive abnormalities in social functioning, including failure to develop adaptive relational functioning, impairments in cooperative and prosocial relational capacity, and instability and poor integration of their mental representations of others and relationships. Such deficits often give rise to interpersonal relationships marred by self-fulfilling prophecies (Carson, 1982), maladaptive transaction cycles (Kiesler, 1991), and deleterious vicious circles (Millon, 1996). Self/Identity problems are characterized by unstable and poorly integrated mental representations of self and others reflected in the subjective experience of chronic emptiness; contradictory self-perceptions; contradictory behavior that cannot be integrated in an emotionally meaningful way; and shallow, flat, impoverished perceptions of others. Difficulties maintaining self-cohesion, a sense of well-being and vitality, and goal-directedness are common (Kohut & Wolf, 1978). Finally, the core beliefs, cognitive schemas, expectancies, and thoughts about the self of individuals with personality disorders are dysfunctional, distressing, or both. While Livesley (2001) did not explicitly link his core features to a system of phenomenological description, the body of his work would suggest that the factor analytically derived lower-order traits of personality disorder he has identified (e.g., Livesley, Jackson, & Schroeder, 1992) would be a reasonable choice.

Switching briefly to Step 2, the task of describing individual differences in personality disorder phenomenology, a number of potential specific descriptive systems could be employed (see Table 6.2). The most common models for describing individual differences in personality and personality disorder are dimensional trait models, which have several advantages including their inherent continuity with normal functioning. Even the SNAP and DAPP personality disorder trait dimensions exhibit continuous distributions across normal and clinical populations. A number of categori-

TABLE 6.2. Some Systems to Describe Individual Differences in Personality Disorder Phenomenology

<u>Dimensional systems</u>

- Personality trait dimensions
  Interpersonal circumplex (IPC)
  Eysenck's three-factor model (P-E-N)
  Five-factor model (FFM)
- Personality disorder trait dimensions
  Schedule for Nonadaptive and adaptive personality (SNAP)
  Dimensional assessment of personality pathology (DAPP)
- Temperament dimensions
  Temperament character inventory (TCI)
- Livesley's convergent dimensions
  Emotional dysregulation, dissocial behavior, inhibitedness, compulsivity

<u>Categorical systems</u>

- Broad classes of evolutionary adaptations
- Constellations of defense mechanisms
- Prototype matching: Shedler–Westen Assessment Procedure—200 (SWAP-200)
- Specific cognitive schemas

cal systems have also been proposed for describing individual differences in personality disorder phenomenology. These include broad classes of evolutionary adaptations (Millon, 1990; Millon & Davis, 1996), constellations of defense mechanisms (McWilliams, 1994; Vaillant & McCullough, 1998), matching patient characteristics to empirically derived clinical prototypes (Westen & Shedler, 2000), and specific sets of cognitive schemas (Pretzer & Beck, 1996; Young, 1990).

CONTEMPORARY INTEGRATIVE INTERPERSONAL THEORY OF PERSONALITY: I. ORIGINS, FOUNDATIONS, AND DESCRIPTIVE SCOPE

I believe Livesley's distillation of the core clinical features of personality disorder—that is, *chronic interpersonal dysfunction* and *problems with self and identity*—provides an excellent starting point for a definition of personality disorder. However, Livesley (2001) lamented that no theory of personality disorder currently exists to link this definition to an empirically based classification system. In terms of the trends discussed in this chapter, a new classification of personality disorders requires a theory that can coordinate the definitional strengths of causal–theoretical approaches and the descriptive strengths of practical–empirical approaches. When considering these core defining features, I was struck by their convergence with Sullivan's (1953a, 1953b, 1954, 1956, 1962, 1964) extremely generative interpersonal theory of psychiatry, which clearly considered interpersonal relations and the self-concept to be the core emphases of normal and abnormal personality. My view is that the interpersonal approach to personality that emerged from Sullivan's work (e.g., Benjamin, 1974; Carson, 1969; Kiesler, 1982, 1983; Leary, 1957; McLemore & Benjamin, 1979; Wiggins, 1979, 1980, 1982) has evolved dramatically in recent years, becoming broader and more integrative in scope (e.g., Benjamin, 2003; Horowitz, 2004; Kiesler, 1996; Moskowitz & Zuroff, 2004; Pincus & Ansell, 2003; Wiggins, 1991, 1997a; Wiggins & Trapnell, 1996; Wiggins & Trobst, 1999). Pincus (in press) noted that the culmination of these advances, CIIT allows the interpersonal tradition in personality theory to provide a coordinated nexus between causal–theoretical approaches and practical–empirical approaches to personality disorder. CIIT provides a basis for the definition of personality disorder for Step 1 and empirically based models and methods to describe personality disorder phenomenology for Step 2. Figure 6.1 presents an overview of the scope of CIIT of personality disorders.

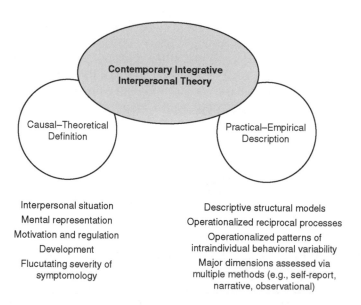

FIGURE 6.1. Contemporary integrative interpersonal theory coordinates definition and description of personality disorders.

CIIT of personality disorders can enhance the explanatory implications of Livesely's core defining features of personality disorder through the application of the "interpersonal situation" as an integrative theoretical concept (Pincus & Ansell, 2003). To fully satisfy the theoretical and personological needs of definition, CIIT must also articulate the motivational and developmental factors influencing disordered self-concepts and maladaptive patterns of relating to others and account for the fluctuating severity of personality disorder symptomology. What makes CIIT a true nexus is that the interpersonal theory of personality also has a long and reciprocally influential history with research programs that have culminated in well-validated, empirically derived models and methods to describe interpersonal behavior (LaForge, 2004; Pincus, 1994; Wiggins, 1996). Thus CIIT of personality disorders also includes multiple methods to assess the fundamental interpersonal dimensions of Agency and Communion (Wiggins, 1991, 1997a, 2003) and associated circumplex structural models (Benjamin, 1996a; Wiggins, 1996), operational definitions of reciprocal interpersonal processes (Benjamin, 1996b, 2003; Kiesler, 1983), and operational definitions of intraindividual variability in interpersonal behavior (Moskowitz & Zuroff, 2004). In addition, the descriptive models and methods are based on personality dimensions that are continuous with normal and disordered functioning. Using the entire scope of CIIT of personality disorders allows for synchronization of the causal–theoretical definition of personality disorder with the practical–empirical description of personality disorder phenomenology needed for scientifically and clinically useful classification and diagnosis.

Some Comments on Theoretical Integration

In their critique of personality disorder theories, Millon et al. (2001) suggested that current theories tend to be aligned with one psychological domain and consider other domains either derivative or peripheral. In contrast, Pincus and Ansell (2003) argued that contemporary interpersonal theory was integrative rather than derivative and noted that explicit efforts have been made toward integration of interpersonal theory and cognitive theories (e.g., Carson, 1982; Safran, 1990a, 1990b), attachment theory (e.g., Bartholomew & Horowitz, 1991; Florsheim, Henry, & Benjamin, 1996; Gallo, Smith, & Ruiz, 2003; Pincus, Dickinson, Schut, Castonguay, & Bedics, 1999), psychodynamic theories (e.g., Benjamin, 1995; Benjamin & Friedrich, 1991; Heck & Pincus, 2001; Mitchell, 1988; Pincus, 1997; Roemer, 1986), evolutionary theory (e.g., Fournier, Moskowitz, & Zuroff, 2002; Hoyenga, Hoyrenga, Walters, & Schmidt, 1998; Zuroff, Moskowtiz, & Cote, 1999), and even neurobiology (Moskowitz, Pinard, Zuroff, Annable, & Young, 2001). In most reviews of personality disorder theory, authors list cognitive, interpersonal, psychodynamic, evolutionary, and neurobiological theories as separate and distinct categories. However, just like DSM Axis II categories of personality disorders, these theoretical approaches to personality disorder really have a number of shared characteristics, making their distinctions fuzzy. For example, all theories of personality disorder address interpersonal functioning; and CIIT would not suggest that cognitive or neurobiological functioning is somehow derivative of or peripheral to relational experience. It simply asserts that when we look at a domain of personality or its substrates, our best bet may be to look at it in relation to interpersonal functioning. Thus, CIIT is also a nexus for bringing together elements across the theoretical spectrum and it can serve as an integrative framework via consideration of the "interpersonal situation."

The Interpersonal Situation

> I had come to feel over the years that there was an acute need for a discipline that was determined to study not the individual organism or the social heritage, but the interpersonal situations through which persons manifest mental health or mental disorder.
> —HARRY STACK SULLIVAN (1953b, p. 18)

> Personality is the relatively enduring pattern of recurrent interpersonal situations which characterize a human life.
> —HARRY STACK SULLIVAN (1953b, pp. 110–111)

Sullivan's emphasis on the interpersonal situation as the focus for understanding both personality and psychopathology has set an elemental course for psychology and psychiatry. CIIT thus begins with the assumption that the most important expressions of personality occur in phenomena involving more than one person. Sullivan (1953a, 1953b) suggested that individuals express "integrating tendencies" which bring them together in the mutual pursuit of satisfactions (generally a large class of biologically grounded needs), security (i.e., anxiety-free functioning), and self-esteem. These integrating tendencies develop into increasingly complex patterns or "dynamisms" of interpersonal experience. From infancy throughout the lifespan, these dynamisms are encoded in memory via age-appropriate learning. According to Sullivan, interpersonal learning of self-concept and social behavior is based on an "anxiety gradient" associated with interpersonal situations. All interpersonal situations range from rewarding (highly secure) through various degrees of anxiety and ending in a class of situations associated with such severe anxiety that they are dissociated from experience. The interpersonal situation underlies genesis, development, maintenance, and mutability of personality through the continuous patterning and repatterning of interpersonal experience in relation to the vicissitudes of satisfactions, security, and esteem. Over time, this gives rise to lasting conceptions of self and other (Sullivan's "personifications") as well as to enduring patterns of interpersonal relating.

Individual variation in learning occurs due to the interaction between the developing person's level of cognitive maturation (i.e., Sullivan's prototaxic, parataxic, and syntaxic modes of experience) and the characteristics of the interpersonal situations encountered. Interpersonal experience is understood differently depending on the developing person's grasp of cause-and-effect logic and the use of consensual symbols such as language. This affects how one makes sense of the qualities of significant others (including their "reflected appraisals" of the developing person), as well as the ultimate outcomes of interpersonal situations characterizing a human life. Pincus and Ansell (2003) summarized Sullivan's concept of the interpersonal situation as "the experience of a pattern of relating self with other associated with varying levels of anxiety (or security) in which learning takes place that influences the development of self-concept and social behavior" (p. 210). This is a very fundamental human experience which can serve as a point for pantheoretical integration and is directly related to the two core clinical features of personality disorder—*chronic interpersonal dysfunction* and *problems with self/identity*.

A False Dichotomy: The Interpersonal and the Intrapsychic

A second major assumption of CIIT is that the term "interpersonal" is meant to convey a sense of primacy, directing theory to a set of fundamental phenomena important for personality development, structuralization, function, and pathology. The term is not meant as a geographical indicator of locale, it does not imply a dichotomy between what is inside the person and what is outside the person, nor does it limit interpersonal theory to a theory of the observable interactions between two proximal people (Pincus & Ansell, 2003).

I believe there has been a tendency to falsely dichotomize the terms interpersonal and intrapsychic from both within and outside of the interpersonal tradition. There appear to be two reasons for this. First, contemporary surveys of psychoanalytic theory (e.g., Greenberg & Mitchell, 1983) tend to portray Sullivan's thinking as a reaction to Freud's emphasis on drive-based aspects of personality. Because of Sullivan's opposition to drives as the source of personality structuralization, there is a risk of simplifying interpretation of interpersonal theory as focusing solely on what occurs outside the person, in the world of observable interaction. Second, the emphasis of initial efforts in the interpersonal tradition in personality and clinical psychology focused heavily on the description of interpersonal behavior (e.g., Freedman, Leary, Ossorio, & Coffey, 1951; LaForge, 2004;

Lorr & McNair, 1963, 1965; Schaefer, 1959, 1961). Although contemporary interpersonalists have indeed proposed many concepts and processes that clearly imply a rich and meaningful intrapsychic life including personifications, selective inattention, and parataxic distortions (Sullivan, 1953a, 1953b); covert impact messages (Kiesler, Schmidt, & Wagner, 1997); expectancies of contingency (Carson, 1982); fantasies and self-statements (Brokaw & McLemore, 1991); and cognitive interpersonal schemas (Safran, 1990a, 1990b; Wiggins, 1982), I have been critical of the underdeveloped nature of interpersonal theory's conceptions of what occurs in the mind (Pincus, 1994; Pincus & Ansell, 2003). I agree with Safran's (1992) conclusion that the "ongoing attempt to clarify the relationship between interpersonal and intrapsychic levels is what is needed to fully realize the transtheoretical implications of interpersonal theory" (p. 105). Much of the field is moving in this direction, as the relationship between the interpersonal and the intrapsychic is a common entry point for current integrative efforts (e.g., Benjamin, 1995, 2003; Florsheim et al., 1996, Pincus; in press).

Mitchell (1988) pointed out that Sullivan was quite amenable to incorporating the intrapsychic into interpersonal theory as he viewed the most important contents of the mind to be the consequence of lived interpersonal experience. For example, Sullivan (1964) asserted that "everything that can be found in the human mind has been put there by interpersonal relations, excepting only the capabilities to receive *and elaborate* the relevant experiences" (p. 302; see also Stern, 1985, 1988). Sullivan clearly viewed the interpersonal situation as equally likely to be found within the mind of the person as it is to be found in the observable interactions between two people. For example, Sullivan (1964) defined psychiatry as "the study of phenomena that occur in configurations of two or more people, all but one of whom may be more or less completely illusory" (p. 33). These illusory aspects of the interpersonal situation involve mental structures (i.e., personifications of self and others). Sullivan (1953b) was forceful in asserting that personifications are elaborated organizations of past interpersonal experience, stating, "I would like to make it forever clear that the relation of the personifications to that which is personified is always complex and sometimes multiple; and that personifications are not adequate descriptions of that which is personified" (p. 167).

To overcome the false dichotomization of the interpersonal and the intrapsychic, CIIT asserts that interpersonal situations occur between proximal interactants and within the minds of those interactants via the capacity for mental representation of self and others (e.g., Blatt, Auerbach, & Levy, 1997). It also allows CIIT to incorporate important pantheoretical representational constructs such as cognitive interpersonal schemas, internalized object relations, and internal working models. CIIT does suggest that the most important personological phenomena are relational in nature, but it does not suggest that such phenomena are limited to contemporaneous, observable behavior. They occur in perceptions of contemporaneous events, memories of past experiences, and fantasies of future experiences. Regardless of the level of accuracy or distortion in these perceptions, memories, and fantasies, the ability to address both internal experiences and external relationships is necessary for a theory of personality disorder as Livesley's two core defining features have both representational and proximal relational implications. Both internal and proximal interpersonal situations continuously influence an individual's learned relational strategies and conception of self/identity.

Agency and Communion

Wiggins (1991, 1997a, 2003) has reviewed the nature and broad application of Bakan's (1966) metaconcepts of "agency" and "communion" and has argued that these two superordinate dimensions have propaeduetic explanatory power across fields as diverse as philosophy, linguistics, anthropology, sociology, psychiatry, gender studies, and the subdisciplines of personality psychology, evolutionary psychology, cross-cultural psychology, social psychology, and clinical psychology. "Agency" refers to the condition of being a differentiated individual, and it is manifested in strivings for power and mastery which can enhance and protect ones' differentiation. "Communion" refers to the condition of being part of a larger social or spiritual entity, and is manifested in strivings for intimacy, union, and solidarity with the larger entity. Bakan (1966) noted that a key issue for understanding human existence is to comprehend how the tensions of this duality in the human condition are managed.

Wiggins (2003) proposed that agency and communion are most directly related to Sullivan's theory in terms of the goals of human relationship: security (communion) and self-esteem (agency). As can be seen in Figure 6.2, these metaconcepts (concepts about concepts) form a superordinate structure which can be used to derive explanatory and descriptive concepts at different levels of specificity. At the broadest and most interdisciplinary level, metaconcepts serve to classify the motives, strivings, conflicts, and goals of human existence. When the structure is applied to the interpersonal situation, we may consider what agentic or communal motives or goals drive human relationship. At this level, they address the nature of relations between self and other (and self and society)—that is, what states of being and fundamental goals are important to the person?

At more specific levels, the structure provides conceptual coordinates for describing and measuring interpersonal traits and behaviors (Wiggins, 1991). The intermediate level can be used to describe interpersonal traits

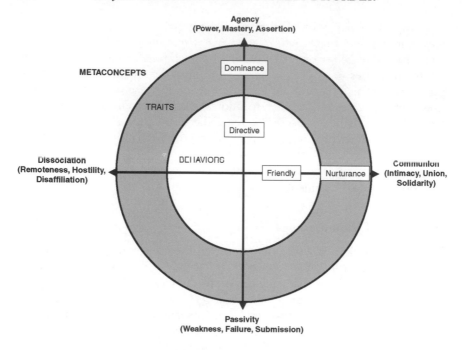

FIGURE 6.2. Agency and communion.

and interpersonal problems, essentially providing a taxonomy of individual differences (Leary, 1957; Wiggins, 1979, 1995). Agentic and communal traits and problems imply consistencies in perceiving, thinking, feeling, and behaving that are probabilistic in nature (Wiggins, 1997b) and describe an individual's interpersonal tendencies aggregated across time, place, and relationships. At the most specific level, the structure can be used to classify the nature and intensity of specific interpersonal behaviors or acts (e.g., Gifford, 1991; Kiesler, 1985; Moskowitz, 1994; Tracey, 1994). Specific interpersonal behaviors can be classified in terms of their varying levels of agentic and communal qualities, and this level of description allows for the specification of reciprocal interpersonal patterns in ongoing relationships and quantification of intraindividual variability in interpersonal behavior. CIIT proposes that (1) agency and communion are the fundamental metaconcepts of personality, providing a superordinate structure for conceptualizing interpersonal situations; (2) explicatory systems derived from agency and communion can be used to understand, describe, and measure interpersonal traits and behaviors; and (3) such systems can be applied equally well to the description of contemporaneous interactions between two or more proximal individuals (e.g., Markey, Funder, & Ozer, 2003) and to interpersonal situations within the mind evoked via memory, fantasy, and mental representation (e.g., Heck & Pincus, 2001).

Interpersonal Description

The emphasis on interpersonal functioning in Sullivan's work led to efforts to develop orderly and lawful conceptual and empirical models describing interpersonal behavior (for reviews of these developments, see LaForge, 2004; LaForge, Freedman, & Wiggins, 1985; Pincus, 1994; Wiggins, 1982, 1996). The goal of such work was to obtain a taxonomy of interpersonal behavior—that is, "to obtain categories of increasing generality that permit description of behaviors according to their natural relationships" (Schaefer, 1961, p. 126). In contemporary terms, these systems are referred to as structural models, which can be used to conceptually systematize observation and covariation of variables of interest. When seen in relation to the metaconcepts of agency and communion, such models can be illuminating nomological nets.

Empirical research into diverse interpersonal taxa including traits (Wiggins, 1979), problems (Alden, Wiggins, & Pincus, 1990); values (Locke, 2000), impact messages (Kiesler et al., 1997), and behaviors (Benjamin, 1974; Gifford, 1991; Moskowitz, 1994; Trobst, 2000) converge in suggesting the structure of interpersonal behavior takes the form of a circle or "circumplex" (Gurtman & Pincus, 2000; Pincus, Gurtman, & Ruiz, 1998; Wiggins & Trobst, 1997). An exemplar of this form based on the two underlying dimensions of dominance–submission (agency) on the vertical axis and nurturance–coldness (communion) on the horizontal axis is often referred to as the Interpersonal Circle (IPC; Kiesler, 1983; Pincus, 1994; Wiggins, 1996) (see Figure 6.3).[1] The geometric properties of circumplex models give rise to unique computational methods for assessment and research (Gurtman, 1994, 1997, 2001; Gurtman & Balakrishnan, 1998; Gurtman & Pincus, 2003; Yik & Russell, 2004) that are not reviewed here. In this chapter, I use the IPC to anchor description of theoretical concepts. The IPC model is a geometric representation of individual differences in a variety of interpersonal domains; thus all qualities of individual differences within these domains can be described as blends of the circle's two underlying dimensions. Blends of dominance and nurturance can be located along the 360-degree perimeter of the circle. Interpersonal qualities close to one another on the perimeter are conceptually and statistically similar, qualities at 90 degrees are conceptually and statistically independent, and qualities 180 degrees apart are conceptual and statistical opposites. While the circular model itself is a continuum without beginning

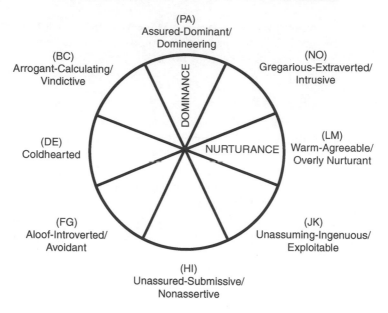

FIGURE 6.3. The interpersonal circumplex.

or end (Carson, 1996; Gurtman & Pincus, 2000), any segmentalization of the IPC perimeter to identify lower-order taxa is potentially useful within the limits of reliable discriminability. The IPC has been segmentalized into sixteenths (Kiesler, 1983), octants (Wiggins, Trapnell, & Phillips, 1988), and quadrants (Carson, 1969).

Intermediate-level structural models derived from agency and communion focus on the description of distinctive consistencies of the individual (e.g., personality traits, interpersonal problems, and interpersonal values) that are assumed to give rise to adaptive and maladaptive behavior that is generally consistent across interpersonal situations (Wiggins, 1997b). Thus, we can use circumplex models to describe a person's typical ways of relating to others and refer to their "interpersonal style" (e.g., Lorr & Youniss, 1986; Pincus & Gurtman, 2003). At the level of behavior, interpersonal description permits microanalytic, or transactional, analyses of interpersonal situations. Because interpersonal situations also occur within the mind, these models can describe the person's typical ways of encoding new interpersonal information and their consistent mental representations of self and others. Using circumplex models to classify individuals in terms of their agentic and communal characteristics is often referred to as "interpersonal diagnosis" (Benjamin, 1996c; Kiesler, 1986; Leary, 1957; McLemore & Benjamin, 1979; Wiggins, Phillips, & Trapnell, 1989).

Implications for Normality and Pathology

Implications of the IPC model for pathological functioning have been based on the concepts of interpersonal rigidity (i.e., displaying a limited repertoire of interpersonal behaviors) and behavioral intensity (i.e., enacting behaviors in extreme forms). Research linking interpersonal traits and problems to particular personality disorder diagnoses (e.g., Pincus & Wiggins, 1990; Wiggins & Pincus, 1989) tended to imply that disorder was reflected in overly rigid and intense agentic and communal expression, such that the press of the interpersonal situation and the needs of others were ignored, unnoticed, or distorted, leading to disrupted interpersonal relations. Adaptivity was assumed to be reflected in flexible expression of agentic and communal behavior around the circle at moderate levels of intensity as called for by the particular interpersonal situation encountered. I have found that these conceptions of adaptive and disordered interpersonal functioning provide limited explanatory power and they do not appear to be sufficient in scope to base a definition of personality disorder. I believe these concepts are better suited to description of individual differences in disordered behavior. This is because trait-like consistency is probabilistic, and clearly even individuals with personality disorders vary in how consistently they behave and in what ways consistency is exhibited. Thus, it does not seem clinically informative to restrict definition of personality disorder to the concepts of interpersonal rigidity and behavioral intensity nor to expect patients with personality disorders to robotically emit the same intense or extreme behaviors without variation. Fortunately, recent developments in the measurement of intraindividual variability of interpersonal behavior (Moskowitz & Hershberger, 2002; Moskowitz & Zuroff, 2004) have added an important dynamic lexicon to enhance the sophistication of description/quantification of interpersonal rigidity and behavioral intensity and increase the utility of these concepts for clinical description.

Interpersonal Flux, Pulse, and Spin

To more accurately describe variability in interpersonal behavior over time using the IPC model, Moskowitz and Zuroff (2004) proposed three variability constructs and demonstrated that they exhibited longitudinal stability in the daily behaviors of individuals. That is, individuals exhibit stable levels of behavioral variability in agentic and communal behaviors that can be described based on the IPC (see Figure 6.4). *Flux* refers to variability about an individual's mean behavioral score on agentic or communal dimensions (e.g., dominant flux, submissive flux, friendly flux, and hostile flux). Describing variability in terms of these basic dimensions provides links with the definitional metaconcepts of agency and communion; how-

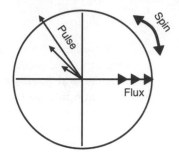

FIGURE 6.4. Interpersonal flux, pulse, and spin.

ever, flux does not incorporate the geometry of the IPC. Moskowitz and Zuroff (2004) also proposed two other forms of variability inherently tied to the circular structure of the IPC, and these provide descriptions of individual differences in the normal and maladaptive behavioral variability that are consistent with traditional interpersonal diagnosis. *Spin* refers to variability of the angular coordinates (i.e., types) of behavior emitted, and *pulse* refers to variability of the overall extremity of an individuals ongoing behavior. Low spin would reflect higher levels of interpersonal rigidity, while low pulse around a high mean would reflect consistent enactment of extreme behaviors of any type classified by the IPC. CIIT proposes that spin and pulse are constructs of behavioral variability that can differentiate phenomenological expression of personality pathology.

Interpersonal Reciprocity and Transaction

Interpersonal behavior is not emitted in an isolated vacuum; rather, it is reciprocally influential in ongoing human transactions. The notion of reciprocity in human relating has been reflected in a wide variety of psychological concepts (Pincus & Ansell, 2003). Within the interpersonal tradition, these have typically been referred to in terms of adaptive and maladaptive transaction cycles (Kiesler, 1991), self-fulfilling prophecies (Carson, 1982), and vicious circles (Millon, 1996). If we assume that an interpersonal situation involves two or more people relating to each other in ways that bring about social and self-related learning, the implication is that something more is happening than mere random activity. Reciprocal relational patterns create an interpersonal field (Wiggins & Trobst, 1999) in which various transactional influences have an impact on both interactants as they resolve, negotiate, or disintegrate the interpersonal situation. Within this field, interpersonal behaviors tend to pull, elicit, invite, or evoke "restricted classes" of responses from the other, and this is a continual, dynamic transactional process. Thus, CIIT emphasizes "field regulatory" processes in addition to "self-regulatory" or "affect regulatory" processes (Mitchell, 1988).

Sullivan (1948) initially conceived of reciprocal processes in terms of basic conjunctive and disjunctive forces that lead to either resolution or disintegration of the interpersonal situation. Later he formally presented his "theorem of reciprocal emotions," which stated that "integration in an interpersonal situation is a process in which (1) complementary needs are resolved (or aggravated); (2) reciprocal patterns of activity are developed (or disintegrated); and (3) foresight of satisfaction (or rebuff) of similar needs is facilitated" (Sullivan, 1953b, p. 129). While this theorem was a powerful interpersonal assertion, it lacked specificity, and "the surviving general notion of complementarity was that actions of human participants are redundantly interrelated (i.e., have patterned regularity) in some manner over the sequence of transactions" (Kiesler, 1983, p. 198).

Leary's (1957) "principle of reciprocal interpersonal relations" further specified the basis for patterned regularity of interpersonal behavior, stating, "Interpersonal reflexes tend (with a probability greater than chance) to initiate or invite reciprocal interpersonal responses from the 'other' person in the interaction that lead to a repetition of the original reflex" (p. 123). Learning in interpersonal situations takes place, in part, because social interaction is reinforcing (Leary, 1957). Carson (1991) referred to this as an interbehavioral contingency process where, "there is a tendency for a given individual's interpersonal behavior to be constrained or controlled in more or less predictable ways by the behavior received from an interaction partner" (p. 191).

Describing Reciprocal Interpersonal Patterns

The IPC provides conceptual anchors and a lexicon to systematically describe the patterned regularity of reciprocal interpersonal processes. The most basic of these processes is "interpersonal complementarity" (Carson, 1969; Kiesler, 1983). Interpersonal complementarity occurs when there is a match between the field regulatory goals of each person. That is, reciprocal patterns of activity evolve where the agentic and communal needs of both persons are met in the interpersonal situation, leading to stability and likely recurrence of the pattern. Carson (1969) first proposed that complementarity could be defined via the IPC. He proposed that complementarity was based on the social exchange of status (agency) and love (communion) as reflected in reciprocity for the vertical dimension (i.e., dominance pulls for submission and submission pulls for dominance) and correspondence for the horizontal dimension (friendliness pulls for friendliness; hostility pulls for hostility). Kiesler (1983) extended this by adapting complementarity to the geometry of the IPC model. Given the continuous nature of the circular model's descriptions of behavior (i.e., all interpersonal behaviors are blends of dominance and nurturance), the principles of reciprocity and correspondence could be employed to specify complementary points along the entire IPC perimeter. Thus, beyond the cardinal points of the IPC, hostile dominance pulls for hostile submission, friendly dominance pulls for friendly submission, and so on, which can be further described by the lower-level taxa in these segments of the model. Kiesler also proposed that complementarity involves behavioral intensity. Reciprocity on dominance, correspondence on nurturance, and equivalent intensity thus define complementary behaviors. While complementarity is not the only reciprocal interpersonal pattern that can be described by the IPC, nor is it proposed as a universal law of interaction, empirical studies consistently find support for its probabilistic predictions (e.g., Gurtman, 2001; Markey et al., 2003; Tracey, 1994). Complementarity is most helpful if considered a common baseline for the field regulatory pulls and invitations of interpersonal behavior. Used this way, deviations from complementary reciprocal patterns may be indicative of pathological functioning.

The two other broad classes of reciprocal interpersonal patterns anchored by the IPC model are referred to as acomplementary and anticomplementary patterns (Kiesler, 1983, 1996). When reciprocal interpersonal patterns meet one of the two rules of complementarity, it is an "acomplementary pattern." In such a case, interactants may exhibit correspondence with regard to nurturance or reciprocity with regard to dominance, but not both. When interactants exhibit neither reciprocity on dominance nor correspondence on nurturance, it is as an "anticomplementary pattern." The patterned regularity in human transaction directly affects the outcomes of interpersonal situations. Complementary reciprocal patterns are considered to promote relational stability; that is, such interpersonal situations are resolved, mutually reinforcing, and recurring. Acomplementary patterns are less stable and instigate negotiation toward or away from greater complementarity. Finally, anticomplementary patterns are the most unstable and lead to avoidance, escape, and disintegration of the interpersonal situation (i.e., disrupted interpersonal relations).

Transaction Cycles and Field Regulation

Table 6.3 summarizes the IPC-based taxonomies of trait and behavioral constructs, reciprocal interpersonal patterns, and forms of intraindividual variability that can be used to describe contemporaneous human transaction (i.e., proximal interpersonal situations). Complementarity is the reciprocal interpersonal pattern that anchors most theoretical discussions of interpersonal interaction. If we are to regard interpersonal behavior as

TABLE 6.3. Foundations for Interpersonal Circumplex Description of Individual Differences in Personality, Interpersonal Behavior, and Personality Disorder Phenomenology

- Assessing agency and communion

  Self-report

  Interpersonal Adjective Scales (IAS; Wiggins, 1995)
  Inventory of Interpersonal Problems (IIP-C: Alden, Wiggins, & Pincus, 1990)
  Circumplex Scales of Interpersonal Values (CSIV; Locke, 2000)
  Impact Message Inventory (IMI-C; Kiesler & Schmidt, 1993)
  Social Behavior Inventory (SBI; Moskowitz, 1994)

  Observational coding

  Checklist of Interpersonal Transactions (CLOIT-R; Kiesler et al., 1991)
  Checklist of Psychotherapy Transactions (CLOPT-R; Kiesler et al., 1991)

  Narrative coding

  Life stories and narratives (McAdams, 1993)
  Free descriptions of self and others (Heck & Pincus, 2001)

- Reciprocal interpersonal processes
  Complementarity, acomplementarity, anticomplementarity (Kiesler, 1983, 1996)

- Intraindividual variability in interpersonal behavior
  Flux, pulse, spin (Moskowitz & Zuroff, 2004)

influential or "field regulatory," there must be some basic goals toward which our behaviors are directed. Sullivan (1953b) viewed the personification of the self to be a dynamism that is built up from the positive reflected appraisals of significant others allowing for relatively anxiety-free functioning and high levels of felt security and self-esteem. The self-dynamism becomes relatively stable over time due to the self-perpetuating influence it has on awareness and organization of interpersonal experience (input) and the field regulatory influences of interpersonal behavior (output). Sullivan proposed that both our perceptions of others' behaviors toward us and our enacted behaviors are strongly affected by our self-concept. When we interact with others, a proximal interpersonal field is created where behavior serves to present and define our self-concept and negotiate the kinds of interactions and relationships we seek from others. Sullivan's (1953b) theorem of reciprocal emotion and Leary's (1957) principle of reciprocal interpersonal relations have led to the formal view that what we attempt to regulate in the interpersonal field are the responses of the other. "Interpersonal behaviors, in a relatively unaware, automatic, and unintended fashion, tend to invite, elicit, pull, draw, or entice from interactants restricted classes of reactions that are reinforcing of, and consistent with, a person's proffered self-definition" (Kiesler, 1983, p. 201; see also Kiesler, 1996). To the extent that individuals can mutually satisfy their needs for interaction that is congruent with their self-definitions (i.e., complementarity), the interpersonal situation remains integrated. To the extent this fails, negotiation or disintegration of the interpersonal situation is more probable.

Interpersonal complementarity (or any other reciprocal pattern) should not be conceived of as some sort of stimulus–response process based solely on overt actions and reactions (Pincus, 1994). A comprehensive account of the contemporaneous interpersonal situation must somehow bridge the gap between the proximal interpersonal situation and the internal interpersonal situation (e.g., Safran, 1992). Kiesler's (1986, 1988, 1991, 1996) "interpersonal transaction cycle" is the most widely applied framework to describe the relations among proximal and internal interpersonal behavior within the interpersonal tradition. He proposes that the basic components of an interpersonal transaction are (1) person X's covert experience of person Y, (2) person X's overt behavior toward person Y, (3) person Y's covert experience in response to Person X's action, and (4) person Y's overt behavioral response to person X. These four components are part of an ongoing transactional chain of events cycling toward resolution, further negotiation, or disintegration. Within this process, overt behavioral output serves the purpose of regulating the proximal interpersonal field via elicitation of complementary overt responses in the other. The IPC specifies the range of descriptive taxa, while the motivational conceptions of interpersonal theory give rise to the nature of regulation of the interpersonal field. For example, dominant interpersonal behavior (e.g., "You have to call your mother") communicates a bid for status (e.g., "I am in charge here") that has an impact on the other in ways that elicit either complementary (e.g., "You're right, I should do that now") or noncomplementary (e.g., "Quit bossing me around!") responses in an ongoing cycle of reciprocal causality, mediated by internal subjective experience.

The Interpersonal and the Intrapsychic Revisited

While there have been a number of proposed constructs related to the covert mediating step in interpersonal transaction cycles (see Pincus, 1994; Pincus & Ansell, 2003, for reviews), CIIT formally proposes that covert reactions reflect internal interpersonal situations that can be described using the same agentic and communal constructs that have been applied to the description of proximal interpersonal situations. Normality may reflect the tendency or capacity to perceive proximal interpersonal situations and their field regulatory influences in generally undistorted forms. That is, the internal interpersonal situation generally is consistent with the proximal interpersonal situation resulting in accurate encoding of the interpersonal "bids" proffered by the interactants. Thus, all goes well, the interpersonal situation is resolved, and the relationship is stable. However, this is clearly not always the case. Psychotherapy with patients with personality disorders provides a clear example. Therapists generally attempt to work in the patient's best interest and promote a positive therapeutic alliance. Patients who are generally free of personality pathology typically enter therapy hoping for relief of their symptoms and are capable of experiencing the therapist as potentially helpful and benign. Thus, the proximal and internal interpersonal situations are consistent with each other and the behavior of therapist and patient is likely to develop into a complementary reciprocal pattern (i.e., a therapeutic alliance). Despite psychotherapists taking a similar stance with patients with personality disorders, the beginning of therapy is often quite rocky as the patients tend to view the therapists with suspicion, fear, contempt, and so on. The internal interpersonal situation is not consistent with the proximal interpersonal situation and the patient and therapist likely begin treatment by experiencing noncomplementary reciprocal patterns requiring further negotiation of the therapeutic relationship.

CIIT proposes that when the internal interpersonal situation is inconsistent with the field regulatory bids communicated in the proximal interpersonal situation, the subjective experience takes precedence. That is, the locus of complementarity (Pincus & Ansell, 2003) is internal and covert experience is influenced to a greater or lesser degree by enduring tendencies to elaborate incoming interpersonal data in particular ways. Interpersonal theory can easily accommodate the notion that individuals exhibit tendencies to organize their experience in certain ways (they have particular interpersonal schemas, expectancies, memories, fantasies, etc.), and CIIT proposes that the best way to characterize these internal interpersonal situations is in terms of their agentic and communal characteristics.

There are now converging literatures that suggest that mental representations of self and other are central structures of personality that significantly affect perception, emotion, cognition, and behavior (Blatt et al., 1997). The fundamental advantage of integrating conceptions of dyadic mental representation into interpersonal theory is the ability to import the proximal interpersonal field (Wiggins & Trobst, 1999) into the intrapsychic world of the interactants (Heck & Pincus, 2001) using a common metric. Thus, an interpersonal relationship is composed of the ongoing participation in proximal interpersonal fields in which overt behavior serves important communicative and regulatory functions, as well as ongoing experiences of internal interpersonal fields that reflect enduring individual differences in covert experience through the elaboration of interpersonal input. The unique and enduring organizational influences that people bring to relationships contribute to their covert feelings, impulses, interpretations, and fantasies in relation to others. CIIT proposes that overt behavior is mediated by such covert processes. Psychodynamic, attachment, and cognitive theories converge with this assertion and suggest that dyadic mental representations are key influences on the subjective elaboration of interpersonal input. Integrating pantheoretical representational constructs may enhance the explanatory power of CIIT by allowing for a developmental account of individuals' enduring tendencies to organize interpersonal information in particular ways. The developmental propositions of CIIT describe the mechanisms that give rise to such tendencies as well as their functional role in personality.

Parataxic Distortions

Sullivan (1953a) proposed the concept of "parataxic distortion" to describe the mediation of proximal relational behavior by internal subjective interpersonal situations and suggested that these occur "when, beside the interpersonal situation as defined within the awareness of the speaker, there is a concomitant interpersonal situation quite different as to its principle integrating tendencies, of which the speaker is more or less completely unaware" (p. 92). The effects of parataxic distortions on interpersonal relations can occur in several forms, including chronic distortions of new interpersonal experiences (input); generation of rigid, extreme, and/or chronically nonnormative interpersonal behavior (output); and dominance of internal interpersonal situations and other affect or self-regulation goals leading to the disconnection of interpersonal input and output.

Normal and pathological personalities may be differentiated by their enduring tendencies to organize interpersonal experience in particular ways, leading to integrated or disturbed interpersonal relations. CIIT proposes that healthy interpersonal relations are promoted by the capacity to organize and elaborate incoming interpersonal input in generally undistorted ways, allowing for the mutual needs of self and other to be met. That is, the proximal interpersonal field and the internal interpersonal field are relatively consistent (i.e., free of parataxic distortion). Maladaptive interpersonal functioning is promoted when the proximal interpersonal field is encoded in distorted or biased ways, leading to behavior (output) that disrupts interpersonal relations due to conflicting or disconnected field regulatory influences. In the psychotherapy context, this can be identified by a preponderance of acomplementary and anticomplementary cycles of transaction between therapist and patient (Kiesler, 1988). Such therapeutic experiences are common in the treatment of personality disorders.

CONTEMPORARY INTEGRATIVE INTERPERSONAL THEORY OF PERSONALITY: II. DEVELOPMENT AND MOTIVATION

A comprehensive theory of personality and personality disorder includes contemporaneous analysis emphasizing present description, as well as developmental analysis emphasizing historical origins and the continuing significance of past experience on current functioning (Millon, 1996). Therefore, beyond contemporaneous description of proximal and internal interpersonal situations based on the metaconcepts of agency and communion, CIIT must account for the development and maintenance of healthy and disordered self-concepts and patterns of interpersonal relating. The basis of an individual's enduring ways of organizing interpersonal experience involves his or her learning history across the recurrent interpersonal situations that characterize his or her life. Early developmental interpersonal situations contribute to the origins of the self-concept and relational patterns, while later the field regulatory influences of interpersonal behavior and the mediation of proximal experience by internal interpersonal situations contribute to the maintenance of personality. CIIT proposes that the process by which interpersonal situations promote enduring influences on personality development is through the internalization and mental representation of reciprocal interpersonal patterns in relationships that are associated with particular developmental motives and regulatory functions. Two necessary conditions must be present for interpersonal situations to have a significant impact on personality development (i.e., for learning to take place that contributes to the development of, or change in, enduring patterns of interpersonal relating and relatively stable conceptions of self/identity). First, a catalyst for internalization must exist. CIIT proposes that those interpersonal situations that involve activation, achievement, or frustration of developmentally salient motives or the impingement of an organismic trauma catalyze internalization of interpersonal experience. Second, the interpersonal situation is associated with one or more regulatory metagoals (i.e., field regulation, affect regulation, or self-regulation).

Internalization and Mental Representation

Since Freud (1923) proposed that the origins of the superego could be found in childrens' early identifications with parents, pantheoretical constructs of mental representation (e.g., cognitive–interpersonal schemas, internal working models, and object relations) all suggest that such structures are a product of interpersonal learning and the internalization of aspects of important proximal interpersonal situations. Internalization is a mechanism for the development of relatively stable mental structures that, when activated, can take the form of internal interpersonal situations.

Benjamin (1996b, 1996c, 2003) has provided the most articulate account of internalization to emerge from the interpersonal tradition, and her concept of interpersonal "copy processes" appears to offer important explanatory power when incorporated into CIIT. Unless or until better concepts emerge, I use these concepts in fairly unmodified form as part of CIIT developmental theory. Benjamin has proposed three developmental "copy processes" that describe the ways in which early interpersonal experiences are internalized. The first is *identification*, which is defined as "treating others as one has been treated." To the extent that individuals strongly identify with early caretakers (typically parents), there will be a tendency to act toward others in ways that copy how important others have acted toward the developing person. When doing so, behavior in proximal interpersonal field is associated with positive reflected appraisals of the self from the representation of the identified-with-other in the internal interpersonal field. This mediates the perception of the proximal situation and may lead to repetition of such behavior regardless of the field regulatory pulls of the other (i.e., noncomplementary reciprocal patterns). The second copy process is *recapitulation*, which is defined as "maintaining a position complementary to an internalized other." This can be described as reacting "as if" the internalized other is still there. In this case, new interpersonal input is likely to be elaborated in a distorted way such that the proximal other is experienced as similar to the internalized other, or new interpersonal input from the proximal other may simply be ignored and field regulation is focused on the dominant internalized other. This again may lead to noncomplementary reciprocal patterns in the proximal interpersonal situation while complementary interpersonal patterns are played out in the internal interpersonal field. The third copy process is *introjection*, which is defined as "treating the self as one has been treated," and is related to Sullivan's conceptions of "reflected appraisals" as a source of self-personification. By treating the self in introjected ways, the internal interpersonal situation may promote security and esteem even while generating noncomplementary behavior in the proximal interpersonal situation.

Identification, recapitulation, and introjection are not incompatible with Kiesler's conception of covert impact messages. In fact, the proposed copy processes can help account for individual differences in covert experience by providing developmental hypotheses regarding the origins of a person's enduring tendencies to experience particular feelings, impulses, cognitions, and fantasies in interpersonal situations. In the initial stages of treatment with patients with personality disorders, it seems that their experience of the therapist is often distorted by strong identifications, recapitulations of relationships with parents and other early caregivers, and the dominance of introjected, often self-destructive, behaviors. This, in turn, leads to parataxic distortions of the proximal interpersonal field in therapy and frequent noncomplementary reciprocal interpersonal patterns in the therapeutic relationship.

Catalysts of Internalization

While forms of internalization and mental representation help to describe possible pathways in which learning in past interpersonal situations gives rise to enduring concepts of self and interpersonal behavior, it is still insufficient to explain "why" early interpersonal situations remain so influential that they can give rise to parataxic distortions of proximal interpersonal situations. The answer to this question requires a discussion of motivation. Sullivan's legacy has led many interpersonal theorists to posit self-confirmation as the core motive underlying human transaction (e.g., Kiesler, 1996). Benjamin (1993) proposed a fundamental shift toward the establishment of attachment as the fundamental interpersonal motivation. In doing so, she provided one mechanism to account for the enduring influence of early interpersonal situations on personality and contemporaneous functioning. Infants and toddlers must form attachments to caregivers in order to survive. Benjamin has suggested that the nature of the early interpersonal environment will dictate what must be done to establish attachments. These early attachment relationships can be described using the IPC model's descriptive taxa (e.g., Bartholomew & Horowitz, 1991; Gallo et al., 2003), reciprocal interpersonal patterns, and forms of intraindividual variability. The primacy of internalized relationships is thus associated with the need to maintain attachment within them even when not immediately present. Benjamin (1993) referred to this as maintaining "psychic proximity" to internalized others. With reference to the CIIT framework, this psychic proximity to attachment figures is one way that internal interpersonal situations mediate contemporaneous transactions, even giving rise to parataxic distortions of the proximal interpersonal situation. The influential primacy of early attachment patterns and their internalized mental representations on current experience is consistent with psychodynamic and attachment theories. Bowlby (1980) suggested that internal working models act conservatively; thus assimilation of new experience into established schemas is typical (see also Stern, 1988).

CIIT seeks to understand why certain reciprocal interpersonal patterns become prominent for an individual. Benjamin has made an important start by suggesting that a basic human motivation is attachment and that the interpersonal behaviors and reciprocal interpersonal patterns that help achieve attachment become fundamental to personality through internalization of relationships. She posited that the wish for attachment and the fear of its loss are universal and that positive early environments lead to secure attachments and culturally normative behavior. If the developing person is faced with achieving attachment in a toxic early environment, behavior will be nonnormative but will develop in the service of attachment needs and be maintained via internalization.

CIIT extends this further in an effort to generate an interpersonal theory of personality (and personality disorder) that more broadly addresses issues of basic human motivation. The maturational trajectory of human life allows us to conceptualize many developmentally salient motives that may function to mediate and moderate current interpersonal experience. That is, *reciprocal interpersonal patterns develop in concert with emerging motives that take developmental priority*, thus expanding the goals that underlie their formation and maintenance (Pincus & Ansell, 2003, pp. 223–224). CIIT posits core issues likely to elicit the activation of mediating internal interpersonal situations, potential developmental deficits associated with early experiences, and unresolved conflicts that continue to influence the subjective experience of self and others. The output of such internal structures and processes for an individual are those consistently sought after relational patterns and their typical strategies for achieving them (i.e., proximal and internal field regulation). These become the basis for the recurrent interpersonal situations that characterize a human life.

CIIT proposes that "catalysts of internalization" (Pincus & Ansell, 2003) fall into two broad classes of developmental experience (see Table 6.4). The interpersonal situations listed in Table 6.4 catalyze and reinforce identification, recapitulation, and introjection due to the organizing power of developmental achievements and traumatic stressors. At different points in personality development certain motives become a priority. Perhaps initially the formation of attachment bonds and security are primary motivations. But later, separation–individuation, self-esteem, mastery of unresolved conflicts, and identity formation may become priorities. If we are to understand the field regulatory strategies individuals employ when such developmental motives or traumas are reactivated, we must learn what interpersonal behaviors and patterns were associated with achievement or frustration of particular developmental milestones or were required to cope with a trauma in the first place.

Identifying the developmental and traumatic catalysts for internalization of reciprocal interpersonal patterns allows for greater understanding

TABLE 6.4. Some Possible Catalysts of Internalization

Developmental achievements	Traumatic learning
Attachment	Early loss of attachment figure
Security	Childhood illness or injury
Separation–individuation	Physical abuse
Positive affects	Sexual abuse
Gender identity	Emotional abuse
Resolution of oedipal issues	Parental neglect
Self-esteem	
Self-confirmation	
Mastery of unresolved conflicts	
Identity formation	

of current behavior. For example, in terms achieving adult attachment relationships, some individuals have developed hostile strategies such as verbally or physically fighting in order to elicit some form of interpersonal connection, whereas others have developed submissive strategies such as avoiding conflict and deferring to the wishes of the other in order to be liked and elicit gratitude. While CIIT asserts that internal interpersonal situations can mediate the perception and encoding of new input, the overt behavior of the other is influential, particularly as it activates a person's expectancies, wishes, fears, and so on, that are associated with important motives or traumas. This will significantly influence their covert experience. Along with unfortunate traumatic experiences, the most important motives of individuals are those associated with the central achievements of personality development that have been identified across the theoretical spectrum.

Regulatory Metagoals

CIIT proposes an additional level of interpersonal learning that takes place concurrently with the association of particular patterns of interpersonal relating to the specific goals associated with emerging developmental achievements and coping with trauma. The second condition necessary for internalization of interpersonal experience is the association of the interpersonal situation with one or more of three superordinate regulatory functions or metagoals: field regulation, emotion regulation, and self-regulation. The concept of regulation has become almost ubiquitous in psychological theory, particularly in the domain of human development. Most theories of personality emphasize the importance of developing mechanisms for emotion regulation and self-regulation. Interpersonal theory is unique in its added emphasis on field regulation (i.e., the processes by which the behavior of self and other transactionally influence each other) (Mitchell, 1988; Sullivan, 1948; Wiggins & Trobst, 1999). CIIT extends this emphasis further by proposing that field regulation may be directed toward a proximal other or an internalized other. Field regulation thus provides a third regulatory metagoal, complementing the important functions of emotion regulation and self-regulation. The emerging developmental achievements and the coping demands of traumas listed in Table 6.4 all have significant implications for emotion regulation, self-regulation, and field regulation. This further contributes to the generalization of interpersonal learning to new interpersonal situations by providing a small number of superordinate psychological triggers to activate internal interpersonal situations.

The importance of distinguishing these three regulatory metagoals is most directly related to understanding the shifting priorities that may be associated with interpersonal behavior. At any given time, the most prominent metagoal may be field regulation as has been emphasized throughout this chapter. However, interpersonal behavior may also be associated with self-regulation such as derogation of others to promote one's self-esteem or emotion regulation such as the use of sexual availability in order to feel more emotionally secure and stable. In such instances, interpersonal behavior may play a central role, even if the priority is not explicitly field regulation. Interpersonal behavior enacted in the service of regulating the self or emotion may reduce the contingencies associated with the behavior of the other person. This is another pathway to parataxic distortion and also helps to account for the fluctuating symptomology of personality disorders.

PERSONALITY DISORDERS

The core clinical features of personality disorder are *chronic interpersonal dysfunction* and *problems with self/identity*. CIIT is in a position to enhance the explanatory power of these clinical features by defining personality disorder and providing a system to describe individual differences in the phenomenological expression of personality disorder. Because the interpersonal tradition views normality and abnormality on a continuum, the entire chapter has addressed both personality and personality disorder concurrently. However, a formal derivation of CIIT's conception of personality disorder for future clinical research and practice can be articulated. Considering the core clinical features of personality disorder, we can propose that healthy personalities exhibit adaptive interpersonal functioning (i.e., healthy relational capacity) and relatively stable and positive self-concepts.

CIIT proposes that the key elements distinguishing the normal and disordered personality involves the capacity to enter into new proximal interpersonal situations without parataxic distortion. In other words, the larger the range of proximal interpersonal situations that can be entered into in which the person exhibits anxiety-free functioning (little need for emotion regulation) and maintains self-esteem (little need for self-regulation), the more adaptive the personality. When this is the case, there is no need to activate mediating internal interpersonal situations and the person can focus on the proximal situation, encode incoming interpersonal input without distortion, respond in adaptive ways that facilitate interpersonal relations (i.e., meet the agentic and communal needs of self and other), and establish complementary patterns of reciprocal behavior by fully participating in the proximal interpersonal field. The individual's current behavior will exhibit relatively strong contingency with the proximal behavior of the other and the normative contextual press of the situation. Adaptive interpersonal functioning is promoted by relatively trauma-free development in a culturally normative facilitating environment that has allowed the person to achieve most developmental milestones in normative ways, leading to full capacity to encode and elaborate incoming interpersonal input without bias from competing psychological needs.

In contrast, when the individual develops in a traumatic or non-normative environment, significant nonnormative interpersonal learning around basic motives such as attachment, individuation, gender identity, and so on may be internalized and associated with difficulties with self-regulation, emotion regulation, and field regulation. In contrast to the healthy personality, personality disorder is reflected in a large range of proximal interpersonal situations that elicit anxiety (activating emotion-regulation strategies), threaten self-esteem (activating self-regulation strategies), and elicit dysfunctional behaviors (nonnormative field-regulation strategies). When this is the case, internal interpersonal situations are activated and the individual is prone to exhibit various forms of parataxic distortion as his or her interpersonal learning history dictates. Thus the perception of the proximal interpersonal situation is mediated by internal experience, incoming interpersonal input is distorted, behavioral responses (output) disrupt interpersonal relations (i.e., fail to meet the agentic and communal needs of self and other), and relationships tend toward non-complementary patterns of reciprocal behavior. The individual's current behavior will exhibit relatively weak contingency with the proximal behavior of the other.

Fluctuating Severity of Personality Disorder Symptomology

It is important for both researchers and clinicians to avoid confusing the stability of personality (e.g., Roberts & DelVecchio, 2000) with the (presumed) stability of personality disorder symptomology. I have been treating patients with personality disorders and supervising their treatment for more than 14 years. Clearly these patients do not walk around emitting the same behaviors over and over again regardless of the situation (or interpersonal situation). As noted by Livesley (2001), many personality disorders exhibit fluctuating courses of acute symptomatic states, crises of all sorts, and oscillating levels of functioning. Many patients with personality disorders can be perfectly appropriate with clinic staff, waiters and waitresses, and others they encounter in daily living situations. Some can maintain employment or even attend university and complete advanced degrees. There is considerable evidence that personality disorder symptomology fluctuates, and that is good news for psychotherapists. If it were otherwise, there would be little sense in treating them. Therapeutic strategies for personality disorder take advantage of stable periods and work toward containment and reestablishing more adaptive functioning during times of dysregulation. The interpersonal approach developed here accounts for this fluctuating severity in terms of interpersonal learning associated with developmentally salient motives and regulatory metagoals. That is, whereas symptoms of patients with personality disorders fluctuate and they exhibit transient capacity for adaptive functioning, when it becomes necessary for them to regulate their sense of self (e.g., cohesion, esteem, identity), their emotions, or the behavior of others, we often see an increase in severity of symptomology. This occurs because such regulatory metagoals are likely to be associated with core motives and the internalized patterns of relating associated with their achievement or frustration. When such metagoals and motives are evoked or thwarted in patients with personality disorders, parataxic distortions dominate functioning. In healthy personalities, only a small number of interpersonal situations require significant regulatory effort, but for individuals with personality disorder, many more interpersonal situations appear to elicit anxiety and self-esteem threat.

Definition of Personality Disorder

In this section I provide the elements for a preliminary contemporary integrative interpersonal definition of personality disorder that elaborates on the core clinical features of *chronic interpersonal dysfunction* and *problems with self or identity*. The elements provide a causal–theoretical definition of personality disorder for Step 1 of a two-step diagnostic process that can be coordinated with practical–empirical approaches to description of individual differences in personality disorder phenomenology through the structural models, operational definitions, and empirical methods of the interpersonal tradition. Personality disorder can be defined by the following:

A. In a large range of situations, the individual exhibits strongly internalized relational patterns associated with (i) activation, achievement, or frustration of salient developmental motives, (ii) traumatic learning, and (iii) regulatory metagoals. These internalized patterns pervade the self-concept and perception of others (via schemas, self-talk, imagery, object relations, internal working models, etc.) leading to parataxic distortions that:

1. Interfere with accurate encoding of new interpersonal experiences (input).
2. Generate inflexible, extreme, and/or non-normative interpersonal behavior leading to vicious circles, self-fulfilling prophecies, and maladaptive transaction cycles (output).
3. Reduce the contingency between the individual's behavior (output) and the behavior of others (input) or the normative situational press (input).

B. Such disturbances typically develop in a toxic social environment at odds with normative developmental experiences, leading to identification, recapitulation, and introjection of maladaptive self-, emotion-, and field-regulatory strategies that generate self-defeating and non-normative interpersonal behavior.

C. Lack of insight is common and may be due to distortion of interpersonal input, dominance of internal field-regulation metagoals, or preoccupation with self-regulation or emotion-regulation metagoals.

Lack of insight is one of the most challenging aspects of treating personality disorders. Such patients are notoriously unaware of their impact on others or the consequences of their behavior for themselves. The underlying causes of poor insight are the various forms of impairment brought about by parataxic distortions. First, distorted input leads to behaviors that make sense to the individuals with a personality disorder but not to others. Second, the priority metagoal may be to regulate the behavior of an internalized other rather than regulation of an actual other in the proximal interpersonal field (e.g., to receive positive reflected appraisals from internalized others for "acting like them"—identification) . Third, the priority metagoal may be regulation of the self or regulation of emotion rather than regulation of an other in the proximal interpersonal field. While self- and emotion-regulation strategies can be largely interpersonal in nature, they typically reduce the contingencies associated with interpersonal input and output.

Describing Individual Differences in Personality Disorders

CIIT proposes that the IPC provides useful taxonomies of individual differences to differentiate the expression of personality disorder defined above. I conclude by sketching out examples of narcissistic and dependent personality disorders from this perspective. These two examples are presented because of their considerable clinical relevance and history. They were not chosen because they appear in the DSM Axis II nosology. My view is that narcissism and dependency are two clear pathological personality patterns that clinicians face today.

Narcissism

Clinical literature (e.g., Cooper, 1998) and empirical research (e.g., Dickinson & Pincus, 2003) on narcissism conclude that there are two forms of pathological expression. Both forms are based on fundamental problems with the self and self-esteem regulation. All narcissistic personalities have difficulty maintaining a stable positive self-image and rely on the provision of narcissistic supplies from their interpersonal relationships. This leads to entitled expectations and exploitative attitudes toward others. The difference between the two forms of expression involves coping responses in light of failure of the proximal interpersonal situation to provide narcissistic supplies to regulate self-esteem. Fundamentally, all narcissistic personalities are prone to experience new interpersonal situations as potential threats to self-esteem and thus are regularly evoking self-regulation strategies which disturb their interpersonal relations via parataxic distortions.

Grandiose narcissists (the only type currently represented in the DSM) regulate self-esteem via self-enhancement strategies that include overly positive assessment of the self and devaluation of others who do not provide needed admiration. Empirical research relating grandiose narcissism to the IPC typically has found it associated with a hostile–dominant interpersonal style reflecting arrogant, calculating, and vindictive behavior (e.g., Pincus & Wiggins, 1990; Wiggins & Pincus, 1989). In Figure 6.5, grandiose narcissism is represented by the solid lines/arrows reflecting a low amount of spin (centered in the BC octant of the IPC) and low pulse around an extreme mean level. Grandiose narcissists tend to be rigidly hostile–dominant in relation to others and to exhibit extreme behavioral expression as in narcissistic rage and chronic devaluation of others. These behaviors are

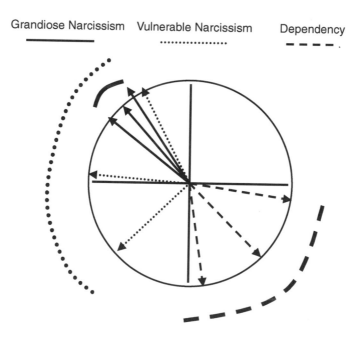

FIGURE 6.5. Interpersonal spin and pulse in grandiose narcissistic personalities, vulnerable narcissistic personalities, and dependent personalities.

often noncomplementary to other interpersonal bids or pulls in the proximal interpersonal situation. Parataxic distortion in grandiose narcissists is activated due to chronic problems with self-regulation, and this reduces the contingencies between their behavior and the behavior of others. Clinically, this parataxic distortion is described as defensive self-enhancement or the successful use of grandiosity to regulate self-esteem. This often gives rise to disrupted interpersonal situations as behavior is often not contingent upon interpersonal input and noncomplementary reciprocal patterns are common.

For example, one such patient grew up in a family where his parents were consistently cold and aloof and he had highly competitive feelings toward his older brother which he was never helped to resolve. To complicate matters, he was frequently treated with allergy medications that left him feeling mentally foggy and disconnected from others. He developed a compensatory grandiose self to regulate self-esteem and was prone to see himself as far more capable, deserving, and powerful than others despite interpersonal feedback to the contrary. His behaviors were often extreme. For example, his apartment had an assigned parking spot in the lot of his building. Despite not driving or owning a car, he would regularly threaten anyone he found parking in "his" spot and even fantasized to his therapist about buying a gun and shooting the next person who parked there. Despite strong efforts on the part of two therapists to form a positive therapeutic alliance with him, he chronically devalued them and insisted they were unable to affect him in any way.

In contrast, the clinical literature clearly describes a second expression of narcissistic personality often labeled the vulnerable, hypersensitive, or closet narcissist. Such individuals have the same fundamental deficits in self-esteem regulation leading to the experience of many new interpersonal situations as threatening to the self. However, they often fail to employ grandiosity to regulate self-esteem. Vulnerable narcissistic personalities are much more labile and their interpersonal behavior and sense of self oscillates from grandiose states to self-critical depression and avoidance of others. In Figure 6.5, vulnerable narcissism is represented by the dotted lines/arrows reflecting significantly greater spin than their grandiose counterparts. Vulnerable narcissists often enter new interpersonal situations with grandiose expectations and exhibit hostile–dominant behavior. However, when needed admiration is not provided, they often spin to a more withdrawn and depressed state of hostile submissiveness. That is, vulnerable narcissists exhibit greater intraindividual variability in interpersonal behavior and greater contingency on the behavior of others than grandiose narcissists. In both self-states, vulnerable narcissists tend to exhibit low pulse around extreme mean levels of hostile–dominant and hostile–submissive behavior.

In contrast to the aforementioned grandiose patient, one such vulnerable patient grew up in a home in which his parents oscillated between being harshly critical and dismissive of him and expecting him to contribute money and status to the family, essentially relying on him to "make things better" for everyone else. The patient's sense of self oscillated between identifications with the neighborhood toughs who had tattoos, stood on the corner, and were feared and respected by everyone on the block and depressive states where he felt like he was "full of shit." He clearly entered most interpersonal situations in grandiose states and was willing to get into conflicts with his spouse, neighbors, and police on a regular basis. However, he also frequently felt disappointed that others did not admire him. At those times, he appeared incapable of devaluing others and would become depressed, self-critical, and punishing. When in such states he destroyed his own stereo equipment, refused to eat, and stayed in his room for days avoiding people. In therapy it was easy to tell which state he was in when he walked through the door. These two states were associated with the divergent interpersonal patterns he experienced in relationships with his family.

Dependency

Dependent personalities typically rely on others for both instrumental support and emotional nurturance, which reflects a core motivation to obtain and maintain nurturant and supportive relationships in the service of emotion regulation and self-regulation (Birtchnell, 1988; Bornstein, 1993). This is not inherently pathological and dependency can take healthy and destructive forms (e.g., Bornstein et al., 2003). For those personalities exhibiting dependent personality disorder, the self is consistently experienced as weak, inept, and needy while others are typically viewed as more capable and powerful than the self (Bornstein, 1996). Dependent personalities are prone to experience new interpersonal situations as potential threats to both emotional well-being and self-esteem if the needed nurturance and instrumental support are not provided. Dependent persons also exhibit intraindividual variability in interpersonal field regulatory behavior emitted to obtain and maintain supportive and nurturant relationships (e.g., Bornstein, 1995; Bornstein, Riggs, Hill, & Calabrese, 1996). Bornstein and colleagues have noted that the types of behaviors dependent individuals emit to evoke support and nurturance from others is contingent upon the interpersonal context. Such strategies may be active or passive or self-denigrating or self-promoting, depending on whether the needed other is a peer or an authority.

A series of studies relating dependency to the IPC suggested that dependency is associated with the entire range of friendly–submissive interpersonal functioning (Pincus, 2002; Pincus & Gurtman, 1995; Pincus & Wilson, 2001). In Figure 6.5, the dependent personality is represented by the dashed lines/arrows reflecting a limited amount of spin centered in friendly–submissiveness and low pulse around an extreme mean level. Beginning with submissiveness and moving counterclockwise toward friendly behaviors, dependency may be expressed via passivity and helplessness, ingratiating deference, or loving approach. At moderate levels of intensity this is not inherently pathological, especially if other forms of interpersonal behavior are easily enacted as interpersonal situations dictate (i.e., large spin). However, when all interpersonal situations become risks to needed support and nurturance and tests of the needed other's availability, parataxic distortions will disrupt interpersonal relations and extreme and rigid dependent behavior will contribute to disturbed interpersonal relations.

While I have seen extremely dependent patients consistently threaten suicide if the other (typically a spouse) did not drop everything and immediately come to their rescue, more typical difficulties involve helplessness, chronic deferential attitudes, and inappropriate efforts to achieve emotional closeness. One such patient had a chronic view of the self as inept, perhaps in response to parents who claimed they "were always right and knew better" than the patient. In addition, her parents were extremely overprotective and chronically punished the patient's developmental efforts to assert autonomy and function independently (see, e.g., Thompson & Zuroff, 1998). When the patient began treatment, she reported that she could not do her own laundry or clean her apartment effectively (and literally left everything piled up until a parent or friend noticed and took action), failed to take her antidepressants on a regular basis, consistently deferred and ingratiated herself to "friends" in hope of it being reciprocated even after repetitive rejections, and occasionally provided sexual favors (typically fellatio) to men she hoped would then "love" her. These types of behaviors persisted despite their lack of success due to parataxic distortions. For example, angry and frustrated parents cleaning her apartment and then demanding she return home to live with them were experienced as supportive. Peers typically made plans without consulting her and then she would passively tag along. She experienced this as being included. She experienced exploitative sexual approaches as caring, even when the men made no further efforts toward relational intimacy. Thus, the patient's interpersonal behavior tended to evoke few true experiences of instrumental support and nurturance. Nonetheless, the patient's self-regulation and emotion-regulation needs were dominant, leading to repetitive maladaptive transactional cycles and noncomplementary interpersonal patterns. In the early phases of psychotherapy, she experienced any effort by the therapist to promote her autonomous functioning (e.g., increase her agency) as a lack of care.

Concluding Comments

These cases were provided to exemplify the potential for CIIT to provide a nexus to coordinate or causal–theoretical definition of personality disorder with a practical–empirical description of individual differences in the phenomenological expression of personality disorder. The descriptive taxonomies of the IPC are neither inherently normal nor pathological. Only when combined with a theory do they provide a potential basis for practical clinical description and differentiation. Currently it remains highly useful to retain as much of the accrued clinical wisdom on abnormal personalities as possible, and thus CIIT currently seeks to account for relevant clinical patterns such as narcissistic and dependent personalities. As theory and classification continue to evolve, relevant forms of personality disorder may be based directly on agentic and communal constructs. In the future, CIIT might retain its basic definition of personality disorder while classification of individual differences in expression could directly reflect individual differences in agentic and communal constructs, representative reciprocal interpersonal patterns, and levels of intraindividual variability. However, such developments are reserved for the next edition of this collection of major theories of personality disorder.

NOTE

1. I consider the IPC model and Benjamin's (1974, 1996a) SASB model to be complementary variants rather than mutually exclusive competitors.

REFERENCES

Abraham, K. (1927). *Selected papers in psychoanalysis.* London: Hogarth Press (Original work published 1921)

Alden, L. E., Wiggins, J. S., & Pincus, A. L. (1990). Construction of circumplex scales for the Inventory of Interpersonal Problems. *Journal of Personality Assessment, 55,* 521–536.

American Psychiatric Association. (1980). *Diagnostic and statistical manual of mental disorders* (3rd ed.). Washington, DC: Author.

American Psychiatric Association. (1987). *Diagnostic and statistical manual of mental disorders* (3rd ed., rev.). Washington, DC: Author.

American Psychiatric Association. (1994). *Diagnostic and statistical manual of mental disorders* (4th ed.). Washington, DC: Author.

American Psychiatric Association. (2000). *Diagnostic and statistical manual of mental disorders* (4th ed., text rev). Washington, DC: Author.

Bakan, D. (1966). *The duality of human existence: Isolation and communion in Western man.* Boston: Beacon Press.

Bartholomew, K., & Horowitz, L.M. (1991). Attachment styles among young adults: A test of a four-category model. *Journal of Personality and Social Psychology, 61*, 226–244.

Beck, A. T., Freeman, A., Davis, D. D., & Associates. (2004). *Cognitive therapy of personality disorders* (2nd ed.). New York: Guilford Press.

Benjamin, L. S. (1974). Structural analysis of social behavior. *Psychological Review, 81*, 392–425.

Benjamin, L. S. (1993). Every psychopathology is a gift of love. *Psychotherapy Research, 3*, 1–24.

Benjamin, L. S. (1995). Good defenses make good neighbors. In H. Conte & R. Plutchik (Eds.), *Ego defenses: Theory and measurement* (pp. 38 -78). New York: Wiley.

Benjamin, L. S. (1996a). A clinician-friendly version of the interpersonal circumplex: Structural Analysis of Social Behavior (SASB). *Journal of Personality Assessment, 66*, 248–266.

Benjamin, L. S. (1996b). An interpersonal theory of personality disorders. In J. F. Clarkin & M. F. Lenzenweger (Eds.), *Major theories of personality disorder* (pp. 141–220). New York: Guilford Press.

Benjamin, L. S. (1996c). *Interpersonal diagnosis and treatment of personality disorders* (2nd ed.). New York: Guilford Press.

Benjamin, L. S. (2003). *Interpersonal reconstructive therapy.* New York: Guilford Press.

Benjamin, L. S. & Friedrich, F. J. (1991). Contributions of Structural Analysis of Social Behavior (SASB) to the bridge between cognitive science and a science of object relations. In M. Horowitz (Ed.), *Person schemas and maladaptive interpersonal patterns* (pp. 379–412). Chicago: Chicago University Press.

Birtchnell, J. (1988). Defining dependency. *British Journal of Medical Psychology, 61*, 111–123.

Blatt, S. J., Auerbach, J. S., & Levy, K. N. (1997). Mental representations in personality development, psychopathology, and the therapeutic process. *Review of General Psychology, 1*, 351–374.

Bornstein, R. F. (1993). *The dependent personality.* New York: Guilford Press.

Bornstein, R. F. (1995). Active dependency. *Journal of Nervous and Mental Disease, 183*, 64–77.

Bornstein, R. F. (1996). Beyond orality: Toward an object relations/interactionist reconceptualization of the etiology and dynamics of dependency. *Psychoanalytic Psychology, 13*, 177–203

Bornstein, R. F. (1997). Dependent personality disorder in the DSM-IV and beyond. *Clinical Psychology: Science and Practice, 4*, 175–187.

Bornstein, R. F. (2003). Behaviorally referenced experimentation and symptom validation: A paradigm for 21st-century personality disorder research. *Journal of Personality Disorders, 17*, 1–18.

Bornstein, R. F., Languirand, M. A., Geiselman, K. J., Creighton, J. A., West, M. A., Gallagher, H. A., & Eisenharet, E. A. (2003). Construct validity of the relationship profile test: A self-report measure of dependency—detachment. *Journal of Personality Assessment, 80*, 64–74.

Bornstein, R. F., Riggs, J. M., Hill, E. L., & Calabrese, C. (1996). Activity, passivity, self-denigration, and self-enhancement: Toward an interactionist model of interpersonal dependency. *Journal of Personality, 64,* 637–673.

Bowlby, J. (1980). *Attachment and loss, Vol. 3. Loss: Sadness and depression.* New York: Basic Books.

Brokaw, D. W., & McLemore, C. W. (1991). Interpersonal models of personality and psychopathology. In D. G. Gilbert & J. J. Connolly (Eds.), *Personality, social skills, and psychopathology: An individual differences approach. Perspectives on individual differences* (pp. 49–83). New York: Plenum Press.

Carson, R. C. (1969). *Interaction concepts of personality.* Chicago: Aldine.

Carson, R. C. (1982). Self-fulfilling prophecy, maladaptive behavior, and psychotherapy. In J. C. Anchin & D. J. Kielser (Eds.), *Handbook of interpersonal psychotherapy* (pp. 64–77). New York: Pergamon Press.

Carson, R. C. (1991). The social-interactional viewpoint. In M. Hersen, A. Kazdin, & A. Bellack (Eds.), *The clinical psychology handbook* (2nd ed., pp. 185–199). New York: Pergamon Press.

Carson, R. C. (1996). Seamlessness in personality and its derangements. *Journal of Personality Assessment, 66,* 240–247.

Clark, L. A. (1993). *Manual for the Schedule for Nonadaptive and Adaptive Personality.* Minneapolis: University of Minnesota Press.

Clark, L. A., Livesley, W. J., & Morey, L. (1997). Personality disorder assessment: The challenge of construct validity. *Journal of Personality Disorders, 11,* 205–231.

Clarkin, J. F., & Lenzenweger, M. F. (1996). *Major theories of personality disorder* (1st ed.). New York: Guilford Press.

Cloninger, C. R. (2000). A practical way to diagnose personality disorder: A proposal. *Journal of Personality Disorders, 14,* 99–108.

Cloninger, C. R., Przybeck, T. R., Svrakic, D., & Wetzel, R. D. (1994). *The Temperament and Character Inventory (TCI): A guide to its development and use.* St. Louis: Washington University, Center for Psychobiology of Personality.

Cooper, A. (1998). Further developments in the clinical diagnosis of narcissistic personality disorder. In E. Ronningstam (Ed.), *Disorders of narcissism: Diagnostic, clinical, and empirical implications* (pp. 53–74). Washington, DC: American Psychiatric Press.

Costa, P. T., Jr., & McCrae, R. R. (1990). Personality disorders and the five-factor model of personality. *Journal of Personality Disorders, 4,* 362–371.

Depue, R. A. (1996). A neurobiological framework for the structure of personality and emotion: Implications for personality disorders. In J. F. Clarkin & M. F. Lenzenweger (Eds.), *Major theories of personality disorder* (1st ed., pp. 347–390). New York: Guilford Press.

Dickinson, K. A., & Pincus, A. L. (2003). Interpersonal analysis of grandiose and vulnerable narcissism. *Journal of Personality Disorders, 17,* 188–207.

Endler, N. S., & Kocovski, N. L. (2002). Personality disorders at the crossroads. *Journal of Personality Disorders, 16,* 487–502.

Florsheim, P., Henry, W. P., & Benjamin, L. S. (1996). Integrating individual and interpersonal approaches to diagnosis: The structural analysis of social behavior and attachment theory. In F. Kaslow (Ed.), *Handbook of relational diagnosis* (pp. 81–101). New York: Wiley.

Fournier, M. A., Moskowitz, D. S., & Zuroff, D. C. (2002). Social rank strategies in hierarchical relationships. *Journal of Personality and Social Psychology*, *83*, 425–433.

Freedman, M. B., Leary, T. F., Ossorio, A. G., & Coffey, H. S. (1951). The interpersonal dimension of personality. *Journal of Personality*, *20*, 143–161.

Freud, S. (1923). The ego and the id. In *Standard Edition* (Vol. 19, pp. 1–53). London: Hogarth Press.

Gallo, L. C., Smith, T. W., & Ruiz, J. M. (2003). An interpersonal analysis of adult attachment style: Circumplex descriptions, recalled developmental experiences, self-representations, and interpersonal functioning in adulthood. *Journal of Personality*, *71*, 141–181.

Gifford, R. (1991). Mapping nonverbal behavior on the Interpersonal Circle. *Journal of Personality and Social Psychology*, *61*, 856–867.

Greenberg, J. R., & Mitchell, S. A. (1983). *Object relations in psychoanalytic theory*. Cambridge, MA: Harvard University Press.

Gurtman, M. B. (1994). The circumplex as a tool for studying normal and abnormal personality: A methodological primer. In S. Strack & M. Lorr (Eds.) *Differentiating normal and abnormal personality* (pp. 243–263). New York: Springer.

Gurtman, M. B. (1997). Studying personality traits: The circular way. In R. Plutchik & H. R. Conte (Eds.), *Circumplex models of personality and emotions* (pp. 81–102). Washington, DC: American Psychological Association.

Gurtman, M. B. (2001). Interpersonal complementarity: Integrating interpersonal measurement with interpersonal models. *Journal of Counseling Psychology*, *48*, 97–110.

Gurtman, M. B., & Balakrishnan, J. D. (1998). Circular measurement redux: The analysis and interpretation of interpersonal circle profiles. *Clinical Psychology: Science and Practice*, *5*, 344–360.

Gurtman, M. B., & Pincus, A. L. (2000). Interpersonal Adjective Scales: Confirmation of circumplex structure from multiple perspectives. *Personality and Social Psychology Bulletin*, *26*, 374–384.

Gurtman, M. B., & Pincus, A. L. (2003). The circumplex model: Methods and research applications. In J. A. Schinka & W. F. Velicer (Eds.), *Comprehensive handbook of psychology, Vol. 2: Research methods in psychology* (pp. 407–428). New York: Wiley.

Hartung, C. M., & Widiger, T. A. (1998). Gender differences in the diagnosis of mental disorders: Conclusions and controversies of the DSM-IV. *Psychological Bulletin*, *123*, 260–278.

Heck, S. A., & Pincus, A. L. (2001). Agency and communion in the structure of parental representations. *Journal of Personality Assessment*, *76*, 180–184.

Horowitz, L. M. (2004). *The interpersonal foundations of psychopathology*. Washington, DC: American Psychological Association.

Hoyenga, K. B., Hoyenga, K. T., Walters, K., & Schmidt, J. A. (1998). Applying the interpersonal circle and evolutionary theory to gender differences in psychopathological traits. In L. Ellis & L. Ebertz (Eds.), *Males, females, and behavior: Towards biological understanding* (pp. 213–241). Westport, CT: Praeger.

Kernberg, O. F. (1984). *Severe personality disorders: Psychotherapeutic strategies.* New Haven: Yale University Press.

Kernberg, O. F. (1996). A psychoanalytic theory of personality disorders. In J. F. Clarkin & M. F. Lenzenweger (Eds.), *Major theories of personality disorder* (1st ed., pp. 106–140). New York: Guilford Press.

Kiesler, D. J. (1982). Interpersonal theory for personality and psychotherapy. In J. C. Anchin & D. J. Kielser (Eds.), *Handbook of interpersonal psychotherapy* (pp. 3–23). New York: Pergamon Press.

Kiesler, D. J. (1983). The 1982 interpersonal circle: A taxonomy for complementarity in human transactions. *Psychological Review, 90,* 185–214.

Kiesler, D. J. (1985). *The 1982 interpersonal circle: Acts version.* Unpublished manuscript, Virginia Commonwealth University, Richmond.

Kiesler, D. J. (1986). The 1982 interpersonal circle: An analysis of DSM-III personality disorders. In T. Millon & G. L. Klerman (Eds.), *Contemporary directions in psychopathology: Toward the DSM-IV* (pp. 571–598). New York: Guilford Press.

Kiesler, D. J. (1988). *Therapeutic metacommunication: Therapist impact disclosure as feedback in psychotherapy.* Palo Alto, CA: Consulting Psychological Press.

Kiesler, D. J. (1991). Interpersonal methods of assessment and diagnosis. In C. R. Snyder & D. R. Forsyth (Eds.), *Handbook of social and clinical psychology* (pp. 438–468). New York: Pergamon Press.

Kiesler, D. J. (1996). *Contemporary interpersonal theory and research: Personality, psychopathology, and psychotherapy.* New York: Wiley.

Kiesler, D. J., Goldston, C. S., & Schmidt, J. A. (1991). *Manual for the Check List of Interpersonal Transactions—Revised (CLOIT-R) and the Check List of Psychotherapy Transactions—Revised (CLOPT-R).* Richmond: Virginia Commonwealth University.

Kiesler, D. J., & Schmidt, J. A. (1993). *The Impact Message Inventory: Form IIA octant scale version.* Palo Alto, CA: Mind Garden.

Kiesler, D. J., Schmidt J. A., & Wagner C. C. (1997). A circumplex inventory of impact messages: An operational bridge between emotion and interpersonal behavior. In R. Plutchik & H. Contes (Eds.), *Circumplex models of personality and emotions* (pp. 221–244). Washington, DC: American Psychological Association.

Kohut, H., & Wolf, E. S. (1978). The disorders of the self and their treatment—An outline. *International Journal of Psycho-Analysis, 59,* 413–425.

Kraepelin, E. (1907). *Clinical psychiatry.* New York: Macmillan.

LaForge, R. (2004). The early development of the interpersonal system of personality (ISP). *Multivariate Behavioral Research, 39,* 359–378.

LaForge, R., Freedman, M. B., & Wiggins, J. S. (1985). Interpersonal circumplex models: 1948–1983. *Journal of Personality Assessment, 49,* 613–631.

Leary, T. (1957). *Interpersonal diagnosis of personality.* New York: Ronald Press.

Lenzenweger, M. F., & Clarkin, J. F. (1996). The personality disorders: History, classification, and research issues. In J. F. Clarkin & M. F. Lenzenweger (Eds.), *Major theories of personality disorder* (pp. 1–35). New York: Guilford Press.

Livesley, W. J. (1998). Suggestions for a framework for an empirically based classification of personality disorder. *Canadian Journal of Psychiatry*, 43, 137–147.

Livesley, W. J. (2001). Conceptual and taxonomic issues. In J. Livesley (Ed.), *Handbook of personality disorders* (pp. 3–38). New York: Guilford Press.

Livesley, W. J., & Jackson, D. N. (in press). *Manual for the dimensional assessment of personality pathology—Basic questionnaire (DAPP)*. Port Huron, MI: Sigma Press.

Livesley, W. J., Jackson, D. N., & Schroeder, M. L. (1992). Factorial structure of traits delineating personality disorders in clinical and general populations samples. *Journal of Abnormal Psychology*, 101, 432–440.

Locke, K. D. (2000). Circumplex scales of interpersonal values: Reliability, validity, and applicability to interpersonal problems and personality disorders. *Journal of Personality Assessment*, 75, 249–267.

Lorr, M., & McNair, D. M. (1963). An interpersonal behavior circle. *Journal of Abnormal and Social Psychology*, 67, 68–75.

Lorr, M., & McNair, D. M. (1965). Expansion of the interpersonal behavior circle. *Journal of Personality and Social Psychology*, 2, 68–75.

Lorr, M., & Youniss, R. P. (1986). *The Interpersonal Style Inventory*. Los Angeles: Western Psychological Services.

Markey, P. M., Funder, D. C., & Ozer, D. J. (2003). Complementarity of interpersonal behaviors in dyadic interactions. *Personality and Social Psychology Bulletin*, 29, 1082–1090.

McAdams, D. P. (1993). *The stories we live by: Personal myths and the making of the self*. New York: Morrow.

McLemore, C. W., & Benjamin, L. S. (1979). Whatever happened to interpersonal diagnosis? *American Psychologist*, 34, 17–34.

McWilliams, N. (1994). *Psychoanalytic diagnosis*. New York: Guilford Press.

Millon, T. (1987). On the nature of taxonomy in psychopathology. In C. Last & M. Hersen (Eds.), *Issues in diagnostic research* (pp. 3–85). New York: Plenum Press.

Millon, T. (1990). *Toward a new personology: An evolutionary model*. New York: Wiley.

Millon, T. (1991). Classification in psychopathology: Rationale, alternatives, and Standards. *Journal of Abnormal Psychology*, 100, 245–261.

Millon, T. (1996). *Disorders of personality: DSM-IV and beyond*. New York: Wiley.

Millon, T. (2000). Reflections on the future of DSM Axis II. *Journal of Personality Disorders*, 14, 30–41.

Millon, T., & Davis, R. (1996). An evolutionary theory of personality disorders. In J. F. Clarkin & M. F. Lenzenweger (Eds.), *Major theories of personality disorder* (pp. 221–346). New York: Guilford Press.

Millon, T., Meagher, S. E., & Grossman, S. D. (2001). Theoretical perspectives. In J. Livesley (Ed.), *Handbook of personality disorders* (pp. 39–59). New York: Guilford Press.

Mitchell, S. A. (1988). The intrapsychic and the interpersonal: Different theories, different domains, or historical artifacts? *Psychoanalytic Inquiry*, 8, 472–496.

Moskowitz, D. S. (1994). Cross-situational generality and the interpersonal circumplex. *Journal of Personality and Social Psychology, 66,* 921–933.

Moskowitz, D. S., & Hershberger, S. L. (2002). *Modeling intraindividual variability with repeated measures data: Methods and applications.* Mahwah, NJ: Erlbaum.

Moskowitz, D. S., Pinard, G., Zuroff, D. C., Annable, L., & Young, S. N. (2001). The effect of trytophan on social interaction in everyday life: A placebo-controlled study. *Neuropsychopharmacology, 25,* 277–289.

Moskowitz, D. S., & Zuroff, D. C. (2004). Flux, pulse, and spin: Dynamic additions to the personality lexicon. *Journal of Personality and Social Psychology, 86,* 880–893.

Paris, J. (2000). The classification of personality disorders should be rooted in biology. *Journal of Personality Disorders, 14,* 127–136.

Parker, G., Both, L., Olley, A., Hadzi-Pavlovic, D., Irvine, P., & Jacobs, G. (2002). Defining personality disordered functioning. *Journal of Personality Disorders, 16,* 503–522.

Pincus, A. L. (1994). The interpersonal circumplex and the interpersonal theory: Perspectives on personality and its pathology. In S. Strack & M. Lorr (Eds.), *Differentiating normal and abnormal personality* (pp. 114–136). New York: Springer.

Pincus, A. L. (1997, August). Beyond complementarity: An object-relations perspective. Paper presented at the symposium on Interpersonal Complementarity: Current Status and Critical Issues, M. B. Gurtman (Chair), annual convention of the American Psychological Association, Chicago.

Pincus, A. L. (2002). Constellations of dependency within the five-factor model of personality. In P. T. Costa, Jr. & T. A. Widiger (Eds.), *Personality disorders and the five-factor model of personality* (2nd ed., pp. 203–214). Washington, DC: American Psychological Association.

Pincus, A. L. (in press). The interpersonal nexus of personality disorders. In S. Strack (Ed.), *Personology and psychopathology.* New York: Wiley.

Pincus, A. L., & Ansell, E. B. (2003). Interpersonal theory of personality. In T. Millon & M. Lerner (Eds.), *Handbook of psychology—Vol. 5: Personality and social psychology* (pp. 209–229). New York: Wiley.

Pincus, A. L., Dickinson, K. A., Schut, A. J., Castonguay, L. G., & Bedics, J. (1999). Integrating interpersonal assessment and adult attachment using SASB. *European Journal of Psychological Assessment, 15,* 206–220.

Pincus, A. L., & Gurtman, M. B. (1995). The three faces of interpersonal dependency: Structural analyses of self-report dependency measures. *Journal of Personality and Social Psychology, 69,* 744–758.

Pincus, A. L., & Gurtman, M. B. (2003). Interpersonal assessment. In J. S. Wiggins, *Paradigms of personality assessment* (pp. 246–261). New York: Guilford Press.

Pincus, A. L., Gurtman, M. B., & Ruiz, M. A. (1998). Structural Analysis of Social Behavior (SASB): Circumplex analyses and structural relations with the Interpersonal Circle and the five-factor model of personality. *Journal of Personality and Social Psychology, 74,* 1629–1645.

Pincus, A. L., & Wiggins, J. S. (1990). Interpersonal problems and conceptions of personality disorders. *Journal of Personality Disorders, 4,* 342–352.

Pincus, A. L., & Wilson, K. R. (2001). Interpersonal variability in dependent personality. *Journal of Personality, 69,* 223–252.

Pretzer, J. L., & Beck, A. T. (1996). A cognitive theory of personality disorders. In J. F. Clarkin & M. F. Lenzenweger (Eds.), *Major theories of personality disorder* (1st ed., pp. 36–105). New York: Guilford Press.

Reich, W. (1949). *Character analysis* (3rd ed.). New York: Farrar, Straus, & Giroux. (Original work published 1933)

Roberts, B. W., & DelVecchio, W. F. (2000). The rank-order consistency of personality traits from childhood to old age: A quantitative review of longitudinal studies. *Psychological Bulletin, 126,* 3–25.

Roemer, W. W. (1986). Leary's circle matrix: A comprehensive model for the statistical measurement of Horney's clinical concepts. *American Journal of Psychoanalysis, 16,* 249–262.

Safran, J. D. (1990a). Towards a refinement in cognitive therapy in light of interpersonal theory: I. Theory. *Clinical Psychology Review, 10,* 87–105.

Safran. J. D. (1990b). Towards a refinement of cognitive therapy in light of interpersonal theory: II. Practice. *Clinical Psychology Review, 10,* 107–121.

Safran, J. D. (1992). Extending the pantheoretical applications of interpersonal inventories. *Journal of Psychotherapy Integration, 2,* 101–105.

Schaefer, E. S. (1959). A circumplex model for maternal behaviors. *Journal of Abnormal and Social Psychology, 59,* 226–235.

Schaefer, E. S. (1961). Converging conceptual models for maternal behavior and child behavior. In J. C. Glidwell (Ed.), *Parental attitudes and child behavior* (pp. 124–146). Springfield, IL: Charles C. Thomas.

Schneider, K. (1950). *Psychopathic personalities.* London: Cassell. (Original work published 1923)

Silk, K. R. (1997). *Biology of personality disorders.* Washington, DC: Amrican Psychiatric Press.

Soldz, S., Budman, S., Demby, A., & Merry, J. (1993). Representation of personality disorders in circumplex and five-factor space: Explorations with a clinical sample. *Psychological Assessment, 5,* 41–52.

Stern, D. N. (1985). *The interpersonal world of the infant.* New York: Basic Books.

Stern, D. N. (1988). The dialectic between the "interpersonal" and the "intrapsychic": With particular emphasis on the role of memory and representation. *Psychoanalytic Inquiry, 8,* 505–512.

Sullivan, H. S. (1948). The meaning of anxiety in psychiatry and life. *Psychiatry, 11,* 1–13.

Sullivan, H. S. (1953a). *Conceptions of modern psychiatry.* New York: Norton.

Sullivan, H. S. (1953b). *The interpersonal theory of psychiatry.* New York: Norton.

Sullivan, H. S. (1954). *The psychiatric interview.* New York: Norton.

Sullivan, H. S. (1956). *Clinical studies in psychiatry.* New York: Norton.

Sullivan, H. S. (1962). *Schizophrenia as a human process.* New York: Norton.

Sullivan, H. S. (1964). *The fusion of psychiatry and social science.* New York: Norton.

Thompson, R., & Zuroff, D. C. (1998). Dependent and self-critical mothers' responses to adolescent autonomy and competence. *Personality and Individual Differences*, 24, 311–324.

Tracey, T. J. G. (1994). An examination of complementarity of interpersonal behavior. *Journal of Personality and Social Psychology*, 67, 864–878.

Trobst, K. K. (2000). An interpersonal conceptualization and quantification of social support transactions. *Personality and Social Psychology Bulletin*, 26, 971–986.

Vaillant, G. E., & McCullough, L. (1998). The role of ego mechanisms of defense in the diagnosis of personality disorders. In J. W. Barron (Ed.), *Making diagnosis meaningful* (pp. 139–158). Washington, DC: American Psychological Association.

Westen, D., & Arkowitz-Westen, L. (1998). Limitations of Axis II in diagnosing personality pathology in clinical practice. *American Journal of Psychiatry*, 155, 1767–1771.

Westen, D., & Shedler, J. (2000). A prototype matching approach to diagnosing personality disorders: Toward DSM-V. *Journal of Personality Disorders*, 14, 109–126.

Widiger, T. A. (1991). Definition, diagnosis, and differentiation. *Journal of Personality Disorders*, 5, 42–51.

Widiger, T. A. (2000). Personality disorders in the 21st-century. *Journal of Personality Disorders*, 14, 3–16.

Widiger, T. A., & Costa, P. T., Jr. (2002). Five-factor model personality disorder research. In P. T. Costa, Jr., & T. A. Widiger (Eds.), *Personality disorders and the five-factor model of personality* (2nd ed., pp. 59–87). Washington, DC: American Psychological Association.

Widiger, T. A., & Sankis, L. M. (2000). Adult psychopathology: Issues and controversies. *Annual Review of Psychology*, 51, 377–404.

Widiger, T. A., & Trull, T. J. (1991). Diagnosis and clinical assessment. *Annual Review of Psychology*, 42, 109–133.

Wiggins, J. S. (1979). A psychological taxonomy of trait descriptive terms: The interpersonal domain. *Journal of Personality and Social Psychology*, 37, 395–412.

Wiggins, J. S. (1980). Circumplex models of interpersonal behavior. In L. Wheeler (Ed.), *Review of personality and social psychology* (Vol. 1, pp. 265–293). Beverly Hills, CA: Sage.

Wiggins, J. S. (1982). Circumplex models of interpersonal behavior in clinical psychology. In P. C. Kendall & J. N. Butcher (Eds.), *Handbook of research methods in clinical psychology* (pp. 183–221). New York: Wiley.

Wiggins, J. S. (1991). Agency and communion as conceptual coordinates for the understanding and measurement of interpersonal behavior. In W. Grove & D. Cicchetti (Eds.), *Thinking clearly about psychology: Essays in honor of Paul E. Meehl* (Vol. 2, pp. 89–113). Minneapolis: University of Minnesota Press.

Wiggins, J. S. (1995). *Interpersonal adjective scales: Professional manual*. Odessa, FL: Psychological Assessment Resources.

Wiggins, J. S. (1996). An informal history of the interpersonal circumplex tradition. *Journal of Personality Assessment*, 66, 217–233.

Wiggins, J. S. (1997a). Circumnavigating Dodge Morgan's interpersonal style. *Journal of Personality, 65,* 1069–1086.

Wiggins, J. S. (1997b). In defense of traits. In R. Hogan, J. Johnson, & S. Briggs (Eds.), *Handbook of personality psychology* (pp. 95–115). New York: Academic Press.

Wiggins, J. S. (2003). *Paradigms of personality assessment.* New York: Guilford Press.

Wiggins, J. S., Phillips, N., & Trapnell, P. (1989). Circular reasoning about interpersonal behavior: Evidence concerning some untested assumptions underlying diagnostic classification. *Journal of Personality and Social Psychology, 56,* 296–305.

Wiggins, J. S., & Pincus, A. L. (1989). Conceptions of personality disorders and dimensions of personality. *Psychological Assessment, 1,* 305–316.

Wiggins, J. S., & Trapnell, P. D. (1996). A dyadic interactional perspective on the five-factor model. In J. S. Wiggins (Ed.), *The five-factor model of personality: Theoretical perspectives* (pp. 88–162). New York: Guilford Press.

Wiggins, J. S., Trapnell, P. D. & Phillips, N. (1988). Psychometric and geometric characteristics of the revised Interpersonal Adjective Scales (IAS-R). *Multivariate Behavioral Research, 23,* 17–30.

Wiggins, J. S., & Trobst, K. K. (1997). When is a circumplex an "interpersonal circumplex"? The case of supportive actions. In R. Plutchik & H. R. Conte (Eds.), *Circumplex models of personality and emotions* (pp. 57–80). Washington, DC: American Psychological Association.

Wiggins, J. S., & Trobst, K. K. (1999). The fields of interpersonal behavior. In L. Pervin & O. P. John (Eds.), *Handbook of personality: Theory and research* (2nd ed., pp. 653–670). New York: Guilford Press.

Yik, M. S. M., & Russell, J. A. (2004). On the relationship between circumplexes: Affect and Wiggins' IAS. *Multivariate Behavioral Research, 39,* 202–229.

Young, J. (1990). *Cognitive therapy for personality disorders: A schema-focused approach.* Sarasota, FL: Professional Resource Exchange.

Zuroff, D. C., Moskowitz, D. S., & Cote, S. (1999). Dependency, self-criticism, interpersonal behaviour and affect: Evolutionary perspectives. *British Journal of Clinical Psychology, 38,* 231–250.

CHAPTER 7

■ ■ ■

Personology: A Theory Based on Evolutionary Concepts

THEODORE MILLON
SETH D. GROSSMAN

Theories that focus their attention on only one level of data (e.g., intrapsychic and cognitive) cannot help but generate formulations that are limited by their narrow preconceptions; moreover, their findings must, inevitably, be incompatible with the simple fact that psychological processes are multidetermined and multidimensional in expression. Those who endorse a single-level approach assert that theories that seek to encompass the totality of personality structure and functions will sink in a sea of data that can be neither charted conceptually nor navigated methodologically. Clearly, those who undertake to propose "integrative" or "holistic" theories are faced with the formidable task not only of exposing the inadequacies of single-level theories but of providing a convincing alternative that is both comprehensive and systematic. The reader must judge whether such theorists possess the intellectual skills and analytic powers necessary, not only to penetrate the vast labyrinths of man's mind and behavior but to chart these intricate pathways in a manner that is both conceptually clear and methodologically testable.

In this chapter, we go beyond current conceptual and research boundaries in personology and incorporate the contributions of past theorists as well as those of our more firmly grounded "adjacent" sciences. Not only may such steps bear new conceptual fruits, but they may provide a foundation that can undergird and guide our own discipline's explorations. Much of psychology as a whole remains adrift, divorced from broader spheres of scientific knowledge, isolated from deeper and more fundamental, if not universal, principles. As the history of psychology amply illustrates, the propositions of our science are not in themselves sufficient to orient its development in a consistent and focused fashion. Consequently, psychology has built a patchwork quilt of dissonant concepts and diverse data domains. Preoccupied with but a small part of the larger pie, or fearing accusations of reductionism, we have failed to draw on the rich possibilities that may be found in both historic and adjacent realms of scholarly pursuit. With few exceptions, cohering concepts that would connect current topics to those of the past have not been developed. We seem repeatedly trapped in (obsessed with?) contemporary fads and horizontal refinements. A search for integrative schemas and cohesive constructs that will link us to relevant observations and laws in other fields of contemporary science is also needed. The goal—albeit a rather "grandiose" one—is to refashion our patchwork quilt into a well-tailored and cohesive tapestry that interweaves the diverse forms in which nature expresses itself.

There is no better sphere within the psychological sciences to undertake such a synthesis than the subject matter of personology, the study of persons. Persons are the only organically integrated system in the psychological domain, evolved through the millennia and inherently created from birth as natural entities, rather than culture-bound and experience-derived gestalts. The intrinsic cohesion of persons is not merely a rhetorical construction but an authentic substantive unity. Personologic features may be differentiated into normal or pathological and may be partitioned conceptually for pragmatic or scientific purposes, but they are segments of an inseparable biopsychosocial entity. Arguing in favor of establishing explicit links between the several domains of personologic science does not call for a reductionistic philosophy, a belief in substantive identicality, or efforts to so fashion such links by formal logic. Rather, one should aspire to their substantive concordance, empirical consistency, conceptual interfacing, convergent dialogues, and mutual enlightenment.

Integrative consonance such as described is not an aspiration limited to ostensibly diverse sciences but is a worthy goal within each science as well. Particularly relevant in this regard are efforts that seek to coordinate the often separate structural and functional domains that comprise a clinical science, namely, its theories, the classification system it has formulated, the diagnostic tools it employs, and the therapeutic techniques it implements. Rather than developing independently and being left to stand in an autonomous and largely unconnected manner, a truly mature clinical science will embody the following:

1. *Theories*, that is, explanatory and heuristic conceptual schemas that are consistent with established knowledge in both its own and related sciences and from which reasonably accurate propositions concerning pathological conditions can be both deduced and understood, enabling thereby the development of a formal,
2. *Taxonomy*, that is, a nosological classification of disorders that has been derived logically from the theory and is arranged to provide a cohesive organization within which its major categories can readily be grouped and differentiated, permitting thereby the development of coordinated,
3. *Instruments*, that is, tools that are empirically grounded and sufficiently sensitive quantitatively to enable the theory's propositions and hypotheses to be adequately investigated and evaluated, and the constructs comprising its nosology to be readily identified (diagnosed) and measured (dimensionalized), specifying therefrom target areas for,
4. *Interventions*, that is, strategies and techniques of therapy, designed in accord with the theory and oriented to modify problematic clinical characteristics consonant with professional standards and social responsibilities.

It is our view that formulas of a psychological nature must not only coordinate with but be anchored firmly to observations derived specifically from modern principles of physical and biological evolution. The polarity model presented in this chapter is grounded in such modern principles, from which a deeper and clearer understanding may be obtained concerning the nature of both normal and pathological functioning. In essence, it seeks to explicate the structure and styles of personality with reference to *deficient*, *imbalanced*, or *conflicted* modes of ecological adaptation and reproductive strategy.

A PHYLOGENETIC MODEL
OF PERSONOLOGIC FUNCTIONS

In the early stages of knowledge, conceptual categories rely invariably on observed similarities among phenomena (Tversky, 1977). As knowledge advances, overt similarities are discovered to be an insufficient if not false basis for cohering categories and imbuing them with scientific meaning (Smith & Medin, 1981). As Hempel (1965) and Quine (1977) have pointed out, it is theory that provides the glue that holds concepts together and gives them both their scientific and clinical relevance. In his discussion of classificatory concepts, Hempel (1965) wrote:

The development of a scientific discipline may often be said to proceed from an initial "natural history" stage . . . to subsequent more and more "theoretical stages. . . . The vocabulary required in the early stages of this development will be largely observational. . . . The shift toward theoretical systematization is marked by the introduction of new, "theoretical" terms . . . more or less removed from the level of directly observable things and events. . . .

   These terms have a distinct meaning and function only in the context of a corresponding theory. (pp. 139–140)

Theory, when properly fashioned, ultimately provides more simplicity and clarity than unintegrated and scattered information. As effectively argued by contemporary philosophers of science (Hempel 1965; Quine 1977), unrelated knowledge and techniques, especially those based on surface similarities, are a sign of a primitive science. All natural sciences have organizing principles that not only create order but also provide the basis for generating hypotheses and stimulating new knowledge. A good theory not only summarizes and incorporates extant knowledge but is heuristic in that it originates and develops new observations and new methods.

   What are the essential elements that distinguish between a true science and an explanatory schema and one that provides a mere descriptive summary of known observations and inferences? Simply stated, the answer lies in its power to generate concepts, propositions, and observations other than those used to construct it. This generative power is what Hempel meant by the "systematic import" of a science. He contrasted what are familiarly known as "natural" (theoretically guided, deductively based) and "artificial" (conceptually barren, similarity based) scientific systems.

   Despite the shortcomings of historical and contemporary theoretical schemas, systematizing principles and abstract concepts can "facilitate a deeper seeing, a more penetrating vision that goes beyond superficial appearances to the order underlying them" (Bowers 1977, p. 130). For example, pre-Darwinian taxonomists such as Linnaeus limited themselves to "apparent" similarities and differences among animals as a means of constructing their categories. Darwin was not "seduced" by appearances. Rather, he sought to understand the principles by which overt features came about. His classifications were based not only on keenly observed descriptive qualities but on genuinely explanatory ones.

   No one argues against the view that theories that float, so to speak, on their own, unconcerned with the empirical domain or clinical knowledge, should be seen as the fatuous achievements they are and the travesty they may make of the virtues of a truly coherent nosological system. Formal theory should not be "pushed" far beyond the data, and its derivations should be linked at all points to established clinical observations. As Millon (1987a) has written elsewhere, structurally weak theories make it impossible to derive systematic and logical nosologies, which results in conflicting derivations and circular reasoning. Most nosological theories of psychopathology have generated brilliant deductions and insights, but few of these ideas can be attributed to their structure, the precision of their concepts, or their formal procedures for hypothesis derivation. Here, of course, is where the concepts and laws of adjacent sciences may come into play, providing models of structure and derivation, as well as substantive theories and data that may undergird and parallel the principles and observations of one's own field.

The adjacent science we have drawn on as a guiding model for our framework of personality studies is that of "evolution" and its many and diverse forms of expression. And the role of evolution may be most clearly grasped when it is paired with the principles of ecology. So conceived, the procession of evolution in physics, chemistry, and biology represents a series of serendipitous transformations in the structure of a phenomenon (e.g., elementary particle, chemical molecule, and living organism) that appear to promote survival in both its current and future environments (Millon, 1990). Such processions usually stem from the consequences of either random fluctuations (such as mutations) or replicative reformations (e.g., recombinant mating) among an infinite number of possibilities—some simpler, others more complex, some more and others less organized, some increasingly specialized, and others not. Evolution is defined, then, when these restructurings enable a natural entity (e.g., a biological species) or its subsequent variants to survive within present and succeeding ecological milieus. It is the continuity through time of these fluctuations and reformations that comprises the sequence we characterize as evolutionary progression.

In recent times, we have seen the emergence of *sociobiology*, a new "science" that explores the interface between human social functioning and evolutionary biology (Cosmides & Tooby, 1987; Daly & Wilson, 1978; Rushton, 1985; Symons, 1992; Wilson 1975, 1978, 1998). Contemporary formulations by psychologists have likewise proposed the potentials and analyzed the problems involved in cohering evolutionary notions, individual differences, and personality traits (e.g., Buss, 1984, 1994). The concept of *personology*, first formulated by Murray (1938), has been extended by Millon's (1990) writings to parallel the concept of sociobiology. It represents a field of science and study that defines and encompasses the broad subject of personality. It is intended to serve as a conceptual model and formal theory that uses evolutionary principles, generates a formal taxonomy, and formulates a basis for clinical assessments and synergistic therapies (Millon, 1997, 1999).

The common goal among personologic scientists is not only the desire to apply common principles across diverse scientific realms but also to reduce the enormous range of personality concepts that have proliferated through history; this might be achieved by exploring the power of evolutionary theory to simplify and order previously disparate features. For example, all organisms seek to avoid injury, find nourishment, and reproduce their kind if they are to survive and maintain their populations. Each species displays commonalities in its adaptive or survival style. Within each species, however, there are differences in style and differences in the success with which its various members adapt to the diverse and changing environments they face. In these simplest of terms, "personality" would be employed as a term to represent the more or less distinctive style of adaptive functioning that a particular organism of a species exhibits as its relates to its typical range of environments. "Normal personalities," so conceived, would signify the utilization of species-specific modes of adaptation that are effective in "average or expectable" environments. "Disorders" of personality, or what we would prefer to term "personality styles" or "patterns of pathology," would represent different ways of maladaptive functioning that can be traced to psychic deficiencies, trait imbalances, or internal conflicts that characterize some members of a species as they relate to the environment they routinely face.

During its life history an organism develops an assemblage of traits that contribute to its individual survival and reproductive success, the two essential components of "fitness" formulated by Darwin. Such assemblages, termed "complex adaptations and strategies" in the literature of evolutionary ecology, are close biological equivalents to what psychologists and psychiatrists have conceptualized as personality styles. In biology, explanations of a life-history strategy of adaptations refer primarily to biogenic variations among constituent traits, their overall covariance structure, and the nature and ratio of favorable to unfavorable ecological resources that have been available for purposes of extending longevity and optimizing reproduction. Such explanations are not appreciably different from those used to account for the development of normal and pathological personality styles.

Bypassing the usual complications of analogies, a relevant and intriguing parallel may be drawn between the *phylogenic evolution* of a species genetic composition and the *ontogenic development* of an individual organism's adaptive strategies (i.e., its "personality style"). At any point in time, a species will possess a limited set of genes that serve as trait potentials. Over succeeding generations the frequency distribution of these genes will likely change in their relative proportions depending on how well the traits they undergird contribute to the species "fittedness" within its varying ecological habitats. In a similar fashion, individual organisms begin life with a limited subset of their species' genes and the trait potentials they subserve. Over time the salience of these trait potentials—not the proportion of the genes themselves—will become differentially prominent as the organism interacts with its environments, "learning" from these experiences which of its traits "fit" best (i.e., are optimally suited to is ecosystem). *In phylogenesis, then, actual gene frequencies change during the generation-to-generation adaptive process, whereas in ontogenesis it is the salience or prominence of gene-based traits that changes as adaptive learning takes place.* Parallel evolutionary processes occur, one within the many generations of life of a species, the other within the limited life of a single organism. What is seen in the individual organism is a shaping of latent potentials in adaptive and manifest styles of perceiving, feeling, thinking, and acting; these learned and distinctive ways of adaptation, engendered by the interaction of biological endowment and social experience, comprise, in our view, the elements of what are termed "personality styles, normal or abnormal." Thus the formative process of a single lifetime parallels gene redistributions among species during their evolutionary history.

In the following section we have established psychological constructs called polarities that are coupled with the principles of evolutionary survival. Later in the chapter we elaborate how these polarities help generate stages of neurodevelopmental ontogenesis and clinical taxonomies that can derive and parallel DSM personalities and syndromes. First, an outline of the phylogenetically based evolutionary polarities.

Existential Aims: The Pain–Pleasure Polarity

The first phase, existence, concerns the survival of integrative phenomena, whether a nuclear particle, virus, or human being, against the forces of entropic decompensation. Evolutionary mechanisms associated with this stage relate to biological survivial processes of life enhancement and life preservation. The former are concerned with orienting individuals toward improving the quality of life; the latter with orienting individuals away from actions or environments that decrease the quality of life or even jeopardize existence itself. These two superordinate processes may be called *existential aims*. At the highest level of abstraction such mechanisms form, phenomenologically or metaphorically, a pleasure–pain polarity. Most humans exhibit both processes, those oriented toward enhancing pleasure and avoiding pain. Some individuals with personality disorders, however, appear to be conflicted in regard to existential aims (e.g., the sadistic), whereas others possess deficits in such aims (e.g., the schizoid). In terms of evolutionary–neurodevelopmental stages (Millon, 1969, 1981, 1990, 2003), orientations on the pleasure–pain polarity are set during a "sensory attachment" developmental stage, the purpose of which is to further mature and selectively refine and focus the largely innate ability to discriminate between pain and pleasure signals.

Every system can be conceptualized on its own terms, as a closed system, existing in and of itself. The most basic of evolutionary functions, that of existence, has a twofold aspect according to Spencer (1870). The first pertains to is the enhancement or enrichment of life—that is, creating or strengthening ecologically survivable organisms. The second is the preservation of life—that is, creating survivability and security by avoiding events that might terminate it. As noted, the former may be seen in life-enhancing acts that enrich existence by what are experientially recorded as "pleasurable" events (positive reinforcers), the latter in life-preserving behaviors oriented to achieve security by repelling or avoiding events that are experientially characterized as "painful" (negative reinforcers).

Existence is literally a to-be or not-to-be issue. In the inorganic world, "to be" is essentially a matter of possessing qualities that distinguish a phenomenon from its surrounding field (i.e., of not being in a state of entropy). Among organic beings, "to be" is a matter of possessing the properties of life as well as being located in ecosystems that facilitate processes that enhance and preserve life, maintaining the integrity of the organism within its surrounding field. As noted, in the phenomenological or experiential world of sentient organisms, events that extend life and preserve it correspond largely to metaphorical terms such as pleasure and pain—that is, recognizing and pursuing life-enriching motivations and rewards, on the one hand, and recognizing and eschewing life-threatening emotions and sensations, on the other.

Numerous theories of psychology and psychiatry a century ago (e.g., Freud 1915/1925) proposed models that referred to affective expressions of this evolutionary bipolarity. In more recent literature, for example, are the factor-analytic dimensions of positive and negative emotionality described by Tellegen (1985) and his students (Clark & Watson, 1988; Watson & Clark, 1984; Watson & Tellegen, 1985). Both positive and negative emotions may display the full quantitative range independent of the other; moreover, low levels of pleasure are not the same as pain, and vice versa; similarly, high and low levels of positive emotionality may coexist with varying levels of negative emotionality.

Related to difficulties associated with the pain–pleasure polarity are affective labilities described as *emotional dysregulation* (Klein & Davis, 1969; Linehan, 1993), a pathological pattern of behavioral disorganization manifested most clearly in unstable and reactive affects, notably and frequently seen in borderline personality disorders. Several theorists associate levels of emotional intensity with the dimension of arousal/activation. In our judgment, however, the active–passive polarity, to be described shortly, relates to a separate evolution-based polarity.

Adaptive Modes: The Active–Passive polarity

Everything which exists, exists in an environment. To come into existence as a surviving particle or living creature is but an initial phase. Once an integrated structure exists, it must maintain its existence through exchanges of energy and information with its environment. This second evolutionary phase relates to what we have termed the "modes of adaptation"; it also is framed as a two-part polarity: a passive orientation (i.e., to be ecologically *accommodating* in one's environmental niche), versus an active orientation (i.e., to be ecologically *modifying* and to intervene in or to alter one's surrounds). These modes of adaptation differ from the first phase of evolution in that they relate to how that which has come to exist, endures. In terms of neuropsychological development, to be discussed shortly, this polarity is ontogenetically expressed as the "sensorimotor-autonomy stage," during which the child typically progresses from an earlier, relatively passive style of accommodation to a relatively active style of modifying his or her physical and social environment.

As noted, passivity may best be characterized as a mode of ecological accommodation, signifying inclinations to passively "fit in," to locate and remain securely anchored in a niche, subject to the vagaries and unpredictabilities of the environment, all acceded to with one crucial proviso: that the elements comprising the surroundings will furnish both the nourishment and the protection needed to sustain existence. Though based on a somewhat simplistic bifurcation among adaptive strategies, this passive accommodating mode is one of the two fundamental instrumental methods that living organisms have evolved as a means of survival. It represents the core process employed in the evolution of what has come to be designated as the plant kingdom, a stationary, rooted, yet essentially pliant and dependent survival mode. By contrast, the other major mode of adaptation is seen in the lifestyle of the animal kingdom. Here we observe a primary inclination toward ecological modification, an instrumentally active tendency to change or rearrange the elements comprising the larger milieu, to intrude upon otherwise quiescent settings, a versatility in shifting from one niche to another as unpredictability arises, a mobile and interventional mode that actively stirs, maneuvers, yields, and, at the human level, substantially transforms the environment to meet its own survival aims.

Both modes—passive and active—have proven impressively capable of nourishing and preserving life. Whether the polarity sketched is phrased in terms of accommodating versus modifying, passivity versus activity, or plant versus animal, it represents, at the most basic level, the two fundamental modes that organisms have evolved to sustain their existence. As noted, this second, modifying–accommodating polarity differs from the first, enhancing–preserving (that concerned with what may be called existential "becoming"), in that it characterizes modes of "being" (i.e., how what has become endures).

Broadening the active–passive polarity model to encompass human experience, we find that the vast range of behaviors engaged in by humans may fundamentally be grouped in terms of whether initiative is taken in altering and shaping life's events or whether behaviors are reactive to and accommodate those events. Often reflective and deliberate, those who are *passive* manifest few overt strategies to gain their ends. They display a seeming inertness, a phlegmatic quality, a tendency toward acquiescence, a restrained attitude in which they initiate little to modify events, waiting for the circumstances of their environment to take their course before making accommodations. Some may be temperamentally ill-equipped to rouse or assert themselves; perhaps past experience has deprived them of opportunities to acquire a range of competencies or confidence in their ability to master the events of their environment; equally possible is a naive confidence that things will come their way with little or no effort on their part. From a variety of diverse sources, then, those at the passive end of the polarity appear to merely sustain their existence, engaging in few direct instrumental activities to intercede in life events or to generate change.

Descriptively, those who are at the *active* end of the polarity are best characterized by their alertness, vigilance, liveliness, vigor, forcefulness, stimulus-seeking energy, and drive. Some plan strategies and scan alternatives to circumvent obstacles or avoid the distress of punishment, rejection, and anxiety. Others are impulsive, precipitate, excitable, rash, and hasty, seeking to elicit pleasures and rewards. Although specific goals vary and change from time to time, actively aroused individuals seek to alter their lives, to intrude on passing events by energetically and busily modifying the circumstances of their environment.

Problematic expressions of the active–passive polarity are seen, for example, in avoidant personality patterns. Here there is an *active restriction* of behavior—what is referred to as the dimension of *inhibitedness*. These individuals display marked intimacy problems, restricted and apprehensive social relationships, constrained inner feelings, and a hesitant anxiousness, fearfulness, and mistrust of close relationships.

As we proceed in evolved complexity to the human species, we cannot help but recognize the almost endless variety of adaptive possibilities that may (and do) arise as secondary derivatives of a large brain possessing an open network of potential interconnections that permit the functions of self-reflection, reasoning, and abstraction. But this takes us beyond this segment of the chapter.

Replicatory Strategies: The Self–Other Polarity

Although organisms may be well-adapted to their environments, the existence of any life form is time-limited. To circumvent this limitation, organisms exhibit patterns of the third polarity, *replicatory strategies,* by which they leave progeny. These strategies relate to what biologists have referred to as an *r*- or *self-propagating* strategy, at one polar extreme, and a *K*- or *other-nurturing* strategy at the second extreme. Psychologically, the former is disposed toward individually oriented actions which are perceived by others as egotistic, insensitive, inconsiderate, and uncaring, whereas the latter is disposed toward nurturant-oriented actions which are seen as affiliative, intimate, protective, and solicitous. Like pleasure–pain, the self–other polarity is not unidimensional. Whereas most humans exhibit a reasonable balance between the two polar extremes, some of those who evince personality pathologies may be conflicted on this polarity, (e.g., the compulsive and negativistic personalities).

Although less profound than the first polarity, which represents the enhancement of order (existence–life–pleasure) and the prevention of disorder (nonexistence–death–pain), or the second polarity, which differentiates the adaptive modes, accommodation (plant–passive) versus those of modification (animal–active), the third polarity, based on distinctions in reproductive strategies (gene replication), is no less fundamental; it contrasts the maximization of reproductive propagation (male-self) from that of the maximization of reproductive nurturance (female-other). In terms of a neuropsychological growth stages, to be discussed in a later section, an individual's orientation toward self and others evolves largely during what we term the "pubertal–gender identity" stage.

Evolutionary biologists (Cole 1954; Trivers 1974; Wilson 1975) have recorded marked differences among species in both the cycle and pattern of their reproductive behaviors. Of special interest is the extreme diversity among and within species in the number of offspring spawned and the consequent nurturing and protective investment the parents make in the survival of their progeny. The r-strategy represents a pattern of propagating a vast number of offspring but exhibiting minimal attention to their survival; the *K*-strategy is typified by the production of few progeny followed by considerable effort to ensure their survival.

Not only do species differ in where they fall on the *r*- to *K*-strategy continuum, but *within* most animal species an important distinction may be drawn between male and female genders. It is this latter differentiation that undergirds what has been termed the self- versus other-oriented polarity, implications of which are briefly elaborated.

Human females typically produce about 400 eggs in a lifetime, of which no more than 20 to 25 can mature into viable infants. The energy investment expended in gestation, nurturing, and caring for each child, both before and during the years following birth, is extraordinary. There appears to be good reason, therefore, to encourage a protective and caring inclination on the part of the female, as evident in a sensitivity to cues of distress and a willingness to persist in attending to the needs and nurturing of her offspring.

Although the male discharges tens of millions of sperm on mating, this is but a small investment, given the ease and frequency with which he can repeat the act. On fertilization, his physical and emotional commitment can end with minimal consequences. Although the protective and food-gathering efforts of the male may be lost by an early abandonment of a mother and an offspring or two, much more may be gained by investing energies in pursuits that achieve the wide reproductive spread of his genes. Relative to the female of the species, whose best strategy appears to be the care and comfort of child and kin (i.e., the K-strategy), the male is likely to be reproductively more prolific by maximizing self-propagation (i.e., adopting the r-strategy).

In sum, males tend to be self-oriented, owing to the fact that competition for reproductive resources maximizes the replicatory advantages of their genes. Conversely, females tend to be other-oriented, owing to the fact that their competence in nurturing and protecting their limited progeny maximizes the replicatory advantages of their genes. As noted previously, the consequences of the male's r-strategy are a broad range of what may be seen as self-advancing as opposed to other-promoting behaviors, such as acting in an egotistic, insensitive, inconsiderate, uncaring, and non-communicative manner. In contrast, females are more disposed to be other-promoting, affiliative, intimate, empathic, protective, and solicitous (Gilligan 1982; Rushton 1985; Wilson 1978). Female relationships demonstrate a horizontal or even reverse hierarchical quality, one founded on equalitarian transactions, or even priority given to others.

Extreme forms in the self-other polarity may be seen in what is termed variously as psychopathy (Millon, Simonsen, Birkit-Smith, & Davis, 1998), DSM's antisocial personality, and the dimension labeled *dissocial* in international classification systems. Here we see a centering at the self polar end, noted by a callous disregard for the feelings and rights of others, as well as tendencies toward cruelty, exploitation, impulsiveness, and, among the young, conduct problems and drug and alcohol misuse.

Also noteworthy are those who struggle ambivalently and unsatisfactorily between the self versus the other focus. Resolved by the tight constraint of self expression are those evidencing *compulsivity* as a trait or disorder, a characteristic in their orderliness, rigidity, conscientiousness, perfectionism, conformity, and an intolerance of ambiguity, disarray, emotionality, and social deviance.

What we have sought in the preceding paragraphs is a theoretical rationale based on concepts derived from evolutionary thinking as a way to account for a frequently studied dimension that contrasts power-oriented, arrogant, impersonal, tough-minded, competitive, ambitious, dominating, and autonomous traits at the one extreme and love-oriented, altruistic, nurturant, intimate, harmony-seeking, warm, trusting, and cooperative behaviors at the other. These two broad trait realms reflect, we believe, a fundamental bipolarity that exists in nature, one that expresses itself in two contrasting attribute clusters that characterize human personality functioning. One is most closely allied with the reproductive strategies exhibited in the male gender, that of self-advancement or what has been termed "individuation," the second connected most centrally to options of reproduction optimal for those of the female gender, that of being other-oriented, or what we see in behaviors called "nurturance."

Abstract Processes: The Thinking–Feeling Polarity

The reflective capacity to transcend the immediate and concrete; to interrelate and synthesize diversity, to represent events and processes symbolically; and to weigh, reason, and anticipate signify a quantum leap in evolution's potential for change and adaptation (Millon, 1990). Emancipated from the real and present, unanticipated possibilities and novel constructions may routinely be created by various styles of abstract processing. It is these capacities that are represented in the neurodevelopmental stage of "intracortical integration," to be described shortly.

The abstract mind may mirror outer realities but reconstructs them in the process, reflectively transforming them into subjective modes of phenomenologic reality, rendering external events subject to individualistic designs (Millon, 2003). Every act of apprehension is transformed by processes of abstract symbolism. Not only are internal and external images emancipated from direct sensory and imaginal realities, allowing them to become entities, but contemporaneous time also loses its immediacy and impact, becoming as much a construction as a substance. Cognitive abstractions bring the past effectively into the present, and their power of anticipation brings the future into the present as well. With past and future embedded in the here and now, humans can encompass, at once, not only the totality of our cosmos but its origins and nature, its evolution, and how they have come to pass. Most impressive of all are the many visions humans have of life's indeterminate future, where no reality as yet exists.

The capacity to sort and to recompose, to coordinate, and to arrange the symbolic representations of experience into new configurations is, in certain ways, analogous to the random processes of recombinant replication, though they are more focused and intentional: To extend this rhetorical liberty, *genetic replication* represents the recombinant mechanism underlying the adaptive progression of phylogeny, whereas *cognitive abstraction* represents the recombinant mechanism underlying the developmental progression of ontogeny. The uses of replication are limited, constrained by the finite potentials inherent in parental genes. In contrast, experiences, internalized and recombined through cognitive processes, are infinite. Over one lifetime, innumerable events of a random, logical, or irrational character transpire, construed and reformulated time and again, some of which proving more and others less adaptive than their originating circumstances may have called forth. Whereas the actions of most subhuman species derive from successfully evolved genetic programs, activating behaviors of a relatively fixed nature suitable for a modest range of environmental settings, the capabilities of both implicit and intentional abstraction give rise to adaptive competencies that are suited to radically divergent ecological circumstances, circumstances which themselves may be the result of far-reaching acts of symbolic and technologic creativity.

AN ONTOGENETIC MODEL OF NEURODEVELOPMENTAL STAGES

A generative theoretical basis for a taxonomy of personality should also be generative with respect to human ontogenetic development. In the pages that follow, we briefly link the evolutionary model to the maturational sequence of personality growth.

The culling of that which we call personality from a universe of possibilities takes place through the addition of successive constraints on system functioning. Each child displays a wide variety of behaviors in the first years of life. Although exhibiting a measure of consistency consonant with his or her constitutional disposition, the way in which the child responds to and copes with the environment tends to be largely spontaneous, changeable, and unpredictable. These seemingly random and capricious behaviors serve an important exploratory function. The child is "trying out" a variety of behavioral alternatives for dealing with his or her environment. Over time the child begins to discern which of these actions enable him to achieve his or her desires and avoid discomforts. Endowed with certain capacities, energies, and temperaments, and through experience with parents, sibs, and peers, the child learns to discriminate which activities are both permissible and rewarding and which are not.

Tracing this sequence over time it can be seen that a shaping process has taken place in which the child's initial range of diverse behaviors gradually becomes narrowed, selective, and, finally, crystallized into preferred ways of relating to others and coping with this world. These learned behaviors not only persist but are accentuated as a result of being repetitively reinforced by a limited social environment. Given continuity in constitutional equipment and a narrow band of experiences for learning behavioral alternatives, the child acquires a pattern of traits that are deeply etched and difficult to modify. These characteristics comprise his or her personality—that is, ingrained and habitual ways of psychological functioning that emerge from the individual's entire developmental history, and which, over time, come to characterize the child's "style."

The *interaction* between biological and psychological factors *is not unidirectional* such that biological determinants always precede and influence the course of learning; the order of effects may be reversed, especially in early development. Biological maturation depends on favorable environmental experience, and the development of the biological substrate itself can be disrupted, even totally arrested, by depriving the maturing organism of stimulation at sensitive periods of neurological growth. Nevertheless, there is an intrinsic continuity throughout life. The authors contend that childhood events are more significant to personality formation than later events, and that later behaviors are related in a determinant way to early experience. Despite an occasional disjunctiveness in development, there is an orderly and sequential continuity, fostered by mechanisms of self-perpetuation and social reinforcement, which links the past to the present.

Deeply embedded behavior patterns may arise as a consequence of psychological experiences that affect developing biological structures so profoundly as to transform them into something substantially different from what they might otherwise have been. Circumstances that exert so profound an effect are usually those experienced during infancy and early childhood, a view articulated in the seminal writings of Freud at the turn of the century. The observations of ethologists on the consequences of early stimulation upon adult animal behaviors add substantial evidence for this position (Rakic, 1985, 1988). Experimental work on early developmental periods also has shown that environmental stimulation is crucial to the neurological maturation of psychological functions. In essence, psychological capacities fail to develop fully if their neurological substrates are subjected to impoverished stimulation; conversely, these capacities may develop to an excessive degree as a consequence of enriched stimulation (Lipton & Kater, 1989).

Maturation refers to the intricate sequence of ontogenetic development in which initially inchoate bodily structures progressively unfold into specific functional units. Early stages of differentiation precede and overlap with more advanced states such that simpler and more diffuse structures interweave and connect into a complex and integrated network of functions displayed ultimately in the adult organism. It was once believed that the course of maturation from diffusion to differentiation to integration arose exclusively from inexorable forces within the genes. Maturation was thought to evolve according to a preset timetable that unfolded independently of environmental conditions. This view is no longer tenable. Neurological maturation follows an orderly progression, but the developmental sequence and level of ultimate neurological capacities and dispositions substantially depend on environmental stimuli and nutritional supplies. Thus, biological maturation does not progress in a fixed course leading to a predetermined level but is subject to numerous variations that reflect the character of environmental experience.

Nutrition should be viewed more broadly than is commonly done; it includes not only obvious components, such as food, but, in addition, what Rapaport (1958) has termed "stimulus nutriment." This concept suggests that the impingement of environmental and psychological stimuli upon the maturing organism has a direct bearing on the chemical composition, ultimate size, and patterns of neural branching within the brain (Lipton & Kater, 1989; Purves & Lichtman, 1985).

The belief that the maturing organism requires periodic psychological nutriments for proper development has led some to suggest that the organism actively seeks an optimum level of stimulation. Thus, just as the infant cries out in search of food when deprived or wails in response to pain, so too may it engage in behaviors that provide it with psychosensory stimulation requisite to maturation (Butler & Rice, 1963; Murphy, 1947). Unless certain chemicals and structures are activated by environmental stimulation, the neurological substrate for a variety of psychological functions may be impaired irrevocably. In turn, deficiencies or abnormalities in functions that normally mature in early life set the stage for progressive constraints on later functioning.

What evidence is there that serious consequences may result from an inadequate supply of early psychological and psychosensory stimulation? Numerous investigators (e.g., Beach & Jaynes, 1954; Killackey, 1990; Melzick, 1965; Rakic, 1985, 1988; Scott, 1968; Thompson & Schaefer, 1961) have shown that *impoverished* early environment results in permanent adaptational difficulties. For example, primates reared in isolation tend to be deficient in traits such as emotionality, activity level, social behavior, curiosity, and learning ability. As adult organisms they possess a reduced capacity to cope with their environments, to discriminate essentials, to devise strategies, and to manage stress.

Conversely, intense levels of early stimulation also appear to have effects, at least as experimentally demonstrated in lower mammalian species. Several investigators have demonstrated that *enriched* environments in early life resulted in measurable changes in brain chemistry and brain weight. Others have found that early stimulation accelerated the maturation of the pituitary–adrenal system, whereas equivalent later stimulation was ineffective. On the behavioral level, enriched environments in animals enhance problem-solving abilities and the capacity to withstand stress. More interesting, however, is the possibility that some kinds of overstimulation may produce detrimental effects. Accordingly, excess stimulation would result in overdevelopments in neurobiological substrates that are disruptive to effective psychological functioning. Just as excess food leads to obesity and physical ill health, so too may the psychostimulation of certain neural substrates, such as those subserving emotional reactivity, dispose the organism to overreact to social situations. Thus, when neurological dispositions that subserve potentially problematic personality traits become prepotent, they may disrupt what would otherwise be a more balanced pattern of psychological functioning.

Another and related question to be posed is whether the *timing* of environmental events have any bearing on their effect? The concept of *sensitive periods* of development states that there are limited periods during which particular stimuli are necessary for the full maturation of an organism, after which they will have minimal or no effects. Without the requisite stimulation, the organism will suffer various maldevelopments which are irremediable and cannot be compensated for at a later date.

Embryological research suggests that the effects of environmental stimuli upon morphological structures are most pronounced when tissue growth is rapid (Killackey, 1990; Rakic, 1985, 1988); the mechanisms that account for the special interaction between stimulation and periods of rapid neural growth are as yet unclear. It appears clear, however, that early psychological stimulation promotes selective growth so that certain neural collaterals establish particular interneuronal connections to the exclusion of others. Once these connections are biologically embedded, the first sets of psychosocial stimuli that traverse them, especially if they are intense or pervasive, appear to preempt the circuit, thereby decreasing the chance that subsequent stimuli will co-opt the circuit for other effects. In cognitive terms, once a cognitive schema is in place for perceiving an objective event in a particular way, these schemas may effectively co-opt future contrary interpretations of a similar event.

The four "neurodevelopmental stages" that individual human organisms progress through are paralleled by a set of four "tasks" that usually must be fulfilled to perform adequately later in life. The first three pairings of stages and tasks, and in part the fourth as well, are shared by all mammalian species; they recapitulate the four polarities of evolution described earlier: existence, adaptation, replication, and abstraction. Each evolutionary component is expressed ontogenetically; that is, each individual organism moves through neurodevelopmental stages which have functional psychological goals related to their respective phases of evolution. Within each stage, every individual acquires personologic dispositions representing a balance or predilection toward one of the two polarity inclinations; which inclination emerges as dominant over time results from the inextricable and reciprocal interplay of intraorganismic and extraorganismic factors. Thus, during early infancy, the primary organismic function is to "continue to exist." Here, evolution has supplied mechanisms that orient the infant toward life-enhancing environments (pleasure) and away from life-threatening ones (pain).

As previously noted, the authors believe that the development of personality should be coordinated with the fundamental polarities embedded in evolutionary theory. These are elaborated next. Although we differentiate four seemingly distinct stages of neurodevelopment in the following section, it is important to state at the outset that all four stages and their related primary processes begin *in utero* and continue throughout life; that is, they proceed simultaneously and overlap throughout the ontogenetic process. For example, the elements that give shape to "gender identity" are underway during the sensory-attachment phase, although at a modest level, as do the elements that give rise to attachment behaviors continue and extend well into puberty. Stages are differentiated only to bring attention to periods of development when certain processes and tasks are prominent and central. The concept of sensitive periods implies that developmental stages are not exclusionary; rather, they merely demarcate a period in life when certain developmental potentialities are salient in their maturation and in their receptivity to relevant life experiences.

Each evolutionary polarity is related to a different stage of ontogenetic development (Millon, 1969). For example, life enhancement–life preservation corresponds to the sensory-attachment stage of development in that the latter represents a period when the young child learns to discriminate between those experiences that are enhancing (pleasurable) and those that are threatening (painful).

Neurodevelopmental Stage 1. Sensory Attachment: The Life Enhancement (Pleasure)–Life Preservation (Pain) Polarity

The first year of life is dominated by sensory processes, functions basic to subsequent development in that they enable the infant to construct some order out of the initial diffusion experienced in the stimulus world, especially that based on distinguishing pleasurable from painful "objects." This period has also been termed "attachment" because infants cannot survive on their own (Fox, Kimmerly, & Schafer, 1991) but must "fasten" themselves to others who will protect, nurture, and stimulate them—that is, provide them with experiences of pleasure rather than those of pain.

Such themes are readily understood through an evolutionary theory of neurodevelopment. While evolution has endowed adult humans with the cognitive ability to project future threats and difficulties as well as potential rewards, human infants are comparably impoverished, being as yet without the benefit of these abstract capacities. Evolution has therefore "provided" mechanisms or substrates that orient the child toward those activities or venues which are life enhancing and away from those which are potentially life threatening. Existence during this highly vulnerable stage is quite literally a to-be or not-to-be matter.

As noted previously, life-enhancing actions or sensations can be subsumed under the rubric of "pleasure," while life-threatening actions or sensations can be subsumed under the metaphorical term "pain." Such a "pleasure–pain polarity" simply recognizes that while the behavioral repertoire of the young child is inchoate, the operational means is manifest and diverse (e.g., smiles, coos, stranger anxiety, and primitive reflexes), and the end, or *existential aim*, is universal and has as its bare minimum the maintenance of life itself. In the normal organism, both pleasure and pain are coordinated toward ontogenetic continuity. However, whether as a result of genetic factors, early experiences, or their interaction, some pathological patterns display aberrations in their orientation toward pleasure or pain. Deficits in the strength of both painful and pleasurable drives, for example, either constitutionally given or experientially derived, are involved in what we refer to clinically, for example, as the schizoid pattern, while a reversed or pleasure–pain orientation might incline toward a masochistic or sadistic pattern.

Development of Sensory Capacities

As noted, the early neonatal period is characterized by undifferentiation. The organism behaves in a diffuse and unintegrated way and perceptions are unfocused and gross. Accordingly, the orientation of the infant is toward sensations that are proportionately broad and undifferentiated, although increasingly the distinction between pleasure and pain becomes central to subsequent refinements. Freud recognized that the mouth region is a richly endowed receptor system through which neonates establish their first significant relationship to the world, but it is clear that this oral unit is merely the focal point of a more diverse system of sensory capacities for making significant distinctions. Through oral and other tactile contacts the infant establishes a sense, or "feel," of the environment which evokes pleasurable or painful responses.

According to our neurodevelopmental evolutionary theory, it would be expected that the amount and quality of tactile stimulation to which the neonate is exposed will contribute significantly to infantile precocities or retardations, depending on whether extreme levels of stimulation occur. The quality and patterning of this stimulation will lead the infant to experience inchoate feelings associated with differing degrees of pleasure–pain. These may form a phenomenological prototype for later-evolving and more distinct emotions such as fear, joy, sadness, and anger.

Development of Attachment Behaviors

The neonate cannot differentiate between objects and persons, both are experienced simply as stimuli. How does this initial indiscriminateness become progressively refined into specific attachments? For all essential purposes, the infant is helpless and dependent on others to avoid pain and supply its pleasurable needs. Separated from the womb, the neonate has lost its physical attachment to the mother's body and the protection and nurturance it provided; it must turn toward other regions or sources of attachment if it is to survive and obtain nourishment and stimulation for further development (Bowlby, 1969/1982; Gewirtz, 1963; Hinde, 1982; Lamb, Thompson, Gardner, & Estes, 1985; Ribble, 1943, Spitz, 1965). Attachment behaviors may be viewed, albeit figuratively, as an attempt to reestablish the unity lost at birth that enhanced and protected life. In fact, recent investigations show that while initial attachments are transformed across stages of development, they remain important across the lifespan (e.g., Sroufe & Fleeson, 1986). Whether the infant's world is conceptualized as a buzz or a blank slate, it must begin to differentiate venues or objects that further its existential aims, supplying nourishment, preservation, and stimulation, from those that diminish, frustrate, or threaten them. These initial relationships, or "internal representational models" (e.g., Crittenden, 1990), apparently "prepared" by evolution, become the context through which other relationships develop.

Task 1: Developing Trust of Others

Trust may be described as a feeling that one can rely on the affections and support of others. There are few periods of life when an individual is so wholly dependent on the goodwill and care of others than during the relatively helpless state of infancy. Nothing is more crucial to the infant's well-being than the nurturance and protection afforded by his or her caretakers. Through the quality and consistency of this support, deeply ingrained feelings of trust are etched within the child. From the evolutionary model presented earlier, trust and mistrust represent facets of the pleasure and pain constructs, generalized to adaptational venues within the physical environment, such as the nursery, as well as to the environment of prototypal social objects. Within the infant's world, of course, trust and mistrust lack their phenomenological and moral dimensions, resembling more global and undifferentiated feelings of soothing calm (pleasure) or tense apprehension (pain) than consciously abstracted states.

Such perceptual indiscriminateness of associations is highly significant. Thus, feelings and expectancies arising from specific experiences become highly generalized and come to characterize the child's image of the entire environment. Because children are unable to make fine discriminations, their early attachments become pervasive and widespread. Nurtured well and given comfort and affection, they will acquire a far-reaching trust of others; they learn that discomfort will be moderated and that others will assist them and provide for their needs. Deprived of warmth and security or handled severely and painfully, they will learn to mistrust their environment, to anticipate further stress, and to view others as harsh and undependable. Rather than developing an optimistic and confident attitude toward the future, they will be disposed to withdraw and avoid people for fear that these persons will recreate the discomfort and anguish that were experienced in the past.

Consequences of Impoverishment

A wealth of clinical evidence is available showing that humans deprived of adequate maternal care in infancy display a variety of pathological behaviors. We cannot, of course, design studies to disentangle precisely which of the complex of variables that compromise maternal care account for these irreparable consequences; the lives of babies cannot be manipulated to meet our scientific needs.

However, extensive reviews of the consequences in animals of early stimulus impoverishment show that sensory neural fibers atrophy and cannot be regenerated by subsequent stimulation (Beach & Jaynes, 1954; Riesen, 1961). Inadequate stimulation in any major receptor function usually results in decrements in the capacity to use these sensory processes in later life. The profound effects of social isolation have been studied thoroughly and show that deprived monkeys are incapable at maturity of relating to peers, of participating effectively in sexual activity, and of assuming adequate roles as mothers. Abstracting to those substrates and pathways that undergird pleasure–pain, we might expect that such underelaboration, if pervasive, might at the least render emotional discriminations of a more refined or narrow character impossible, or worse, might result in the wholesale impoverishment of all affective reactions, as seen in the schizoid pattern.

Consequences of Enrichment

Data on the consequences of too much, or enriched, early sensory stimulation are few and far between; researchers have been concerned with the effects of deficit, rather than excess, stimulation. A not unreasonable hypothesis, however, is that excess stimulation during the sensory-attachment stage would result in overdevelopments among associated neural structures (Rosenzweig, Krech, & Bennett, 1962); these may lead to oversensitivities which might, in turn, result in potentially maladaptive dominance of sensory functions or pleasurable substrates. Along this same line, Freud hypothesized that excess indulgence at the oral stage was conducive to fixations at that period. Eschewing both oral and fixation notions, the authors propose that excess sensory development in childhood will require a high level of maintenance in adulthood, as seen in persistent sensory-seeking or pleasure-seeking behaviors. These individuals might be characterized by their repetitive search for excitement and stimulation, their boredom with routine, and their involvement in incidental and momentarily gratifying adventures. Excess stimulation, especially if anchored exclusively to a parental figure, might result in an overattachment to him or her. This is demonstrated most clearly in the symbiotic child, where an abnormal clinging to the mother and a persistent resistance to stimulation from other sources often result in overwhelming feelings of isolation and panic, as when they are sent to nursery school or "replaced" by a newborn sibling.

Neurodevelopmental Stage 2. Sensorimotor Autonomy: The Ecologically Accommodating (Passive)–Ecologically Modifying (Active) Polarity

Not until the end of the first year has the infant matured sufficiently to engage in actions independent of parental support. Holding the drinking cup, the first few steps, or a word or two, all signify a growing capacity to act autonomously. As the child develops the functions that characterize this stage, he or she begins to comprehend the attitudes and feelings communicated by stimulative sources. No longer is rough parental handling merely excess stimulation, undistinguished from the playful tossing of an affectionate father; the child now discerns the difference between harshness and good-natured roughhousing.

In the sensorimotor-autonomy stage the focus shifts from existence in itself to existence within an environment. From an evolutionary perspective, the child in this stage is learning a *mode of adaptation*, an *active* tendency to modify its ecological niche, versus a *passive* tendency to accommodate to whatever the environment has provided. The former reflects a disposition toward taking the initiative in shaping the course of life events; the latter a disposition to be quiescent, placid, unassertive, to react rather than act, to wait for things to happen, and to accept what is given. Whatever alternative is pursued, it is, of course, a matter of degree rather than an all-or-none decision.

Development of Sensorimotor Capacities

The unorganized movements of the neonate progressively give way to focused muscular activity. As the neural substrate for muscular control unfolds, the aimless motor behavior of the infant is supplanted by focused movements. These newly emergent functions coordinate with sensory capacities to enable the child to explore, manipulate, play, sit, crawl, babble, throw, walk, catch, talk, and otherwise intervene in its ecological milieu as desired. The maturing fusion between the substrates of sensory and motor functions is strengthened by the child's exploratory behavior. Manipulative play and the formation of babbling sounds are methods of self-stimulation that facilitate the growth of action-oriented interneuronal connections; the child is building a neural foundation for more complicated and refined skills such as running, handling utensils, controlling sphincter muscles, and articulating precise speech.

Development of Autonomous Behaviors

Perhaps the most significant aspect of sensorimotor development is that it enables children to begin to take an active stance in doing things for themselves, to influence their environment, to free themselves from domination, and to outgrow the dependencies of their first years. Children become aware of their increasing competence and seek new ventures. Conflicts and restrictions arise as they assert themselves (Erikson, 1959; White, 1960). These are seen clearly during toilet training, when youngsters often resist submitting to the demands of their parents. A delicate exchange of power and cunning often ensues. Opportunities arise for the child to actively extract promises or deny wishes; in response, parents may mete out punishments, submit meekly, or shift inconsistently. Important precedents for attitudes toward authority, power, and autonomy are generated during this period of parent–child interaction.

Task 2: Acquiring Adaptive Confidence

Children become progressively less dependent on their caretakers during the sensorimotor-autonomy stage. By the second and third years they are ambulatory and possess the power of speech and control over many elements in their environment. They have acquired the manipulative skills to venture forth and test their competence to handle events on their own (Erikson, 1959; White, 1960). In terms of the evolutionary model, this stage concerns the active–passive polarity. Here children struggle to break out of the inherently dependent and passive mode of infancy. Rather than remain a passive receptacle for environmental forces, clay to be molded, they acquire competencies that enlarge their vistas and allow them to become legitimate actors in their environments.

However, subtle, as well as obvious, parental attitudes shape children's confidence in their ability to exercise their competencies. These attitudes markedly influence behavior because it is not only what the children can do that determines their actions but how they feel about what they can do. The rewards and punishments to which they are exposed and the degree of encouragement and affection surrounding their first performances will contribute to their confidence in themselves. Conversely, faced with rebuffs and ridicule, children learn to doubt their competence and adequacy. Whether they actually possess the skills to handle events is no longer the issue; they simply lack the confidence to try, to venture out, or to compete. Believing their efforts will be ineffectual and futile, these children often adopt a passive, wait-and-see attitude toward their environment and their future.

Consequences of Impoverishment

A lack of stimulation of sensorimotor capacities can lead to retardations in the functions necessary to the development of autonomy and initiative, causing children to remain within a passive adaptational mode. This is seen most clearly in children of overprotective parents. Spoon-fed, excused from "chores," restrained from exploration, curtailed in friendships, and protected from "danger"—all illustrate controls that restrict growing children's opportunities to exercise their sensorimotor skills and develop the means for autonomous behavior. A self-perpetuating cycle often unfolds.

Consequences of Enrichment

The consequences of excessive enrichment during the sensorimotor-autonomy stage are found most often in children of excessively lax, permissive, or overindulgent parents. Given free rein with minimal restraint, stimulated to explore and manipulate things to their suiting without guidance or control, these children often become irresponsibly undisciplined in their behaviors. Their active style compels these children to view the entire ecological milieu as a playground or medium to be modified according to their whims. Carried into the wider social context, these behaviors run up against the desires of other children and the restrictions of less permissive adults. Unless the youngsters are extremely adept, they will find that their actively self-centered and free-wheeling tactics fail miserably. For the few who succeed, however, a pattern of egocentrism, unbridled self-expression, and social arrogance may become dominant.

Neurodevelopmental Stage 3. Pubertal Gender Identity: The Progeny Nurturance (Other)–Individual Propagation (Self) Polarity

Somewhere between the 11th and 15th years a rather sweeping series of hormonal changes unsettle the psychic state that had been so carefully constructed in preceding years. These changes reflect the onset of puberty and the instantiation of sexual and gender-related characteristics which are preparatory for the emergence of the r- and K- strategies—strong sexual impulses and adult-like features of anatomy, voice, and bearing. Erratic moods, changing self-images, reinterpretations of one's view of others, new urges, hopeful expectancies, and a growing physical and social awkwardness all upset the relative equanimity of an earlier age. Disruptive as it may be, this turbulent stage of growth bifurcates and focuses many of the remaining elements of the youngster's biological potential. Not only is it a preparatory phase for the forthcoming independence from parental direction, but it is when the psychological equivalent of the r- and K- strategies, self (male) and other (female) orientations, begin to diverge and then coalesce into distinct gender roles.

With the unsettling influences of adolescence, both physiological and social, and the emergence of the individual as a being of genuine reproductive potential, the r- and K- strategies begin to take on an implicitly criterial role in the selection of the behaviors of the moment, as well as future goals, from a universe of implicit alternatives. These strategies are psychologically expressed, at the highest level of abstraction, in an orientation toward self and an orientation toward others. Here the male can be prototypally described as more dominant, imperial, and acquisitive and the female more communal, nurturant, and deferent.

Development of Pubertal Maturation

Pubescence is characterized by the rapidity of body growth, genital maturity, and sexual awareness. A series of transformations take place that are qualitatively different from those developed earlier in childhood. They create an element of discontinuity from prior experiences, confronting the youngster not only with an internal "revolution" of a physiological nature but also with a series of psychological tasks that are prompted by emergent sexual feelings. Much effort is invested both consciously and unconsciously to incorporate these new bodily impulses into one's sense of self and one's relationship to others. Youngsters must establish a gender identity that incorporates physiological changes and the powerful libidinal feelings with which they are associated. The increase in pubertal libidinal drives requires a reorganization of one's sense of adolescent identity. Developed in a satisfactory manner, the adolescent is enabled to search out relevant extra-familial love objects.

Development of Gender Identity

Developing a gender identity is not so much acquiring a means for satisfying libidinal impulses as it is a process of refining the youngster's previously diffused and undifferentiated sense of self. This is achieved most effectively by reflecting the admiration of a beloved other. The feedback received in real and fantasized love relationships assists the teenager to revise and define their gender identity. It serves also to clarify and further develop a new self-concept that encompasses relationships with peer companions of both genders, rather than parents or siblings.

Task 3: Assimilating Sexual Roles (Self–Other Polarity)

The many crushes and infatuations experienced during the pubertal period serves as a genuine source of development. Gender roles emerge in significant ways by interacting with others, especially as enacted in peer-group relationships. Adhering to the models of peer behaviors helps the youngster find and evaluate how certain gender roles fit. The high school clique, the neighborhood gang, and the athletic team all aid the teenager in discovering his or her gender identity, providing both useful role models and instant social feedback. The "bull" session among boys and the endless phone and e-mail conversations between girls serve significant goals by providing evaluative feedback as the youngster searches to define him- or herself. It is particularly during the time of rapid body changes when genital impulses stimulate sexual fantasies that the adolescent learns to rely on peers as important guides and sounding boards.

Security is found in peer relationships in that youngsters share a code as to what constitutes appropriate gender behaviors. No less important is the mutuality they experience in struggling through the same pubertal issues. The importance of the influence of the peer group is perhaps nowhere more significant than in the realm of sexual behaviors. For the most part, the adolescent finds security in accepting the peer-gender norms as preliminary guides regarding how one can regulate one's impulses, feelings and sexual inclinations.

Consequences of Impoverishment

The goal of the adolescent is in part to achieve a libidinous extrafamilial object, an aim ultimately resulting in a richer and more mature emotional life. As noted, with the onset of puberty, parental identification declines and is replaced by identifications with valued peers, both real friendships and romanticized heroes. The lack of such identifications and role models during adolescence may culminate in imaginary infatuations, unreal and ineffectual substitutes for the desirable qualities that usually emerge from everyday personal relationships.

Without direct tuition from his elders, the teenager will be left to his own devices to master the complexities of a varied world, to control intense aggressive and sexual urges that well up within him, to channel his fantasies and to pursue the goals to which he aspires. He may become a victim of his own growth, unable to discipline his impulses or fashion acceptable means for expressing his desires. Scattered and unguided, he cannot get hold of a sense of personal identity, a consistent direction and purpose to his existence. Borderline personality disorders often characterize this pattern of gender diffusion (Millon, 1996). Their aimlessness and disaffiliation from the mainstream of traditional sociocultural life may be traced, in part, to the failure of experience to provide a coherent set of gender role models and values around which they can focus their lives and orient themselves toward a meaningful future.

Consequences of Enrichment

In contrast to the problems that arise from a deficiency of gender role models, we frequently observe excessive dependency on peer-group sexual habits and values. Some adolescents who have been ill-disposed to the values of problematic peer groups may find themselves isolated and avoided, if not ridiculed and ostracized. To protect themselves against this discomforting possibility, the teenager may submerge his identity to fit the roles given him by others. He may adopt gender models that have been explicitly or implicitly established by group customs. They act, dress, use language, and enact their gender roles in terms of peer-group standards.

Neurodevelopmental Stage 4. Intracortical Integration: The Intellective Reasoning (Thinking)–Affective Resonance (Feeling) Polarity

The intracortical–integration stage coordinates with the fourth phase of the evolutionary progression, the thinking–feeling polarity (Millon, 2003). The peak period of neurological maturation for certain psychological functions generally occurs between the ages of 4 and 18. The amount and kind of intrapsychic and contextual stimulation at these times of rapid growth will have a strong bearing on the degree to which these functions mature. Thinking and feeling are broad and multifaceted constructs with diverse manifestations. While the focus in the first three stages of development was on the child's existential aims, modes of adaptation, and gender identification, here the focus shifts to the individual as a being-in-time.

Initially, the child must acquire abstract capacities that enable it to transcend the purely concrete reality of the present moment and project the self-as-object into myriad futures contingent upon its own style of action or accommodation. Such capacities are both cognitive and emotional, and may have wide-ranging consequences for the personality system if they fail to cohere as integrated structures, as in the more severe personality disorders (e.g., borderline and schizotypal).

Development of Intracortical Capacities

Progressively more complex arrangements of neural cells become possible as children advance in maturation. Although these higher-order connections begin in early infancy, they do not form into structures capable of rational foresight and adult-level planning until the youngsters have fully developed their more basic sensorimotor skills and pubertal maturations. With these capacities as a base, they are able to differentiate and arrange the objects of the physical world. As verbal skills unfold, they learn to symbolize concrete objects; soon they are able to manipulate and coordinate these symbols as well as, if not better than, the tangible events themselves. Free of the need to make direct reference to the concrete world, they are able to recall past events and anticipate future ones. As increasingly complex cortical connections are established, higher conceptual abstractions are formulated, enabling the children to transfer, associate, and coordinate these symbols into ideas of finer differentiation, greater intricacy, and broader integration. These internal representations of reality, the product of symbolic thought, the construction of events past, present, and future, take over as the primary elements of the representational world. Especially significant at this period is a fusion between the capacities to think and to feel.

Development of Integrative Processes

When the inner world of symbols is mastered, giving objective reality an order and integration, youngsters are able to create some consistency and continuity in their lives. No longer are they buffeted from one mood or action to another by the swirl of changing events; they now have an internal anchor, a nucleus of cognitions that serves as a base and imposes a sense of sameness and continuity upon an otherwise fluid environment. As they grow in their capacity to organize and integrate their world, one configuration becomes increasingly differentiated and begins to predominate. Accrued from experiences with others and their reactions to the child, an image or representation of self-as-object has taken shape. This highest order of abstraction, the sense of individual identity as distinct from others, becomes the dominant source of stimuli that guides the youngster's thoughts and feelings. External events no longer have the power they once exerted; the youngster now has an ever present and stable sphere of internal representations, transformed by rational and emotional reflections, which govern one's course of action and from which behaviors are initiated.

Task 4: Balancing Reason and Emotion

The emergence of this final developmental stage—with its capacities for thinking, feeling, evaluating, and planning—leads children to formulate a clear image of themselves as a certain "kind of adult," an identity discernible from others, one capable of having independent judgments and of fashioning their own course of action. Healthy children must acquire a coherent system of internalized values that will guide them through a changing and varied environment. They must find their own anchor and compass by which to coordinate both their feelings and ideas about life. Equipped by successful efforts toward autonomy, they will have confidence that they possess a direction in life that is valued by others and one that can safely withstand the buffeting of changing events. In terms of the evolutionary model, such children are capable of integrating their feelings and thoughts, setting their own agendas, and becoming masters of their own fate.

Consequences of Impoverishment

The task of integrating a consistent self–other differentiation, as well as consolidating the divergencies of thought and feeling, is not easy in a world of changing events and pluralistic values. From what sources can a genuine balance betweeen reason and emotion be developed? The institutions that interweave to form the complex fabric of society are implicitly designed to shape the assumptive world of its younger members. Family, school, and church transmit implicit values and explicit rules by which the child is guided in behaving and thinking in a manner consonant with those of others. The youngster not only is subject to cultural pressures but requires them to give direction to his or her proliferating capacities and impulses. Without them, potentials may become overly diffuse and scattered; conversely, too much guidance may narrow the child's potentials and restrict his or her adaptiveness. In either case, the sense of self and other, as well as the relationship of thought and emotion, is no longer expressed in personally elaborated and multifaceted forms.

What are the effects of inadequate or erratic stimulation during the peak years of intracortical integration? Without direct tuition from elders, youngsters are left to their own devices to master the complexities of a varied world, to control intense urges, to channel fantasies, and to pursue the goals to which they aspire. They may become victims of their own growth, unable to orient their impulses or fashion acceptable means for expressing their desires, unable to construct a sense of internal cohesion or a consistent direction and purpose to their existence, a feature most prominently seen in borderline personality patterns. They may vacillate at every turn, overly responsive to fleeting stimuli, shifting from one erratic course to another.

Without an inner core or anchor to guide their future, they may flounder or stagnate.

Consequences of Enrichment

The negative consequences of overenrichment at the fourth stage usually occur when parents are controlling and perfectionistic. The overly trained, overly disciplined, and overly integrated youngster is given little opportunity to shape his own destiny. Whether by coercion or enticement, the child who, too early, is led to control his emergent feelings, to focus his thoughts along narrowly defined paths and to follow the prescriptions of parental demands, has been subverted into adopting the identities of others. Whatever individuality he may have acquired is drowned in a model of adult orderliness, propriety, and virtue, features most clearly observed among compulsive personality patterns. Such oversocialized and rigid youngsters lack the spontaneity, flexibility, and creativeness we expect of the young; they have been overly trained before their time, too narrow in perspective to respond to excitement, variety, and the challenge of new events. Overenrichment at this stage has fixed them on a restrictive course and has deprived them of the rewards of being themselves.

Comment

As evident in the foregoing, it would have been an error to leave the discussion of evolutionary–neuropsychological development with the impression that personality growth was merely a function of stimulation at sensitive maturational periods. Impoverishment and enrichment have their profound effects, but the *quality* or *kind of stimulation* the youngster experiences is often of greater importance. The impact of parental harshness or inconsistency, of sibling rivalry or social failure, is more than a matter of stimulus volume and timing. Different dimensions of experience take precedence as the meaning conveyed by the source of stimulation becomes clear to the growing child. Although the basic architecture of the nervous system is laid down in a relatively fixed manner, refinements in this linkage system do not develop without the aid of psychosocial experiences. These experiences not only activate the growth of neural collaterals but alter these structures in such ways as to preempt them for similar subsequent experiences. Early stimulus experiences not only construct new neural pathways but, in addition, selectively prepare these pathways to be receptive to "later stimuli" which are qualitatively similar. This second consequence of stimulus experience, representing a selective lowering of the threshold for the neural transmission of similar subsequent stimuli, is described in the conceptual language of psychology as the process of *learning*; it reflects the observation that perceptions and behaviors that have been subjected to prior psychosocial experience and training are reactivated with relative ease.

Both neurological and learning concepts can be used to describe changes in response probabilities arising from prior stimulus exposure. But, because learning concepts are formulated in terms of behavior–environment interactions, it is reasonable, when discussing the specific properties of qualitatively discriminable stimulus events, to use the conceptual language of learning. Moreover, the principles derived from learning theory and research describe subtle features of psychological behavior which cannot begin to be handled intelligently in neurological terms. Moreover, further reason for the stage-specific significance of experience is the observation that children are exposed to a succession of social *tasks* that they are expected to fulfill at different points in the neurodevelopmental sequence. These stage-specific tasks are timed to coincide with periods of rapid neurological growth (e.g., the training of bladder control is begun when the child possesses the requisite neural equipment for such control; similarly, children are taught to read when intracortical development has advanced sufficiently to enable a measure of consistent success). In short, a reciprocity appears between periods of rapid neurological growth and exposure to related experiences and tasks. To use Erikson's (1950) terms, the child's newly emerging neurological potentials are challenged by a series of "crises" with the environment. Children are especially vulnerable at these critical stages because experience both shapes their neurological patterns and results in learning a series of fundamental attitudes about themselves and others. As noted in prior paragraphs, during the sensory-attachment stage, when pleasure and pain discriminations are central, the critical attitude learned dealt with one's "trust of others." The sensorimotor–autonomy stage, when the progression from passive to active modes of adaptation occurs, was noted by learning attitudes concerning "adaptive confidence." During the pubertal–gender identity stage, when the separation between self and other roles is sharpened, we saw the development of reasonably distinct "sexual roles." The intracortical–integrative stage, when the coordination between intellectual and affective processes develops, was characterized by the acquisition of a balance between "reason and emotion."

A DEDUCTIVE THEORY OF NORMAL AND PATHOLOGICAL PERSONALITY PATTERNS

A taxonomic system will go awry if its major categories encompass too diverse a range of clinical conditions; there is a need to subdivide pathological phenomena in terms of certain fundamental criteria. For this reason we have stressed an integrative perspective, which differentiates among DSM

Axis I syndromes and Axis II patterns on the basis of the formal deductive properties of our evolutionary system. Such an innovation distinguishes pathologies that would otherwise be seen as simply lying alongside each other, on the same plane so to speak, according to their presumed proto-typal characteristics, either linear or hierarchical, deriving from one or another level of organization, or circular, possessing a qualitative organiza-tion which cuts across and is anchored at all levels of organization (Millon, 1987a, 1991).

Pathological Personality Patterns (Axis II) and Classical Psychiatric Syndromes (Axis I)

Any conception of clinical personality patterns must distinguish these pat-terns not only from their more normal variants but also from the classical psychiatric disorders. Personality disorders are not medical illnesses for which some discrete pathogen can be found, or for which exists some underlying unitary cause. The use of such language as "disorder" is indeed unfortunate, for personality disorders are not disorders at all in the medical sense in that a healthy organism has been upset or undermined. Personality disorders are best conceptualized as an intrinsic and enduring pattern com-prising the entire matrix of the person that functions maladaptively in an "average, expectable" environment. Hence, we prefer the terms "pattern" or "style" rather than the implicitly misleading "disorder." This mislabel-ing tends to nullify the logic of the multiaxial model, encouraging the view that clinical syndromes and personality "disorders" exist alongside each the other in a horizontal relationship. The essence of the multiaxial model reflects its *structural* innovation; that is, it has been specifically composed to encourage the view that classical psychiatric syndromes are a disabling outcome when the overarching personality patterns, from which they arise, has been upset or "disordered." *That is, clinical syndromes (Axis I) signify a disordered state, whereas personality pathologies (Axis II) are pervasive and enduring maladaptations.*

The multiaxial model may be more formally represented with the aid of general systems concepts and the idea of levels of organization. *Both axes represent prototypal expressions of systemic dysfunctioning, but the causal nature of the dysfunction is different for each axis.* With the Axis I pathologies, etiology flows from one or more levels of organization. Prototypally, these are distinctly vertical pathologies whose manifest symp-tomatology reflects the interaction of biological, psychological, and social inputs. Major depression, for example, may be driven primarily by an endogenous neurochemical substrate or may be precipitated by grief fol-lowing the death of a family member but then complicated by psychic trait dispositions.

Personality pathologies do not stem from systemically dysregulating inputs from any one level of organization. They are distinctly horizontal in that they reflect qualitative inputs that drive from multiple sources and thus have referents in every level of biopsychosocial organization. The organization of personality pathologies is as integrative as those of so-called normal personalities, which is why personality pathologies are so tenacious. These integrative personality patterns are sustained by causal pathways which are invariably circular or reflexive, whereas Axis I disorders, although they may also be multidetermined, are typically linear in nature (Millon, Blaney, & Davis 1999). That is, all functional and structural clinical domains (biological, cognitive) can be equipotent in the degree to which they constrain system functioning (Millon, 1996). Most often, the behavior of "real patients" is typically highly constrained in only certain clinical domains (interpersonal, intrapsychic, cognitive) and not in others, such that the expressions of each patient's pathology may be manifested in limited and not all spheres. Further, dysregulating inputs from any of the several domains of maladaptation will create systemic reverberations which lend each individual's pathology and adaptive capacity its unique coloration. Each person's pathology thus forms a dynamic–organizational or integrated whole which may be decomposed clinically and theoretically according to the separate two axes for purposes which are diagnostic or heuristic, rather than real. No one really believes that the individual "exists" as an entity dismembered on the two separate axes, I and II. Nevertheless, the multiaxial model recognizes that certain taxonomic structural boundaries can be established to accord with the formal properties of the diagnostic system, irrespective of issues of individuality. As noted later, there are numerous *personality subtypes* of each of the classical (DSM) personality pathologies (Millon, 1996); these represent frequent variants seen in "real patients" that comprise nonidenticals subsumed in one or another of the DSM's broad categories.

Personality Patterns, Complex Syndromes, and Simple Reactions

For taxonomic purposes, we may distinguish three prototypal kinds of clinical pathologies—*personality patterns, complex syndromes,* and *simple reactions*—depending on the character of their constituents (see Millon, 1999, for a full discussion of these taxonomic distinctions). Although behavior is always the product of an individual by environment transaction at multiple levels of both organism and context, we must nevertheless average over certain elements in order to place in high relief certain broad classes of clinical phenomena, which then serve as structural definitions for a proposed taxonomy.

With *personality patterns*, behavioral constraints are assumed to lie primarily within the person. Clinical patterns of personality pathology result when these personalities are dysfunctional in "average or expectable environments" (Hartmann, 1939). In the *complex syndromes*, difficulties are conceived as disruptions in a patient's characteristic (personality pattern) style of functioning; they are viewed as a pathological response to a situation for which the individual's psychic makeup is notably vulnerable. Hysterical conversions and fugue states would be dramatic examples of complex syndromes in that they usually arise in response to situations that appear rather trivial or innocuous when viewed objectively. Nevertheless, vulnerable patients with a pathology of personality style feel and respond in a manner similar to those of so-called normal persons who face a realistically distressing situation. As a consequence, complex syndromes may fail to "make sense" and often appear irrational and strangely complicated. To the experienced clinician, however, the response signifies the presence of an unusual vulnerability on the part of the patient; in effect, a seemingly neutral stimulus apparently has touched a painful hidden memory or emotion. Viewed in this manner, complex syndromes arise among individuals encumbered with adverse past experiences. They reflect the upsurge of deeply rooted feelings that press to the surface, override present realities, and become the prime stimulus to which the individual responds. It is this flooding into the present of the reactivated past that gives complex syndromes much of their symbolic, bizarre, and hidden meaning.

At the furthest end of the clinical continuum are *simple reactions*, defined as highly specific pathological responses that are precipitated by and largely attributable to circumscribed external events or endogenous biochemical dispositions. These clinical responses result when an otherwise "normal person" is faced with situations to which almost anyone would react pathologically, the demise of one's entire family in a natural disaster, for example. In contrast to complex syndromes, simple reactions are uncomplicated and straightforward. They do not "pass through" a chain of intricate and circuitous transformations before emerging in manifest form. Uncontaminated by the intrusion of personality vulnerabilities (e.g., distant memories or intrapsychic transformations), simple reactions tend to be rational and understandable in terms of a precipitating external stimulus or endogenous biological weakness. Isolated from a problematic past, a defensive manipulation, or a neurochemical susceptibility, they are expressed in a direct and understandable fashion—unlike complex syndromes, whose features tend to be highly fluid, wax and wane, taking on different forms at different times.

Traits that comprise *personality patterns* have an inner momentum and autonomy; they are expressed with or without inducement or external precipitation. In contrast, responses comprising simple reactions are stimulus specific; that is, they are linked to external or internal precipitants, operating independently of the individual's personality, elicited by events that are "objectively" troublesome. *Complex syndromes* are similar to simple reactions in that they are prompted also by distinct external events or unseen biological vulnerabilities, but their interaction with personality weaknesses results in the intrusion of enduring traits that complicate what might otherwise be a response to the environment within the nonclinical range.

Normal and Clinical Personality Patterns

Numerous attempts have been made to develop definitive criteria for distinguishing psychological normality from abnormality. Some of these criteria focus on features that characterize the so-called normal, or ideal, state of mental health, as illustrated in the writings of Offer and Sabshin (1974, 1991). Central to our understanding of normality and abnormality is the recognition that these terms exist as relative concepts; they represent arbitrary points on a continuum or gradient. No sharp line divides normal from pathological behavior. Not only is personality so complex that certain areas of psychological functioning operate normally while others do not, but environmental circumstances change such that behaviors and strategies that prove adaptive at one time fail to do so at another. Moreover, features differentiating normal from abnormal functioning must be extracted from a complex of signs that not only wax and wane but often develop in an insidious and unpredictable manner. Pathological personality patterns, as previously remarked, are not disorders or diseases at all in the medical sense. Rather, personality pathologies are reified constructs employed to represent varied styles or patterns in which the personality system functions *maladaptively* in relation to its environment and over time.

The interactional aspect of such a conception is an important one, because it is informed by general systems concepts: Normal persons exhibit flexibility in their transactions with their environment, meaning that their responses or behaviors are appropriate to a given situation and over time. If person and environment are conceptualized as a dynamic system, an intercoupled person–environment unit, then the evolution of the unit through its successive states is said to be subject to constraints that lie both in the person and in the environment. When environmental constraints dominate, the behavior of individuals tends to converge, regardless of their prepotent dispositions: Almost everyone stops when traffic lights are red. When environmental constraints are few or not well-defined, however, there is opportunity for flexibility, novelty, and the expression of individual differences in behavior, such as seen in the varied responses to the ambiguous inkblots of the Rorschach test.

When alternative strategies employed to achieve goals, relate to others, and cope with stress are few in number and rigidly practiced (*adaptive inflexibility*), when habitual perceptions, needs, and behaviors perpetuate and intensify preexisting difficulties (*vicious circles*), and when the person tends to lack resilience under conditions of stress (*tenuous stability*), we speak of a pathological personality pattern. We keep in mind that personality is an interactional concept which admits of degrees, shading gently from normality to clinicality, and has at a latent level no single underlying cause or pathogenicity but instead is as multidetermined as the personality system itself is multifaceted. The three aforementioned disorder criteria are intimately related to the personality pathology taxonomy we propose later. However, before proceeding to the clinical realm we discuss several criteria we deem significant in appraising normality.

NORMAL PERSONALITY CRITERIA

In the following sections we draw on the first three of the evolutionary polarities described previously. The fourth polarity is also worthy of note and relevant to an understanding of personality traits; however, to include this polarity in the following section will take us somewhat afield in this already overly long chapter. Interested readers wishing to review the details of this fourth and cognitively oriented polarity may look into the manual for the Millon Index of Personality Styles (MIPS; Millon, Weiss, Millon, & Davis, 1994; 2004) or another recent elaboration (Millon, 2003).

Aims of Existence: Pain–Pleasure Polarity

An interweaving and shifting balance between the two extremes that comprise the pain–pleasure bipolarity typifies normality. Both of the following criteria should be met in varying degrees as life circumstances require. In essence, a synchronous and coordinated personal style should have developed to answer the question of whether the person should focus on experiencing only the pleasures of life versus concentrating his or her efforts on avoiding its pains.

Life Preservation: Avoiding Danger and Threat

One might assume that a criterion based on the avoidance of psychic or physical pain would be sufficiently self-evident not to require specification. As is well known, debates have arisen in the literature as to whether mental health/normality reflects the absence of mental disorder, being merely the reverse side of the mental illness or abnormality coin. That there is a relationship between health and disease cannot be questioned; the two are intimately connected, conceptually and physically. On the other hand, to define health solely as the absence of disorder will not suffice. As a single criterion among several, however, features of behavior and experience that signify both the lack of (e.g., anxiety and depression) and an aversion to (e.g., threats to safety and security) pain in its many and diverse forms provide a necessary foundation on which other, more positively constructed criteria may rest. Substantively, positive normality must comprise elements beyond mere nonnormality or abnormality. And despite the complexities and inconsistencies of personality, from a definitional point of view normality does preclude nonnormality.

It may be of interest next to record some of the psychic pathologies of personality that can be traced to aberrations in meeting this first criterion of normality. For example, among those termed "avoidant personalities" (Millon 1969, 1981, 1996), we see an excessive preoccupation with threats to one's psychic security, an expectation of and hyperalertness to the signs of potential rejection that leads these persons to disengage from everyday relationships and pleasures. At the other extreme of the criterion we see a risk-taking attitude, a proclivity to chance hazards and to endanger one's life and liberty, a behavioral pattern characteristic of those we label antisocial personalities. Here there is little of the caution and prudence expected in the normality criterion of avoiding danger and threat; rather, we observe its opposite, a rash willingness to put one's safety in jeopardy, to play with fire and throw caution to the wind.

Life Enhancement: Seeking Rewarding Experiences

At the other end of the "existence polarity" are attitudes and behaviors designed to foster and enrich life; to generate joy, pleasure, contentment, and fulfillment; and thereby to strengthen the capacity of the individual to remain vital and competent physically and psychically. This criterion asserts that existence/survival calls for more than life preservation alone; beyond pain avoidance is pleasure enhancement.

This criterion asks us to go at least one step further than Freud's parallel notion that life's motivation is chiefly that of "reducing tensions" (i.e., avoiding/minimizing pain), maintaining thereby a steady state, if you will, a homeostatic balance and inner stability. In accord with our view of evolution's polarities, we would assert that normal humans are driven also by the desire to enrich their lives, to seek invigorating sensations and challenges, to venture and explore, all to the end of magnifying if not escalating the probabilities of both individual viability and species replicability.

As before, a note or two should be recorded on the pathological consequences of a failure to meet a criterion. These are seen most clearly in the personality disorders labeled schizoid and avoidant. In the former there is a marked hedonic deficiency, stemming either from an inherent deficit in affective substrates or the failure of stimulative experience to develop either or both attachment behaviors or affective capacity (Millon 1981, 1996). Among those designated avoidant personalities, constitutional sensitivities or abusive life experiences have led to an intense attentional sensitivity to psychic pain and a consequent distrust in either the genuineness or durability of the "pleasures," such that these individuals can no longer permit themselves to experience them. Both of these personalities tend to be withdrawn and isolated, joyless and grim, neither seeking nor sharing in the rewards of life.

Modes of Adaptation: Passive–Active Polarity

To maintain their unique structure, differentiated from the larger ecosystem of which they are a part, to be sustained as a discrete entity among other phenomena that comprise their environmental field, requires good fortune and the presence of effective modes of functioning. The vast range of behaviors engaged in by humans may fundamentally be grouped in terms of whether initiative is taken in altering and shaping life's events or whether behaviors are reactive to and accommodate those events.

"Normal" or optimal functioning, at least among humans, appears to call for a flexible balance that interweaves both polar extremes. In the first evolutionary stage, that relating to existence, behaviors encouraging both life enhancement (pleasure) and life preservation (pain avoidance) are likely to be more successful in achieving survival than actions limited to one or the other alone. Similarly, regarding adaptation, modes of functioning that exhibit both ecological accommodation and ecological modification are likely to be more successful than either by itself. Normality calls for a synchronous and coordinated personal style that weaves a balanced answer to the question of whether one should accept what the fates have brought forth or take the initiative in altering the circumstances of one's life.

Ecological Accommodation: Abiding Hospitable Realities

On first reflection, it would seem to be less than optimal to submit meekly to what life presents, to "adjust" obligingly to one's destiny. As described earlier, however, the evolution of plants is essentially grounded in environmental accommodation, in an adaptive acquiescence to the ecosystem. Crucial to this adaptive course, however, is the capacity of these surroundings to provide the nourishment and protection requisite to the thriving of a species.

To the extent that the events of life have been and continue to be caring and giving, is it not perhaps wisest, from an evolutionary perspective, to accept this good fortune and "let matters be"? This accommodating or passive life philosophy has worked extremely well in sustaining and fostering those complex organisms that comprise the plant kingdom. Hence passivity, the yielding to environmental forces, may be in itself not only unproblematic but, where events and circumstances provide the "pleasures" of life and protect against their "pains," positively adaptive and constructive.

Where do we find clinical nonnormality that reflects failures to meet the accommodating/abiding criterion?

One example of an inability to leave things as they are is seen in what the DSM terms the "histrionic personality disorder." Their persistent and unrelenting manipulation of events is designed to maximize the receipt of attention and favors as well as to avoid social disinterest and disapproval. They show an insatiable if not indiscriminate search for stimulation and approval. Their clever and often artful social behaviors may give the appearance of an inner confidence and self-assurance; but beneath this guise lies a fear that a failure on their part to ensure the receipt of attention will, in short order, result in indifference or rejection, and hence their desperate need for reassurance and repeated signs of approval. As they are quickly bored and sated, they keep stirring up things, becoming enthusiastic about one activity and then another. There is a restless stimulus-seeking quality in which they cannot leave well enough alone.

At the other end of the polarity are personality pathologies that exhibit an excess of passivity, failing thereby to give direction to their own lives. Several Axis II disorders demonstrate this passive style, although their passivity derives from and is expressed in appreciably different ways. Dependents typically are average on the pleasure–pain polarity. Passivity for them stems from deficits in self-confidence and competence, leading to deficits in initiative and autonomous skills as well as a tendency to wait passively while others assume leadership and guide them. Passivity among obsessive–compulsive personalities stems from their fear of acting independently, owing to intrapsychic resolutions they have made to quell hidden thoughts and emotions generated by their intense self–other ambivalence. Dreading the possibility of making mistakes or engaging in disapproved behaviors, they became indecisive, immobilized, restrained, and passive.

Ecological Modification: Mastering One's Environment

The active end of the bipolarity signifies the taking of initiative in altering and shaping life's events. As stated previously, such persons are best characterized by their alertness, vigilance, liveliness, vigor, and forcefulness, their stimulus-seeking energy and drive.

White (1960), in his concept of effectance, sees it as an intrinsic motive that activates persons to impose their desires upon environments. In a similar vein, Fromm (1955) proposed a need on the part of man to rise above the roles of passive creatures in an accidental if not random world. To him, humans are driven to transcend the state of merely having been created; instead, humans seek to become the creators, the active shapers of their own destiny. Rising above the passive and accidental nature of existence, humans generate their own purposes and thereby provide themselves with a true basis of freedom.

Strategies of Replication: Other–Self Polarity

If an organism merely duplicates itself prior to death, then its replica is "doomed" to repeat the same fate it suffered. However, if new potentials for extending existence can be fashioned by chance or routine events, the possibility of achieving a different and conceivably superior outcome may be increased. And it is this co-occurrence of random and recombinant processes that does lead to the prolongation of a species' existence. This third hallmark of evolution's procession also undergirds another of nature's fundamental polarities, that between self and other.

As before, we consider both of the following criteria necessary to the definition and determination of normality. We see no necessary antithesis between the two. Humans can be both self-actualizing and other-encouraging, although most persons are likely to lean toward one or the other side. A balance that coordinates the two provides a satisfactory answer to the question of whether one should be devoted to the support and welfare of others or fashion one's life in accord with one's own needs and desires.

Progeny Nurturance: Constructively Encouraging Others

As described earlier, recombinant replication achieved by sexual mating entails a balanced though asymmetric parental investment in both the genesis and nurturance of offspring.

Before we turn to some of the indices and views of the self–other polarity, let us be mindful that these conceptually derived extremes do not evince themselves in sharp and distinct gender differences. Such proclivities are matters of degree, not absolutes, owing not only to the consequences of recombinant "shuffling" and gene "crossing over" but to the influential effects of cultural values and social learning. Consequently, most "normal" individuals exhibit intermediate characteristics on this as well as on the other two polarity sets.

Eloquent proposals related to this criterion have been formulated by the noted psychologist Gordon Allport. One of Allport's (1961) criteria of the "mature" personality, which he terms a "warm relating of self to others," refers to the capability of displaying intimacy and love for a parent, child, spouse, or close friend. Here the person manifests an authentic oneness with the other and a deep concern for his or her welfare. Beyond one's intimate family and friends, there is an extension of warmth in the mature person to humankind at large, an understanding of the human condition and a kinship with all peoples.

The pathological consequences of a failure to embrace the polarity criterion of "others" are seen most clearly in the personality pathologies termed "antisocial" and "narcissistic." Both personalities exhibit an imbalance in their replication strategy; in this case, however, there is a primary reliance on self rather than others. They have learned that reproductive success as well as maximum pleasure and minimum pain is achieved by turning primarily to themselves.

The tendency to focus on self follows two major lines of development. In the narcissistic personality, development reflects the acquisition of a self-image of superior worth, learned largely in response to admiring and doting parents. Providing self-rewards is highly gratifying if one values oneself or possesses either a "real" or inflated sense of self-worth. They display manifest confidence, arrogance, and an exploitative egocentricity in social contexts, blithely assuming that others will recognize their specialness. Those exhibiting the antisocial personality act to counter the expectation of pain at the hand of others; this is done by actively engaging in duplicitous or illegal behaviors in which they seek to exploit others for self-gain. Skeptical regarding the motives of others, they desire autonomy and wish revenge for what are felt as past injustices. Many are irresponsible and impulsive, actions they see as justified because they judge others to be unreliable and disloyal. Insensitivity and ruthlessness with others are the primary means they have learned to head off abuse and victimization.

Individual Propagation: Actualizing Self

The converse of progeny nurturance is not progeny propagation but rather the lack of progeny nurturance. Thus, to fail to encourage others constructively does not enure the actualization of one's potentials. Both may and should exist in normal/healthy individuals.

Perhaps it was the senior author's own early mentor, Kurt Goldstein (1939, 1940), who first coined the concept under review with the self-actualization designation. As he phrased it, "There is only one motive by which human activity is set going: the tendency to actualize oneself" (p. 196). In like manner, Rogers (1963) posited a single, overreaching motive for the normal/healthy person—maintaining, actualizing, and enhancing one's potential. The goal is not that of maintaining a homeostatic balance or a high degree of ease and comfort but, rather, to move forward in becoming what is intrinsic to self and to enhance further that which one has already become. Believing that humans have an innate urge to create, Rogers stated that the most creative product of all is one's own self.

Where do we see failures in the achievement of self-actualization, a giving up of self to gain the approbation of others? One personality disorder may be drawn on to illustrate forms of self-denial. Those with dependent personalities have learned that feeling good, secure, confident, and so on—that is, those feelings associated with pleasure or the avoidance of pain—is provided almost exclusively in their relationship with others. Behaviorally, these persons learn early that they themselves do not readily achieve rewarding experiences; the experiences are secured better by leaning on others. They learn not only to turn to others as their source of nurturance and security but to wait passively for others to take the initiative in providing safety and sustenance.

A TAXONOMY
OF PATHOLOGICAL PERSONALITY PATTERNS

This section turns to a formulation that employs the evolutionary-based theoretical concepts for deducing and coordinating pathological personality patterns. The full scope of this schema has been published by the senior author in earlier texts. First identified as a *biosocial–learning theory* (Millon, 1969), it is now cast, as indicated in prior pages, in evolutionary terms (Millon, 1990, 1996) and serves to establish the DSM personality categories through formal deduction as well as to show their covariation with other mental disorders.

Forgotten as a metapsychological speculation by most, the scaffolding comprising the evolutionary polarities was fashioned by Millon (1969). Unacquainted with Freud's seminal proposals at the time, and first employing a Skinnerian learning model, Millon constructed a framework similar to Freud's "great polarities that govern all of mental life" (Freud, 1915/ 1925). Phrased in the terminology of learning concepts, the model comprised three polar dimensions: positive versus negative reinforcement (pleasure–pain); self–other as reinforcement source; and the instrumental styles of active versus passive. Millon (1969) stated:

> By framing our thinking in terms of what reinforcements the individual is seeking, whether he is looking to find them and how he performs we may see more simply and more clearly the essential strategies which guide his coping behaviors. These reinforcements [relate to] whether he seeks primarily to achieve positive reinforcements (pleasure) or to avoid negative reinforcements (pain).

Some patients turn to others as their source of reinforcement, whereas some turn primarily to themselves. The distinction [is] between *others* and *self* as the primary reinforcement source.

On what basis can a useful distinction be made among instrumental behaviors? A review of the literature suggests that the behavioral dimension of activity-passivity may prove useful. . . . Active patients [are] busily intent on controlling the circumstances of their environment. Passive patients wait for the circumstances of their environment to take their course reacting to them only after they occur. (pp. 193–195)

Using the threefold polarity framework as a foundation, Millon (1969) formulated a series of personality "coping strategies" that corresponded in significant detail to each of the "official" personality disorders that were subsequently introduced in DSM-III (American Psychiatric Association, 1980). Coping strategies were viewed as complex forms of instrumental behavior (i.e., ways of achieving positive reinforcements and avoiding negative reinforcements). As noted, these strategies reflected what kinds of reinforcements individuals learned to seek or avoid (pleasure–pain), where individuals looked to obtain them (self–others), and how individuals learned to behave in order to elicit or escape them (active–passive). Eight basic personality patterns and three severe variants were derived by combining the *nature* (positive or pleasure vs. negative or pain), the *source* (self vs. others), and the *instrumental behaviors* (active vs. passive) engaged in to achieve various reinforcements.

Though the taxonomy of personality patterns to follow is combinatorially generated, the personologic consequences of a single polar extreme should first be noted. A high standing on the pain pole—a position typically associated with a disposition to experience anxiety—will be used for this purpose. The upshot of this singular sensitivity takes different forms depending on a variety of factors which lead to the learning of diverse styles of anxiety coping. For example, *avoidants* learn to deal with their pervasively experienced anxiety sensitivity by removing themselves "across the board," that is, actively withdrawing from most relationships unless strong assurances of acceptance are given. The *compulsive*, often equally prone to experience anxiety, has learned that there are sanctioned but limited spheres of acceptable conduct; the compulsive reduces anxiety by restricting activities only to those which are permitted by more powerful and potentially rejecting others, as well as to adhere carefully to rules so that unacceptable boundaries will not be transgressed. And the anxiety-prone *paranoid* has learned to neutralize pain by constructing a semidelusional pseudocommunity (Cameron, 1963), one in which environmental realities are transformed to make them more tolerable and less threatening, albeit not very successfully. In sum, a high standing at the pain pole leads not to one but to diverse personality outcomes.

Another of the polar extremes is selected here to illustrate the diversity of forms that coping styles may take as a function of covariant polarity positions; in this case reference is made to a shared position on the passivity pole. Five primary Axis II disorders demonstrate the passive style, but their passivity derives from and is expressed in appreciably different ways that reflect disparate polarity combinations. *Schizoids*, for example, are passive owing to their relative incapacity to experience pleasure and pain; without the rewards these emotional valences normally activate, they will be devoid of the drive to acquire rewards, leading them to become rather indifferent and passive observers. *Dependents* typically are average on the pleasure and pain polarity, yet they are usually no less passive than schizoids. Strongly oriented to "others," they are notably weak with regard to "self." Passivity for them stems from deficits in self-confidence and competence, leading to deficits in initiative and autonomous skills, as well as to a tendency to wait passively while others assume leadership and guide them. Passivity among *compulsives*, as noted previously, stems from their fear of acting independently, owing to intrapsychic resolutions they have made to quell hidden thoughts and emotions generated by their intense self–other ambivalence. Dreading the possibility of making mistakes or engaging in disapproved behaviors, they became indecisive, immobilized, restrained, and passive. High on pain and low on both pleasure and self, *self-defeating* (masochistic) personalities operate on the assumption that they dare not expect, nor do they deserve, to have life go their way; giving up any efforts to achieve a life that accords with their "true" desires, they passively submit to others' wishes, acquiescently accepting their fate. Finally, *narcissists*, especially high on self and low on others, benignly assume that "good things" will come their way with little or no effort on their part; this passive exploitation of others is a consequence of the unexplored confidence that underlies their self-centered presumptions.

Specifically, each of the DSM disorders is described and interpreted briefly in terms of the polarity model. Also noted briefly are a number of the several *subtypes* of each personality pathology prototype. The effort is made here in recognition of the fact that each "pure prototype" is merely an anchoring referent about which "real patients" vary.

Schizoid Personalities

On what basis can pathology in the level or capacity of either the pain or pleasure polarity be seen as relevant to personality disorders? Several possibilities present themselves. Schizoid patients are those in whom *both* polarity systems are deficient; that is, they lack the capacity, relatively speaking, to experience life's events either as painful or pleasurable. They tend to be apathetic, listless, distant, and asocial. Affectionate needs and emotional feelings are minimal and the individual functions as a passive observer detached from the rewards and affections as well as from the demands of human relationships. Among the subtypes we find the *affectless* schizoid, noted by his or her partial compulsive traits and lackluster and passionless characteristics, the *languid* schizoid, with limited depressive features, as evident in his or her phlegmatic behaviors, as well as *remote* and *depersonalized* subtype variants.

Avoidant Personalities

The second clinically meaningful combination based on problems in the pleasure–pain polarity comprises patients with a diminished ability to experience pleasure but with a foreboding anticipation and responsiveness to psychic pain. To them, life is vexatious, possessing few rewards and much anxiety. Among the major subtypes of the avoidant we find the *phobic* variant with dependent personality features such as general apprehensiveness and seeking of institutional supports; also, there are *hypersensitive* subtypes who evidence paranoid features such as suspiciousness and a general timorousness. Among other subtypes are the *self-deserting* and the *conflicted*.

Depressive Personalities

Akin to both the schizoid and avoidant personalities, as well as the soon-to-be discussed self-defeating (masochistic) type, is the newly introduced DSM depressive personality disorder. All four disorders share a deficiency in their ability to experience pleasure. Avoidants, depressives, and self-defeating types also share an overreactivity to pain. The avoidant, however, actively eschews pain, anticipates it, and, as best as possible, attempts to distance from its occurrence. Avoidant personalities display a vigorous effort to elude and circumvent the pain they envisage, resulting in their perennial state of anguished expectation. By contrast, the depressive's difficulty reflects hopeless resignation, a giving up, a sense that something of significance has been lost and can no longer be retrieved. The subtypes we find (Millon, 1996) are the *self-derogating* variant with dependent traits, evident in a tendency to be self-deriding and self-discrediting. Another variant is the *ill-humored* depressive, noted by negativistic features seen as irritability and general discontent. Other subtypes include the *voguish*, the *restive*, and the *morbid*.

Self-Defeating (Masochistic) Personalities

This disorder stems largely from a reversal of the pain–pleasure polarity. These persons interpret events and engage in relationships in a manner that is not only at variance with this deeply rooted polarity but is contrary to the associations these life-promoting emotions usually acquire through learning. To the self-defeating personality, pain may be a preferred experience, tolerantly accepted if not encouraged in intimate relationships. It is often intensified by purposeful self-denial, and blame acceptance may be aggravated by acts that engender difficulties as well as by thoughts that exaggerate past misfortunes and anticipate future ones. Among the subtypes are the *virtuous* masochistic, possessing histrionic features, noted by being proudly unselfish and self-sacrificial. Also notable is the *possessive* subtype with negativistic features such as being overprotective and jealous. Two other subtypes are recorded, namely, the *self-undoing* and the *oppressed* variants.

Aggressive (Sadistic) Personalities

There are other patients in whom the usual properties associated with pain and pleasure are conflicted or reversed. As with the self-defeating, these patients not only seek or create objectively "painful" events but experience them as "pleasurable." This second variant of pain-pleasure reversal, what we term "the aggressive personality" (DSM-III-R [American Psychiatric Association, 1987] sadistic, deleted from DSM-IV [American Psychiatric Association, 1994]), considers pain (stress, fear, cruelty) rather than pleasure to be the preferred mode of relating to others; in contrast to the self-defeating, this individual assumes an active role in controlling, dominating, and abusing others. Acts that humiliate, demean, if not brutalize are experienced as pleasurable. Among the sadistic subtypes are the *spineless* variant with avoidant, cowardly, and scapegoating characteristics. Also common among these subtypes is the *tyrannical* sadist, with paranoid features, and noted by accusatory and abusive behaviors. Other subtypes include the *explosive* and *enforcing* variants.

Dependent Personalities

Following the polarity model, one must ask whether particular clinical consequences occur among individuals who are markedly imbalanced by virtue of turning almost exclusively either toward others or toward themselves as a means of experiencing pleasure and avoiding pain. Such persons differ from the two detached and the two discordant types discussed previously; for example, neither detached type experiences pleasure from self or others. Personalities whose difficulties are traceable to the pathology of choosing one or the other polar end of the self–other dimension do experience both pain and pleasure and do experience them in a consonant, nonreversed manner; their pathology arises from the fact that they are tied almost exclusively *either* to others or to themselves as the source of these experiences.

Those with a dependency pathology have learned that feeling good, secure, confident, and so on—that is, those feelings associated with pleasure or the avoidance of pain—is provided almost exclusively in their relationship with others. Behaviorally, these persons display a strong need for external support and attention; should they be deprived of affection and nurturance they will experience marked discomfort, if not sadness and anxiety. Among the five subtypes recorded in Millon (1996), we find the *disquieted* variant with avoidant features, as seen in their fretful and foreboding behaviors. Notable also is the *accommodating* subtype with histrionic traits and their compliant and agreeable features. Among the others we noted the *ineffectual, immature* and *selfless* subtypes.

Histrionic Personalities

Also turning to others as their primary strategy is a group of personalities who take an "active" dependency stance. They achieve their goal of maximizing protection, nurturance, and reproductive success by engaging busily in a series of manipulative, seductive, gregarious, and attention-getting maneuvers. This active dependency *imbalance* in particular characterizes the behavior of the DSM histrionic personality, according to the theory. Six subtypes variants are noted, among them the *vivacious*, with narcissistic features, evident in their charming, impulsive, and ebullient behaviors. Notable also is the disingenuous type, with antisocial, calculating and deceitful behaviors and the *tempestuous* variant with negativistic features, as seen in moody complaints, sulking, and turbulent behaviors. Others found are the *infantile, appeasing* and *theatrical* types.

Narcissistic Personalities

Patients falling into the "independent" personality pattern also exhibit an *imbalance* in their replication strategy; in this case, however, there is a primary reliance on self rather than others. They have learned that an individuation focus, as well as maximum pleasure and minimum pain, is achieved by turning exclusively to themselves. The tendency to focus on self follows two major lines of development. In the first, the narcissistic personality, it reflects the acquisition of a self-image of superior worth, learned largely in response to admiring and doting parents. Providing self-rewards is highly gratifying if one values oneself or possesses either a real or an inflated sense of self-worth. Displaying manifest confidence, arrogance, and an exploitive egocentricity in social contexts, this self-orientation is termed "the passive–independent" style in the theory, because the individual "already" has all that is important—him- or herself. The four subtypes of the narcissist include *elitists*, who fancy themselves as demigods, flaunt their status, and engage in self-promotion. Other notable variants are the *compensatory* type with covert avoidant features, underlying feelings of inferiority, and illusions of superiority. Noteworthy too are the *amorous* and *unprincipled* subtypes.

Antisocial Personalities

Those whom we characterize as exhibiting the active–independent orientation resemble the outlook, temperament, and socially unacceptable behaviors
of the DSM antisocial personality disorder. They act to counter the expectation of pain at the hand of others; by actively engaging in duplicitous or illegal
behaviors in which they seek to exploit others for self-gain. Skeptical regarding the motives of others, they desire autonomy and wish revenge for what are
felt as past injustices. There are five subtypes of the antisocial; most common
is the *covetous* variant, noted by enviousness, retribution seeking, and a
greedy avariciousness. Also prevalent is the *risk-taking* type, seen in their
recklessness, impulsivity, and heedless behaviors; other variants include
reputation-defending, *nomadic*, and *malevolent* subtypes.

Negativistic (Passive–Aggressive) Personalities

Certain pathological personalities, those whom we shall speak of as
"ambivalent," also are oriented both toward self and others, but they are in
intense conflict between one or the other. A number of these patients, those
represented in the DSM negativistic personality, vacillate between others
and self, behaving obediently one time and reacting defiantly the next. Feeling intensely yet unable to resolve their ambivalence, they weave an erratic
course from voicing their self-deprecation and guilt for failing to meet the
expectations of others to expressing stubborn negativism and resistance
over having submitted to the wishes of others rather than their own.
Patients whose conflicts are overt, worn on their sleeves, so to speak, are
characterized in the theory as actively ambivalent, a richer and more varied
lot than the early DSM portrayals of the passive–aggressive. There are four
common negativistic subtypes, the *circuitous*, with dependent traits prevalent, as seen in their inefficiency, forgetfulness, and procrastination. Also
common is the *discontented* variant, frequently with depressive traits, and
noted by their grumbling, petty, complaining, and embittered feelings. The
other subtypes include the *abrasive* and *vacillating* variants.

Obsessive–Compulsive Personalities

Another major conflicted pattern, the DSM obsessive–compulsive personality disorder, displays a picture of distinct other-directedness, a consistency
in social compliance and interpersonal respect: Their histories usually indicate their having been subjected to constraint and discipline, but only when
they transgressed parental strictures and expectations. Beneath the con-
forming other-oriented veneer they exhibit are intense desires to rebel and
assert their own self-oriented feelings and impulses. Five subtypes of the
obsessive–compulsive are notable. The pure type is termed the "conscien-

tious," noted by being earnest, meticulous, but also inflexible and indecisive. Also noteworthy is the *bureaucratic* subtype with modest narcissistic features who acts in an officious, petty-minded, mettlesome, and close-minded manner. The other three variants include the *parsimonious*, the *bedeviled*, and the *puritanical*.

We turn next to the severe personality patterns. Dysfunctional or decompensated levels differ from their less severe parallel patterns by several criteria, notably deficits in social competence and frequent (but readily reversible) psychotic episodes. As noted, they almost invariably coexist with and are more intense variants of the basic 11 personality patterns discussed previously—for example, schizotypals tend to exhibit more problematic features also seen among schizoids and/or avoidants. Less integrated in terms of their personality organization and less effective in coping than their milder counterparts, they are especially vulnerable to decompensate when faced with the strains of everyday life. All three of the more severe patterns are adaptively problematic, difficult to relate to socially, and often isolated, hostile, or confused. Hence, they are not likely to elicit the interpersonal support that could bolster their flagging defenses and orient them to a more effective and satisfying lifestyle. A clear breakdown in the cohesion of personality organization is seen in the first two of these patterns—the borderline and schizotypal: the converse is evident in the third, the paranoid, where there is an overly rigid and narrow focus to the personality structure. In the former pair, there has been a dissolution or diffusion of ego capacities; in the latter pattern there is an inelasticity and constriction of personality, giving rise to a fragility and an inadaptability of psychological functions.

Borderline Personalities

Although the borderline personality has been referred to previously it may be helpful to describe it further. The cardinal feature of this pattern is that its hierarchical control structures are poorly differentiated—modular rather than integrated. In the relative absence of higher self-regulatory processes wrought by a consistent view of the world and self, there is intense lability between competing cognitive–affective–behavioral structures as one and then another co-opts control of the personality system on the basis of fleeting and idiosyncratic associations with the current environment. Several subtypes are notable among the borderline pattern. Common are the *self-destructive* variants with their depressive traits and their high-strung, inward-turning, and moody behaviors. Also prevalent is the *impulsive* type with histrionic and/or antisocial features, evident in their capricious, agitated, irritable, and potentially suicidal behaviors. The other two variants are the *discouraged* and *petulant* subtypes.

Schizotypal Personalities

This personality disorder represents a cognitively dysfunctional and mal-adaptively detached orientation in the polarity theory. Schizotypal person-alities may experience minimal pleasure and have difficulty consistently dif-ferentiating between self and other strategies, as well as active and passive modes of adaptation. Many prefer social isolation with minimal personal attachments and obligations. Inclined to be either autistic or confused cognitively, they think tangentially and often appear self-absorbed and ruminative. Behavioral eccentricities are notable and the individual is often perceived by others as strange or different. Two major subtypes are found among the schizotypals. One is an outgrowth of the schizoid pattern and is noted by its sluggish, imexpressive behavior and its vague and obscure thinking; it is called the *insipid* subtype. The second, the *timorous* variant, is warily apprehensive, alienated from self, and disqualifies one's own thoughts; it is a more severe or decompensated form of the basic avoidant pattern.

Paranoid Personalities

Here are seen a vigilant mistrust of others and an edgy defensiveness against anticipated criticism and deception. Driven by a high sensitivity to pain (rejection–humiliation) and oriented strongly to the self polarity, these patients exhibit a touchy irritability and a need to assert themselves, not necessarily in action but in an inner world of self-determined beliefs and assumptions. They are "prepared" to provoke social conflicts and fractious circumstances as a means of gratifying their confused mix of pain sensitiv-ity and self-assertion. Among the five subtypes of the paranoid described by Millon (1996), we find the *fanatic*, inhibiting narcissistic features, and clini-cal signs such as grandiose delusions, an arrogant expansiveness, and extravagant fantasies. Also typical is the *insular* variant with avoidant fea-tures, exhibiting a reclusive, hypervigilant, and defensive lifestyle. Other subtypes include the *querulous*, *obdurate*, and *malignant* variants.

PERSONOLOGIC ASSESSMENT

Personality may be usefully conceptualized and measured with a variety of approaches and methodologies. Five instruments—the Millon Clinical Multiaxial Inventory (MCMI), the Millon Adolescent Clinical Inventory (MACI), the Millon Behavioral Medicine Diagnostic (MBMD), the Millon Personality Diagnostic Checklist (MPDC), and the Millon Index of Person-ality Styles (MIPS)—have been created to operationalize the constructs of the theoretical model presented herein. These instruments vary according to their intended populations and all but one, the MPDC, follows the self-report format. Only two of these are briefly discussed, the MCMI and the MIPS; readers interested in the other instruments may be provided with relevant details by reading their manuals and either or both Millon (1997) and Strack (2002).

Millon Clinical Multiaxial Inventory–III (MCMI-III): Assessment of "Pathological Personality Patterns" and "Clinical Syndromes"

A 175-item true–false self-report inventory, the MCMI and its subsequent revisions, MCMI-II (Millon, 1987b) and MCMI-III (Millon, Millon, & Davis, 1997), include 14 personality disorder scales (all the personality disorders in both the main texts and appendices of DSM-III, DSM-III-R, and DSM-IV), nine clinical syndrome scales (e.g., anxiety and major depression), and three "modifying indices" to appraise problematic response tendencies.

Within the restrictions on validity set by the limits of the self-report mode, the narrow frontiers of psychometric technology, and the slender range of consensually shared diagnostic knowledge, all steps were taken to maximize the MCMI's concordance with its generative theory and the official classification system. Pragmatic and philosophical compromises were made where valued objectives could not be simultaneously achieved (e.g., instrument brevity vs. item independence; representative national patient norms vs. local base rate specificity; theoretical criterion considerations vs. empirical data).

Separate scales of the MCMI have been constructed in line with DSM to distinguish the more enduring personality characteristics of patients (Axis II) from the acute clinical disorders they display (Axis I), a distinction judged to be of considerable use by both test developers and clinicians (Dahlstrom, 1972). This distinction should enable the clinician to separate those syndrome features of psychopathological functioning that are persistent and pervasive from those that are transient or circumscribed. Moreover, profiles based on all 23 clinical scales illuminate the interplay between long-standing characterological patterns and the distinctive clinical symptomatology a patient manifests under psychic stress.

Validation data with a variety of populations (e.g., outpatients and inpatients and alcohol and drug centers) suggest that the MCMI can be used with a reasonable level of confidence in most clinical settings. Its recognition as one of only four assessment instruments (the others being the Rorschach, Thematic Apperception Test, Minnesota Multiphasic Personality Inventory), and the only one developed in the last five decades to be considered necessary tools by more than half of those who train Ph.D and Psy.D psychologists, attests to its level of acceptance and utility. As of this writing, some 650 research studies including the MCMI as a measure have been published in the literature (see Millon, 1997; Strack, 2002; Choca, 2003).

Millon Index of Personality Styles—Revised (MIPS-R): Assessment of Normal Personality

Beyond breaking down the theory's manifest personality types into their constituent latent constructs, the theory as described in previous pages has been expanded substantially. Whereas the three polarities of the theory are crucial elements of the model as a gauge of personality pathology, they are now judged to be insufficient as a scaffold for encompassing the many varieties of normal personality styles. This is not the chapter to elaborate both the full rationale and specifics of the expanded model; a recent essay on this theme may be found in the MIPS-R manual (Millon, Weiss, & Millon, 2004).

Briefly, we should note that cognitive differences among individuals and the manner in which they are expressed have not been a sufficiently appreciated domain for generating personality traits. We have added a set of four polarities that reflect different "styles of thinking" (e.g., realistic–imaginative) to the MIPS. These follow the initial three polarity pairs (e.g., self–other), which are termed "motivating styles." Similarly, we have added a third domain of polarities to those of "motivating" and "thinking," that of "behaving styles" (e.g., submissive–dominant). This third domain, comprising five interpersonal relating polarities, concludes the MIPS test form. The tripartite structure of the MIPS scales divides the test in the manner in which organisms function in their environment, one which we believe may be a useful theory-based schema for purposes of normal personologic analysis.

Research with the MIPS was conducted to assess its usefulness in applied settings, as well as its cross validity with other established "normal" personality inventories, such as the Myers-Briggs Type Inventory (Myers, 1962), the Sixteen-Personality Factor Inventory (Cattell, Eber, & Tatsuoka, 1970), the California Personality Inventory (Gough, 1987), and the NEO Personality Inventory (Costa & McCrae, 1985), among others.

SYNERGISTIC PERSONOLOGIC THERAPY

This chapter has advocated integrative and organizational conceptions not only of the personality construct but also of clinical science itself. We have noted in earlier publications (Millon, 1996, 1999) that the polarity schema and clinical domains can serve as useful points of focus for corresponding modalities of therapy, the final element of a mature clinical science, as noted in the opening pages of this chapter. In a way, everything that went before was done in order to arrive at this *summum bonum* of an applied clinical science. A good theory not only should allow us to conceive nature in its esthetic glory but also should serve as a basis on which to *do* something; that is, a good theory should also be a theory of action. If the principles and variables are where they have been assumed to be, the theory should allow us to help others identify and create more flexible and adaptive psychological styles of functioning, if the tactics of therapy can be specific and properly selected.

Before turning to substantive therapeutic matters, a brief comment on a few philosophical issues is necessary. These issues bear on a rationale for developing theory-based treatment techniques and methods, that is, methods that transcend the merely empirical (e.g., electroconvulsive therapy for depressives) (see Millon, 1999). However, what differentiates our treatment approach has little to do with either its theoretical underpinnings or its empirical support. While personality is an integrative construct, what differentiates the behavioral, cognitive, psychodynamic, and biological orientations is merely the fact that they limit their attention to different clinical domains.

Integrative psychotherapy, or what we have termed "synergistic therapy," at least as it should be applied to the personality pathologies, must make specifications of both form and substance. Synergistic therapy is more than eclecticism; perhaps it should be termed "posteclecticism," if we may borrow a characterization of modern art a century ago. Eclecticism, of course, is not a matter of choice. We all must be eclectics, engaging in differential (Frances, Clarkin, & Perry, 1984) and multimodal (Lazarus, 1981) therapeutics, selecting the techniques that are empirically the most efficacious for the problems at hand. However, synergistic treatment is more than the coexistence of two or three previously discordant orientations or techniques.

The synergistic integration, labeled "personality-guided therapy" (Millon, 1988, 1999), insists on the primacy of an overarching gestalt that gives coherence, provides an interactive framework, and creates an organic order among otherwise discrete methodologies and techniques. While it is eclectic in the sense that it pulls from here and there, it does so to *create a coherent treatment approach that parallels the patient's psychic configuration*; it is synthesized from a comprehensive and coherent pattern of techniques whose overall focus and orientation derives from that old chestnut: The whole is greater than the sum of its parts. As we know well, the personality problems our patients bring to us are an inextricably linked nexus of interpersonal behaviors, cognitive styles, regulatory processes, and so on. They flow through a tangle of feedback loops and serially unfolding concatenations that emerge at different times in dynamic and changing configurations. Each component of these configurations has its role and significance altered by virtue of its place in these continually evolving constellations. In parallel form, so should synergistic therapy be conceived as an integrated configuration of strategies and tactics that mirror patient's configuration of pathological attributes; moreover, each intervention technique is selected *not only* for its efficacy in resolving particular pathological attributes but also for its contribution to the overall constellation of treatment procedures of which it is but one.

Synergistic therapists must take cognizance of the person from the start, for the parts and the contexts take on different meanings and call for different interventions in terms of the person to whom they are anchored. To focus on one social structure (family, job) or one psychic form of expression, that is, to advocate any single domain approach (intrapsychic, cognitive, behavioral) without understanding its embeddedness in substantively whole persons, is to engage in potentially misguided, if not random, therapeutic techniques.

Relevant to this section of the chapter would be a reading of *Personality-Guided Therapy* (Millon, 1999), which analyzes well over 100 complex syndrome and personality pattern cases and details the several strategies and tactics employed to remediate their difficulties. This clinical text argues for a psychologically designed composite and progression among diverse techniques. In a "catalytic sequence," for example, one might seek first to alter a patient's humiliating and painful stuttering by direct *behavior modification* procedures, which, if achieved, may facilitate the use of *cognitive methods* in producing self-image changes in confidence, which may, in turn, foster the utility of *interpersonal techniques* in effecting improvements in relationships with others. In "potentiated pairing" one may simultaneously combine, as is commonly done these days, both behavioral and cognitive methods to overcome problematic interactions with others and conceptions of self that might be refractory to either technique if employed alone.

CONCLUDING COMMENT

Our aims in this chapter were (1) to connect the conceptual structure of both normal and abnormal personalities and their stages of neurodevelopment to what we judge to be the omnipresent principles of evolution, a theoretical ambition; (2) to use the evolutionary theory to create a deductively derived clinical taxonomy, also a conceptual goal; (3) to link the taxonomy to newly developed assessment instruments; and (4) to outline prescriptions for an integrative or synergistic model of psychotherapy, the latter two practical and utilitarian purposes. And it is on these foundations that we see a framework for a systematic clinical science of personology and psychopathology.

REFERENCES

Allport, G. (1961). *Pattern and growth in personality.* New York: Holt, Rinehart & Winston.

American Psychiatric Association. (1980). *Diagnostic and statistical manual of mental disorders* (3rd ed.). Washington, DC: Author.

American Psychiatric Association. (1987). *Diagnostic and statistical manual of mental disorders* (3rd ed., rev.). Washington, DC: Author.

American Psychiatric Association. (1994). *Diagnostic and statistical manual of mental disorders* (4th ed.). Washington, DC: Author.

Bandura, A. (1969). *Principles of behavior modification.* New York: Holt. Rinehart & Winston.

Beach, F., & Jaynes, J. (1954). Effects of early experience upon the behavior of animals. *Psychological Bullein, 51,* 239–262.

Beck, A. T. (1976). *Cognitive therapy and the emotional disorders.* New York: International Universities Press.

Bowers, K. S. (1977). There's more to Iago than meets the eye: A clinical account of personality consistency. In D. Magnusson & N. S. Endler (Eds.). *Personality at the crossroads.* Hillsdale, NJ: Erlbaum.

Bowlby, J. (1982). *Attachment and loss: Vol 1: Attachment.* New York: Basic Books. (Original work published 1969)

Buss, D. M. (1984). Evolutionary biology and personality psychology. *American Psychologist, 39,* 1135–1147.

Buss, D. M. (1994). *The evolution of desire: Strategies of human mating.* New York: Basic Books.

Butcher, J. N. (Ed.). (1972). *Objective personality assessment.* New York: Academic Press.

Butler, J. M., & Rice, L. N. (1963). Adience, self-actualization, and drive theory. In J. I. Wepman & R. Heine (Eds.), *Concepts of personality.* Chicago: Aldine.

Cameron, N. (1963). *Personality development and psychopathology.* New York: Houghton Mifflin.

Cattell, R. B., Eber, H. W., & Tatsuoka, M. M. (1970). *Handbook for the Sixteen Personality Factor Questionnaire (16PF).* Champaign, IL: Institute for Personality and Ability Testing.

Choca, J. P. (2003). *Interpretive Guide to the Millon clinical inventories* (3rd ed.). Washington, DC: American Psychological Association.

Clark, L., & Watson, D. (1988). Mood and the mundane: Relations between daily life events and self-reported mood. *Journal of Personality and Social Psychology, 54,* 296–308.

Cole, L. C. (1954). The population consequences of life history phenomena. *Quarterly Review of Biology*, 29, 103–137

Cosmides, L., & Tooby, J. (1987). From evolution to behavior: Evolutionary psychology as the missing link. In J. Dupre (Ed.), *The latest on the best: Essays on evolution and optimality*. Cambridge, MA: MIT Press.

Costa, P. T., & McCrae, R. R. (1985). *The NEO Personality Inventory manual*. Odessa, FL: Psychological Assessment Resources.

Crittenden, P. M. (1990). Internal representational models of attachment. *Infant Mental Health Journal*, 11, 259–277.

Dahlstrom, W. G. (1972). Whither the MMPI? In J. N. Butcher (Ed.), *Objective personality assessment*. New York: Academic Press.

Daly, M., & Wilson, M. (1978). *Sex, evolution and behavior*. Boston: Grant Press.

Ellis, A. (1970). *The essence of rational psychotherapy: A comprehensive approach to treatment*. New York: Institute for Rational Living.

Erikson, E. (1950). *Childhood and society*. New York: Norton.

Erikson, E. (1959). Growth and crises of the healthy personality. In G. S. Klein (Ed.), *Psychological issues*. New York: International Universities Press.

Fox, N. A., Kimmerly, N. L., & Schafer, W. D. (1991). Attachment to mother/attachment to father: A meta-analysis. *Child Development*, 62, 210–225.

Frances, A., Clarkin, J., & Perry, S. (1984). *Differential therapeutics in psychiatry*. New York: Brunner/Mazel.

Freud, S. (1925). The instincts and their vicissitudes. In *Collected papers* (vol. 4). London: Hogarth. (Original work published 1915)

Fromm, E. (1955). *The sane society*. New York: Holt, Rinehart, & Winston.

Gewirtz, J. L. (1963). A learning analysis of the effects of normal stimulation upon social and exploratory behavior in the human infant. In B. M. Foss (Ed.), *Determinants of infant dehavior II*. New York: Wiley.

Gilligan, C. (1982). *In a different voice*. Cambridge, MA. Harvard University Press.

Goldstein, K. (1939). *The organism*. New York: American Books.

Goldstein, K. (1940). *Human nature in the light of psychopathology*. Cambridge, MA: Harvard University Press.

Gough, H. G. (1987). *California Psychological Inventory: Administrator's guide*. Palo Alto, CA: Consulting Psychologists Press.

Hartmann, H. (1939). *Ego psychology and the problem of adaptation*. New York: International Universities Press.

Hempel, C. G. (1965). *Aspects of scientific explanation*. New York: Free Press.

Hinde, R. A. (1982). Attachment: Some conceptual and biological issues. In J. Stevenson-Hinde & C. P. Parkes (Eds.), *The place of attachment in human behavior*. New York: Basic Books.

Killackey, H. P. (1990). Neocortical expansion: An attempt toward relating phylogeny and ontogeny. *Journal of Cognitive Neuroscience*, 2, 1–17.

Klein, D. F., & Davis, J. (1969). *Diagnosis and drug treatment of psychiatric disorders*. Baltimore: Williams and Wilkins.

Lamb, M. E., Thompson, R. A., Gardner, W., & Estes, D. (1985). *Infant–mother attachment*. Hillsdale, NJ: Erlbaum.

Lazarus, A. A. (1981). *The practice of multimodal therapy*. New York: McGraw-Hill.

Linehan, M. M. (1993). *Cognitive-behavioral therapy of borderline personality disorder.* New York: Guilford Press.

Lipton, S. A., & Kater, S. B. (1989). Neurotransmitter regulation of neuronal outgrowth, plasticity, and survival. *Trends in Neuroscience, 12,* 265–269.

Meichenbaum, D. (1977). *Cognitive-behavioral modification.* New York: Plenum Press.

Melzick, R. (1965). Effects of early experience upon behavior: Experimental and conceptual considerations. P. In Hoch & J. Zubin (Eds.), *Psychopathology of perception.* New York: Grune & Stratton.

Millon, T. (1969). *Modern psychopathology: A biosocial approach to maladaptive learning and functioning.* Philadelphia: Saunders.

Millon, T. (1981). *Disorders of personality: DSM-III; Axis II.* New York: Wiley-Interscience.

Millon, T. (1987a). On the nature of taxonomy in psychopathology. In C. Last & M. Hersen (Eds.), *Issues in diagnostic research.* New York: Plenum Press.

Millon, T. (1987b). *Millon Clinical Multiaxial Inventory-II (MCMI-II).* Minneapolis, MN: National Computer Systems.

Millon, T. (1988). Personologic psychotherapy: Ten commandments for a post-eclectic approach to integrative treatment. *Psychotherapy, 25,* 209–219.

Millon, T. (1990). *Toward a new personology: An evolutionary model.* New York: Wiley-Interscience.

Millon, T. (1991). Normality: What can we learn from evolutionary theory? In D. Offer & M. Sabshin (Eds.), *Normality: Context and theory.* New York: Basic Books.

Millon, T. (with Davis, R.). (1996). *Disorders of personality: DSM-IV and beyond.* New York: Wiley-Interscience.

Millon, T. (1997). *The Millon inventories: Clinical and personality assessment.* New York: Guilford Press.

Millon, T. (1999). *Personality-guided therapy.* New York: Wiley-Interscience.

Millon, T. (2003). Evolution: A generative source for conceptualizing the attributes of personality. In T. Millon & M. Lerner (Eds.) *Handbook of psychology: Personality and social psychology* (vol. 5). New York: Wiley.

Millon, T., Blaney, P., & Davis, R. (Eds.). (1999). *Oxford textbook of psychopathology.* New York: Oxford University Press.

Millon, T., Millon, C., & Davis, R. (1997). *Millon Clinical Multiaxial Inventory—III (MCMI-III) manual.* Minneapolis, MN: National Computer Systems.

Millon, T., Simonsen, E., Birket-Smith, M., & Davis, R. (Eds.). (1998). *Psychopathy: Antisocial, criminal, and violent behavior.* New York: Guilford Press.

Millon, T., Weiss, L., & Millon, C., & Davis, R. (1994). *Millon Index of Personality Styles (MIPS) manual.* San Antonio, TX: Psychological Corporation.

Millon, T., Weiss, L., & Millon, C. (2004). *Millon Index of Personality Styles—Revised (MIPS-R) manual.* Minneapolis, MN: Pearson Assessments.

Murphy, G. (1947). *Personality: A biosocial approach to origins and structures.* New York: Harper.

Myers, I. B. (1962). *The Myers–Briggs type indicator.* Palo Alto, CA: Consulting Psychologist Press.

Murray, H. A. (Ed.). (1938). *Explorations in personality*. New York: Oxford University Press.

Offer, D., & Sabshin, M. (Eds.). (1974). *Normality*. New York: Basic Books.

Offer, D., & Sabshin, M. (Eds.). (1991). *The diversity of normality*. New York: Basic Books.

Purves, D., & Lichtman, J. W. (1985). *Principles of neural development*. Sunderland, MA: Sinauer.

Quine, W. V. O. (1977). Natural kinds. In S. P. Schwartz (Ed.), *Naming, necessity, and natural groups*. Ithaca, NY: Cornell University Press.

Rakic, P. (1985). Limits of neurogenesis in primates. *Science, 227,* 154–156.

Rakic, P. (1988). Specification of cerebral cortical areas. *Science, 241,* 170–176.

Rapaport, D. (1958). The theory of ego-autonomy: A generalization. *Bulletin of the Menninger Clinic, 22,* 13–35.

Ribble, M. A. (1943). *The rights of infants*. New York: Columbia University Press.

Riesen, A. H. (1961). Stimulation as a requirement for growth and function in behavioral development. In D. Fiske & S. Maddi (Eds.), *Functions of varied experience*. Homewood, IL: Dorsey.

Rogers, C. R. (1963). Toward a science of the person. *Journal of Humanistic Psychology, 3,* 79–92.

Rosenzweig, M. R., Krech, D., & Bennett, E. L. (1962). Effect of environmental complexity and training on brain chemistry and anatomy: A replication and extension. *Journal of Comparative Physiological Psychology, 55,* 429–437.

Rushton, J. P. (1985). Differential K theory: The sociobiology of individual and group differences. *Personality and Individual Differences, 6,* 441–452.

Scott, J. P. (1968). *Early experience and the organization of behavior*. Belmont, CA: Brooks/Cole.

Smith, E. E., & Medin, D. L. (1981). *Categories and concepts*. Cambridge, MA: Harvard University Press.

Spencer, H. (1870). *The principles of psychology*. London: Williams and Norgate.

Spitz, R. A. (1965). *The first year of life*. New York: International University Press.

Sroufe, L. A., & Fleeson, J. (1986). Attachment and the construction of relationships. In W. Hartup & Z. Rubin. (Eds.), *Relationships and development*. Hillsdale, NJ: Erlbaum.

Strack, S. (Ed.). (2002). *Essentials of Millon inventories assessment* (2nd ed.). New York: Wiley.

Symons, D. (1992). On the use and misuse of Darwinism in the study of human behavior. In J. Barkow, L. Cosmides, & J. Tooby (Eds.), *The adapted mind*. New York: Oxford University Press.

Tellegen, A. (1985). Structures of mood and personality and relevance to assessing anxiety, with an emphasis on self-report. In A. H. Tuma & J. Maser (Eds.). *Anxiety and the anxiety disorders*. Hillsdale, NJ: Erlbaum.

Thompson, W. R., & Schaefer, T. (1961). Early environmental stimulation. In D. Fiske & S. Maddi (Eds.), *Functions of varied experience*. Homewood, IL: Dorsey.

Trivers, R. L. (1974). Parental investment and sexual selection. In B. Campbell (Ed.), *Sexual selection and the descent of man 1871–1971*. Chicago: Aldine.

Tversky, A. (1977). Features of similarity. *Psychological Review, 84*, 327–352.

Watson, D., & Clark, L. (1984). Negative affectivity: The disposition to experience aversive emotional states. *Psychological Bulletin, 96*, 465–490.

Watson, D., & Tellegen, A. (1985). Toward a consensual structure of mood. *Psychological Bulletin, 98*, 219–235.

White, R. W. (1960). Competence and the psychosexual stages of development. In M. R. Jones (Ed.), *Nebraska Symposium on Motivation*. Lincoln: University of Nebraska Press.

Wilson, E. O. (1975). *Sociobiology: The new synthesis*. Cambridge, MA: Harvard University Press.

Wilson, E. O. (1978). *On human nature*. Cambridge, MA: Harvard University Press.

Wilson, E. O. (1998). *Consilience: The unity of knowledge*. New York: Knopf.

CHAPTER 8

■ ■ ■

A Neurobehavioral
Dimensional Model
of Personality Disturbance

RICHARD A. DEPUE
MARK F. LENZENWEGER

THE PROBLEM OF MODELING NONENTITIES

From a scientific perspective, it is really no longer possible to accept the notion that personality disorders represent distinct, categorical diagnostic entities. The behavioral features of personality disorders are not organized into discrete diagnostic entities, and multivariate studies of behavioral criteria fail to identify factors that resemble existing diagnostic constructs (Block, 2001; Ekselius, Lindstrom, von Knorring, Bodlund, & Kullgren 1994; Livesley, 2001; Livesley, Schroeder, Jackson, & Jang, 1994). Indeed, just the opposite is observed: The behavioral features of personality disorders merge imperceptibly in a continuous fashion across diagnostic categories, resulting in (1) significant overlap of behavioral features across categories and hence diagnostic comorbidity within individuals, and (2) symptom heterogeneity within categories and hence frequent (and most common in some studies) application of the ambiguous diagnosis of *personality disorder not otherwise specified* (Livesley, 2001; Saulsman & Page, 2004). Moreover, aside from schizotypy/schizotypical disorders, the existing latent class and taxometric analysis literature on personality disorders generally does *not* provide support for distinct entities in the personality disorder realm in any compelling fashion, and some provisional taxonic findings for

391

borderline and antisocial personality disorders are open to doubt. It is, accordingly, not surprising that diagnostic membership is not significantly associated with predictive validity as to prognosis nor psychological or pharmacological treatments (Livesley, 2001). Such a state of affairs recently led Livesley (2001) to declare that "evidence on these points has accumulated to the point that it can no longer be ignored" (p. 278).

Such a state of affairs supports proponents of a dimensional approach to personality disorders, who note that (1) the behavioral features of personality disorders not only overlap diagnostic categories but also merge imperceptibly with normality (Livesley, 2001; Saulsman & Page, 2004); and (2) the factorial structure of behavioral traits associated with personality disorders is similar in clinical and nonclinical samples (Livesley, Jackson, & Schroeder, 1992; Reynolds & Clark, 2001). Furthermore, the higher-order structure of personality disorder traits resembles four of the five major traits identified in the higher-order structure of normal personality (Clark & Livesley, 1994; Clark, Livesley, Schroeder, & Irish, 1996; Reynolds & Clark, 2001). These findings suggest that personality disorders may be better understood as emerging at the extremes of personality dimensions that define the structure of behavior in the normal population (for reviews of this position, see Costa & Widiger, 1994; Depue & Lenzenweger, 2001; Lenzenweger & Clarkin, 1996; Livesley, 2001; Reynolds & Clark, 2001; Saulsman & Page, 2004; Widiger, Trull, Clarkin, Sanderson, & Costa, 1994).

This realization has led to innumerable attempts to illustrate the association of personality traits to personality disorder diagnostic categories. Most of these studies have relied on the so-called five-factor model of personality, which defines a structure characterized by the five higher-order traits of extraversion, neuroticism, agreeableness, conscientiousness, and openness to experience. Although Reynolds and Clark (2001) demonstrated that four of these traits (openness shows no consistent relation to personality disorders; Saulsman & Page, 2004) account for a substantial proportion of the variance in interview-based ratings of personality disorder diagnoses according to the fourth edition of *Diagnostic and Statistical Manual of Mental Disorders* (DSM-IV; American Psychiatric Association, 1994), a recent meta-analysis of similar studies demonstrated the limitation of the approach of correlating four traits with personality disorders (Saulsman & Page, 2004). The meta-analysis showed what most such studies illustrate: (1) the correlation of these four traits with personality disorder categories is moderate to weak, (2) the complex "entity" of a personality disorder category is defined by as little as one trait but never by four traits in a significant way, and (3) single traits (e.g., neuroticism) characterize more than one, sometimes several, putatively distinct personality disorders. For example, how helpful is it to know that histrionic personality disorder is characterized by moderately high extraversion but by no other trait; or, similarly, that dependent personality disorder is associated with moderately high neuroticism but by no other trait. To what line of research or clinical intervention does that knowledge lead? Moreover, the traits relate more highly to personality disorder categories that are studied in nonclinical samples, indicating that the traits may be less valuable in defining clinical entities. What the meta-analysis did reveal is that most personality disorders manifest, in common, higher trait levels of neuroticism and lower trait levels of agreeableness, meaning that most individuals with personality disorders are subject to negative emotionality and impaired affiliative or interpersonal behavior. Thus, again, when personality disorder categories serve as the outcome variable, personality traits provide little in the way of power to discriminate between such categories. Overall, then, it is probably not unfair to conclude that such correlational studies have done little to inform the issue of continuity from personality systems to states of disorder, most of them having merely specified correlates of personality disorders and nothing more, and most of these studies lacked an underlying framework for understanding both personality and personality disorders.

The paradox in all of this is that, despite knowing that the personality disorder diagnostic categories are unreliable and lack compelling construct and predictive validity, researchers cling to the approach of relating major personality traits, typically considered at the conceptual level of analysis one trait at a time, to *nonentities* of personality disorders. How can one learn something substantive by relating four higher-order traits to heterogeneous behavioral phenomena that are clustered conceptually (not statistically or theoretically) into diagnostic entities? As Livesley (2001) aptly notes, because personality disorder diagnoses are so fundamentally flawed, it is not important to know whether each personality disorder diagnosis can be accommodated by a dimensional model. Furthermore, the problem in this approach does not appear to be explained simply by use of a small number of broad traits. When the 30 facet scales of the NEO-PI were correlated with personality disorder categories, only modest gains were achieved relative to the use of the four major traits (mean difference in $R^2 \sim .04$) (Dyce & O'Connor, 1998; Millon, 1997).

Perhaps one of the most crucial issues associated with a dimensional personality approach to personality disorders is that the substantive meaning of the four major traits is not clear and generally has been a neglected topic (Block, 2001). Put differently, there is no clear understanding as to which underlying neurobehavioral systems these traits reflect, which the behavioral genetic literature implies they must (Tellegen et al., 1988). Accordingly, in this chapter we attempt to promote an alternative empirical and theoretical approach to personality disorders. First, we embrace the fact that personality disorders do not exist as *distinct entities*, and, therefore, we refer to the behavioral manifestations that emerge at the extremes of personality dimensions as *personality disturbance* rather than disorders. We exclude schizotypal and paranoid personality disorders from our model because there is evidence that they may be genetically related to schizophrenia (e.g., Kendler et al., 1993; Lenzenweger & Loranger, 1989), representing an alternative manifestation of schizophrenia liability (Lenzenweger, 1998), and studies of the latent class structure of schizotypy show evidence that its underlying nature is more likely of a taxonic or qualitative nature (Lenzenweger & Korfine, 1992; Korfine & Lenzenweger, 1995). The term "disorder," though less formal and regimented than the term "disease," nevertheless connotes a relatively coherent symptomatic entity that, with only more empirical attention, will be characterized by distinct boundaries and underlying dysfunction. We do not believe that, as personality disorders are currently conceived, such a state of scientific credibility will be achieved and hence warrant the use of the terms "syndrome," "disorder," or "disease." Second, we attempt to delineate the nature of the neurobehavioral systems that we postulate underlie the four major traits of personality. In so doing, we hope to provide a substantive meaning to the four major personality traits that supersedes the extant variation in trait labels and psychological concepts.

The implications of defining personality traits in terms of neurobehavioral systems leads to a third aspect of the chapter, where we derive a model of personality disturbance based on the *interaction* of these neurobehavioral systems. Though genetically speaking it may be possible to conceive of the neurobiological variables associated with neurobehavioral systems as subject to independent influences, it is impossible to imagine that neurobehavioral systems are independent at a functional level. Similarly, it is impossible to imagine that personality traits can be associated in an independent manner with personality disorders. Neurobehavioral systems, and the personality traits that reflect their influence, interact to produce complex behavior patterns—personality as a whole—in a multivariate fashion. Therefore, our model of personality disturbance rests on a foundation of multivariate interaction of neurobehavioral systems. Such an interaction may yield a phenotypical clustering of behavioral signs or symptoms that could be taken to suggest a demarcation, perhaps indicative of latent threshold effects in the neurobehavioral systems, but the observed clustering represents the end product of underlying continuous dimensional neurobehavioral systems. Furthermore, while it is true that our model is dimensional in nature, where personality disturbance lies at the extreme of normal, interacting personality dimensions, it is worth noting that no assumption is made herein that phenotypical dimensions of personality are genetically continuous. The phenotypical continuity could well represent several underlying *distinct* genotypical distributions (Gottesman, 1997), as may be the case even within the normal range of variation of some personality traits (Benjamin et al., 1996; Ebstein et al., 1996).

NEUROBEHAVIORAL SYSTEMS
UNDERLYING HIGHER-ORDER PERSONALITY TRAITS

The higher-order structure of personality is converging on three to seven factors that account for the phenotypical variation in behavior (Digman, 1997; Tellegen & Waller, in press). Although there is considerable agreement on the robustness of at least four higher-order traits, there is nevertheless substantial variation in the definition of these traits because researchers emphasize different characteristics depending on their trait concepts. Our model focuses on four higher-order traits that are robustly identified in the psychometric literature, and which we define with reference to coherent neurobehavioral systems. Higher-order traits resembling *extraversion* and *neuroticism* (anxiety) are identified in virtually every taxonomy of personality. Affiliation, termed "agreeableness" (Costa & McCrae, 1992; Goldberg & Rosolack, 1994) or "social closeness" (Tellegen & Waller, in press), has emerged more recently as a robust trait and consists of affiliative tendencies, cooperativeness, and feelings of warmth and affection (Depue & Morrone-Strupinksy, in press). Finally, some form of impulsivity, more recently termed "constraint" (Tellegen & Waller, in press) or "conscientiousness" (due to an emphasis on the unreliability, unorderliness, and disorganization accompanying an impulsive disposition [Costa & McCrae, 1992; Goldberg & Rosolack, 1994]), frequently emerges in factor studies.

Agentic Extraversion and Affiliation

Trait Complexities Related to Interpersonal Behavior

Interpersonal behavior is not a unitary characteristic but rather has two major components. One component, *affiliation*, reflects enjoying and valuing close interpersonal bonds and being warm and affectionate; the other component, *agency*, reflects social dominance, assertiveness, exhibitionism, and a subjective sense of potency in accomplishing goals. These two components are consistent with the two independent major traits identified in the theory of interpersonal behavior: warm–agreeable vs. assured–dominant (Wiggins, 1991). Recent studies have consistently supported a two-component structure of interpersonal behavior in joint factor analyses of multidimensional personality questionnaires (Church, 1994; Church & Burke, 1994; Digman, 1997; Morrone, Depue, Scherer, & White, 2000;

Morrone-Strupinsky & Depue, 2004; Tellegen & Waller, in press), where two general traits were identified in each case as affiliation and agency (Depue & Collins, 1999). Lower-order traits of social dominance, achievement, endurance, persistence, efficacy, activity, and energy all loaded much more strongly on agency than on affiliation, whereas traits of sociability, warmth, and agreeableness showed a reverse pattern. Such findings have led trait psychologists to propose that affiliation and agency represent distinct dispositions (Depue & Collins, 1999; Depue & Morrone-Strupinsky, in press; Tellegen & Waller, in press): Whereas affiliation is clearly interpersonal in nature, agency represents a more general disposition that is manifest in a range of achievement-related, as well as interpersonal, contexts (Costa & McCrae, 1992; Goldberg & Rosolack, 1994; Tellegen & Waller, in press; Watson & Clark, 1997; Wiggins, 1991).

Association of Agentic Extraversion and Affiliation with Two Neurobehavioral Systems

Behavioral systems may be understood as behavior patterns that evolved to adapt to stimuli critical for survival and species preservation (Gray, 1973, 1992; MacLean, 1986; Schneirla, 1959). As opposed to specific behavioral systems that guide interaction with very specific stimulus contexts, *general* behavioral systems are more flexible and have less immediate objectives and more variable topographies (Blackburn, Phillips, Jakubovic, & Fibiger, 1989; MacLean, 1986). General systems are activated by broad *classes* of stimulus (Depue & Collins, 1999; Gray, 1973, 1992) and regulate general emotional–behavioral dispositions, such as desire–approach, fear–inhibition, or affiliative tendencies, that modulate goal-directed activity. It is the general systems that directly influence the structure of mammalian behavior at higher-order levels of organization, because, like higher-order personality traits, their pervasive modulatory effects on behavior derive from frequent activation by broad stimulus classes. *Thus, the higher-order traits of personality, which are general and few, most likely reflect the activity of the few, general neurobehavioral systems.*

We have suggested that the two traits of agentic extraversion and affiliation reflect the activity of two neurobehavioral systems involved in guiding behavior to *rewarding* goals (Depue & Collins, 1999; Depue & Morrone-Strupinsky, in press). Reward involves several dynamically interacting neurobehavioral processes occurring across two phases of goal acquisition: appetitive and consummatory. Although both phases are elicited by unconditioned incentive (reward-connoting) stimuli, their temporal onset, behavioral manifestations, and putative neural systems differ (Berridge, 1999; Blackburn et al., 1989; Depue & Collins, 1999; DiChiara

& North, 1992; Wyvell & Berridge, 2000) and are dissociated in factor-analytic studies based on behavioral characteristics of animals (Pfaus, Smith, & Coopersmith, 1999).

An appetitive, preparatory phase of goal acquisition represents the first step toward attaining biologically important goals (Blackburn et al., 1989; Hillard, Domjan, Nguyen, & Cusato, 1998). It is based on a mammalian behavioral system that is activated by, and serves to bring an animal in contact with, unconditioned and conditioned rewarding incentive stimuli (Depue & Collins, 1999; Gray, 1973; Schneirla, 1959). This system is consistently described in all animals across phylogeny (Schneirla, 1959), and we define this system as "behavioral approach based on incentive motivation" (Depue & Collins, 1999).

The nature of this behavioral system, as well as the system associated with a consummatory phase of reward (discussed next), can be most efficiently described by using an affiliative object (e.g., a potential mate) as the rewarding goal object. Thus, an affiliative goal is used throughout this and the next sections. In the appetitive phase of affiliation (see Figure 8.1), specific, *distal* affiliative stimuli of potential bonding partners (e.g., facial features and smiles, friendly vocalizations and gestures, and bodily features [Porges, 1998]) serve as unconditioned incentive stimuli based on their distinct patterns of sensory properties, such as smell, color, shape, and temperature (DiChiara & North, 1992; Hilliard et al., 1998). For instance, Breiter, Aharon, Kahneman, Dale, and Shizgal (2001) and Aharon et al. (2001) have shown that even passive viewing of attractive female faces unconditionally activates the anatomical areas that integrate reward, incentive motivation, and approach behavior in heterosexual males. These incentives are inherently evaluated as positive in valence and activate incentive motivation, increased energy through sympathetic nervous system activity, and forward locomotion as a means of bringing individuals into close proximity (DiChiara & North, 1992). Moreover, the incentive state is inherently rewarding but in a highly activated manner, and animals will work intensively to obtain that reward without evidence of satiety (Depue & Collins, 1999).

In humans, the incentive state is associated with subjective feelings of desire, wanting, excitement, elation, enthusiasm, energy, potency, and self-efficacy that are distinct from, but typically co-occur with, feelings of pleasure and liking (Berridge, 1999; Watson & Tellegen, 1985). This subjective experience is concordant with the nature of the lower-order traits of social dominance, achievement, endurance, persistence, efficacy, activity, and energy that all load strongly on the *agency* personality factor (see earlier), and with the adjectives that define the subjective *state* of positive affect that is so closely associated with agentic extraversion (activated, peppy, strong,

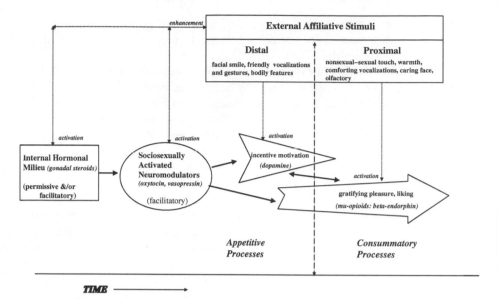

FIGURE 8.1. The development and maintenance of affiliative bonds across two phases of reward. Distal affiliative stimuli elicit an incentive-motivated approach to an affiliative goal, accompanied by strong emotional–motivational feelings of wanting, desire, and positive activation. The approach phase not only ensures sociosexual interaction with an affiliative object but also acquisition of a memory ensemble or network of the context in which approach, reward, and goal acquisition occur. Next, proximal affiliative stimuli emanating from interaction with the affiliative object elicit strong feelings of consummatory reward, liking, and physiological quiescence, all of which become associated with these stimuli as well as the context predictive of reward. As discussed below, dopamine encodes the incentive salience of contextual stimuli predictive of reward during the approach phase and, in collaboration with μ-opiate mediated consummatory reward, encodes the incentive salience of proximal stimuli directly linked to the affiliative object. The end result of this sequence of processes is an incentive-encoded affiliative memory network that continues to motivate approach toward and interaction with the affiliative object. Specialized processes ensure that affiliative stimuli are weighted as significant elements in the contextual ensembles representing affiliative memory networks. These specialized processes include the construction of a contextual ensemble via affiliative stimulus-induced opiate potentiation of dopamine processes, and the influence of permissive and/or facilitatory factors such as gonadal steroids, oxytocin, and vasopressin on (1) sensory, perceptual, and attentional processing of affiliative stimuli and (2) formation of social memories. See Depue and Morrone-Strupinsky (in press) for details.

enthused, energetic; Watson & Tellegen, 1985). Therefore, we have proposed that agentic extraversion reflects the activity of a behavioral approach system based on *positive incentive motivation.*

When close proximity to a rewarding goal is achieved, incentive–motivational approach gives way to a consummatory phase of goal acquisition (Herbert, 1993). In this phase, specific *interoceptive* and *proximal exteroceptive* stimuli related to critical primary biological aims elicit behavioral patterns that are relatively specific to those conditions (e.g., sexual, social, or food-related) (Blackburn et al., 1989; Hilliard et al., 1998; MacLean, 1986; Timberlake & Silva, 1995). Performance of these behavioral patterns is inherently rewarding (Berridge, 1999). In the case of potential mate acquisition, examples of affiliative behavioral patterns are courtship, gentle stroking and grooming, mating, and certain maternal patterns such as breastfeeding, all of which may include facial, caressive tactile, gestural, and certain vocal behaviors (Polan & Hofer, 1998). Tactile stimulation may be particularly effective in activating affiliative reward processes in animals and humans (Fleming, Korsmit, & Deller, 1994). Significantly, light, pleasant touch, that occurs to caress-like, skin-to-skin contact between individuals is transmitted by different afferents than hard or unpleasant touch (Olausson et al., 2002): light, pleasant touch is transmitted by slow-conducting unmyelinated afferents which project to the insular cortex but not to somatosensory areas S1 and S2, whereas hard, unpleasant touch is transmitted by fast-conducting myelinated afferents to S1 and S2 (anterior parietal). The insular cortex is a paralimbic region known to integrate several sensory modalities, including autonomic, gustatory, visual, auditory, and somatosensory, in order to characterize the emotional nature of sensory input (Damasio, 2003; Mesulam, 1990).

As opposed to an incentive motivational state of activation, desire, and wanting, the expression of *consummatory* behavioral patterns elicits intense feelings of pleasure, gratification, and liking, plus physiological quiescence characterized by rest, sedation, anabolism, and parasympathetic nervous system activity, thereby reinforcing the production and repetition of those behaviors (Berridge, 1999; DiChiara & North, 1992; Porges, 1998, 2001). Thus, whereas appetitive approach processes bring an individual into contact with unconditioned incentive stimuli, consummatory processes bring behavior to a gratifying conclusion (Hilliard et al., 1998). Whether the pleasurable state generated in affiliative interactions shares a common neurobiology with the pleasure generated by other consummatory behaviors (e.g., feeding) is not certain but is assumed by some to be so (DiChiara & North, 1992; Panksepp, 1998).

The core content of affiliation scales seems to reflect the operation of neurobehavioral processes that (1) create a warm, affectionate, gratifying subjective emotional state elicited by others, which (2) motivate close interpersonal behavior. Our hypothesis is that the subjective experience of warmth and affection reflects the *capacity to experience consummatory reward that is elicited by a broad array of affiliative stimuli* (Depue & Morrone-Strupinsky, in press). This capacity is viewed as providing the key element used in additional psychobiological processes that permit the development and maintenance of longer-term affective bonds—defined as long-term selective social attachments observed most intensely between infants and parents and between adult mates, and that are characteristic of social organization in human and other primate societies (Gingrich, Liu, Cascio, Wang, & Insel, 2000; Wang et al., 1999). It is important to emphasize that a core capacity for affiliative reward and bonding is not viewed as a sufficient determinant of close social relationships, only as a necessary one, a *sine qua non*. Such affiliative reward is hypothesized to underlie all human social relationships having a positive affective component. Other interpersonal constructs of sociability, attachment, and separation anxiety are accordingly viewed as either broader than affiliation as defined here and/or as based on different neurobehavioral systems (see Depue & Morrone-Strupinsky, in press, for a full discussion).

Through Pavlovian associative learning, the experience of reward generated throughout appetitive and consummatory phases is associated with previously affectively neutral stimulus contexts (objects, acts, events, places) in which pleasure occurred, thereby forming conditioned incentive stimuli that are predictive of reward and that have gained the capacity to elicit anticipatory pleasure and incentive motivation (Berridge, 1999; Ostrowski, 1998; Timberlake & Silva, 1995). Because of the predominance of symbolic (conditioned) processes in guiding human behavior in the absence of unconditioned stimuli, conditioned incentives are likely to be particularly important elicitors of *enduring* reward processes (Fowles, 1987). Thus, the acquisition and maintenance of a mate relationship, for example, depends closely on Pavlovian associative learning that links the experience of reward with (1) the salient contextual cues that predict reward during the appetitive phase (e.g., features of a laboratory cage), and (2) a mate's individualistic cues associated directly with consummatory reward (e.g., individual characteristics of a sexually receptive female rate) (Domjan, Cusato, & Villarreal, 2000). Taken together, the foregoing processes support acquisition of affiliative memories, where contextual ensembles are formed and weighted in association with the reward provided by interaction with the potential mate.

Neurobiology of Incentive Motivation and Affiliative Reward

By drawing an association between traits and behavioral systems (i.e., agentic extraversion and incentive motivation and affiliation and affiliative reward), we are able to use the behavioral neurobiology animal literature to discern the neurobiology associated with these behavioral systems and, by analogy, with the personality traits of agentic extraversion and affiliation. As reviewed recently (Depue & Collins, 1999), animal research demonstrates that the positive incentive motivation and experience of reward that underlies a behavioral system of approach is dependent on the functional properties of the midbrain ventral tegmental area (VTA) dopamine (DA) projection system. DA agonists or antagonists in the VTA or nucleus accumbens (NAS), which is a major terminal area of VTA DA projections, in rats and monkeys facilitate or markedly impair, respectively, a broad array of incentive motivated behaviors. Furthermore, dose-dependent DA receptor activation in the VTA–NAS pathway facilitates the acute rewarding effects of stimulants, and the NAS is a particularly strong site for intracranial self-administration of DA agonists (Le Moal & Simon, 1991; Pich et al., 1997). DA agonists injected in the NAS also modulate behavioral responses to *conditioned* incentive stimuli in a dose-dependent fashion (Cador, Taylor, & Robbins, 1991; Robbins, Cador, Taylor, & Everitt, 1989; Wolterink, Cador, Wolterink, Robbins, & Everitt, 1989). In single-unit recording studies, VTA DA neurons are activated preferentially by appetitive incentive stimuli (Schultz, Dayan, & Montague, 1997). DA cells, most numerously in the VTA, respond vigorously to and in proportion to the magnitude of both conditioned and unconditioned incentive stimuli and in anticipation of reward (Schultz et al., 1997).

Finally, incentive motivation is associated in humans with both positive *emotional* feelings such as elation and euphoria and *motivational* feelings of desire, wanting, craving, potency, and self-efficacy. In humans, DA-activating psychostimulant drugs induce both sets of feelings (Drevets et al., 2001). Also, neuroimaging studies of cocaine addicts found that during acute administration the intensity of a subject's subjective euphoria increased in a dose-dependent manner in proportion to cocaine binding to the DA uptake transporter (and hence to DA levels) in the striatum (Volkow et al., 1997). Moreover, cocaine-induced activity in the NAS was linked equally strongly (if not more strongly) to motivational feelings of desire, wanting, and craving, as to the emotional experience of euphoric rush (Breiter et al., 1997). And the degree of amphetamine-induced DA release in healthy human ventral striatum assessed by positron emission tomography (PET) was correlated strongly with feelings of euphoria (Drevets et al., 2001). Hence, taken together, the animal and human evidence demonstrates that the VTA DA–NAS pathway is a primary neural circuit for incentive motivation and its accompanying subjective state of reward.

With respect to consummatory reward and affiliative behavior, a broad range of evidence suggests a role for endogenous opiates. Endogenous opiate release or receptor binding is increased in rats, monkeys, and humans by lactation and nursing, sexual activity, vaginocervical stimulation, maternal social interaction, brief social isolation, and grooming and other nonsexual tactile stimulation (Depue & Morrone-Strupinsky, in press; Keverne, 1996; Silk, Alberts, & Altmann, 2003). Opiate receptor (OR) antagonists naltrexone or naloxone in small doses apparently reduce the reward derived from social interactions because they enhance attempts to obtain such reward, manifested as increases in (1) the amount of maternal contact by young monkeys, and (2) solicitations for grooming and frequency of being groomed in mature female monkeys, which has been associated with increased cerebrospinal fluid levels of beta-endorphin (Graves, Wallen, & Maestripieri, 2002; Martel, Nerison, Simpson, & Keverne, 1995). In addition, the endogenous opiate beta-endorphin stimulates play behavior and grooming in juvenile rats, whereas naltrexone leads to reduced grooming of infants and other group members in monkeys and rats, and to maternal neglect in monkeys and sheep that is similar to the neglect shown by human mothers who abuse opiates (Keverne, 1996; Martel et al., 1995). Similarly, human females administered the opiate antagonist naltrexone showed an increased amount of time spent alone, a reduced amount of time spent with friends, and a reduced frequency and pleasantness of their social interactions relative to placebo. Such findings suggest that opiates provide a critical part of the neural basis on which primate sociality has evolved (Nelson & Panksepp, 1998). Particularly important is the relation between μ-opiates and grooming, because the primary function of primate grooming may well be to establish and maintain social bonds (Matheson & Bernstein, 2000).

Perhaps most relevant to affiliative reward is the mu (μ)OR OR family, which is the main site of exogenously administered opiate drugs (e.g., morphine) and of endogenous endorphins (particularly, beta-endorphin) (La Buda, Sora, Uhl, & Fuchs, 2000; Schlaepfer et al., 1998; Shippenberg & Elmer, 1998; Stefano et al., 2000; Wiedenmayer & Barr, 2000). μORs also appear to be the main site for the effects of endogenous beta-endorphins and endogenous morphine on the subjective feelings in humans of *increased* interpersonal warmth, euphoria, well-being, and peaceful calmness, as well as of *decreased* elation, energy, and incentive motivation (Schlaepfer et al., 1998; Shippenberg & Elmer, 1998; Stefano et al., 2000; Uhl, Sora, & Wang, 1999).

The facilitatory effects of opiates on affiliative behavior are thought to be exerted by fibers that arise mainly from the hypothalamic arcuate nucleus and terminate in brain regions that typically express μORs. μORs may facilitate the rewarding effects associated with many motivated behaviors (Nelson & Panksepp, 1998; Niesink, Vanderschuen, & van Ree, 1996; Olive, Koenig, Nannini, & Hodges, 2001; Olson, Olson, & Kastin, 1997;

Stefano et al., 2000; Strand, 1999). For instance, whereas DA antagonists block appetitive behaviors in pursuit of reward but not the acutal consumption of reward (e.g., sucrose; Ikemoto & Panksepp, 1996), μOR-antagonists block rewarding effects of sucrose and sexual behavior, and in neonatal rats persistently impair the response to the inherently rewarding properties of novel stimulation (Herz, 1998). Rewarding properties of μOR-agonists are directly indicated by the fact that animals will work for the prototypical μ-agonists morphine and heroin, and that they are dose-dependently self-administered in animals and humans (Di Chiara, 1995; Nelson & Panksepp, 1998; Olson et al., 1997; Shippenberg & Elmer, 1998). There is a significant correlation between an agonist's affinity at the μOR and the dose that maintains maximal rates of drug self-administration behavior (Shippenberg & Elmer, 1998).

The rewarding effect of opiates may be especially mediated by μORs located in the NAS and VTA, both of which support self-administration of μOR-agonists that is attenuated by intracranially administered μOR-antagonists (David & Cazala, 2000; Herz, 1998; Schlaepfer et al., 1998; Shippenberg & Elmer, 1998). When opiate and DA specific antagonists were given prior to cocaine or heroin self-administration, the opiate antagonist selectively altered opiate self-administration, while DA antagonists selectively altered the response to the DA agonist cocaine (Shippenberg & Elmer, 1998). Destruction of DA terminals in the NAS also showed that opiate self-administration is independent of DA function, at least at the level of the NAS (Dworkin, Guerin, Goeders, & Smith, 1988). Furthermore, NAS DA functioning was specifically related to the incentive salience of reward cues but was unrelated to the hedonic state generated by consuming the rewards (Wyvell & Berridge, 2000). *Thus, DA and opiates appear to functionally interact in the NAS, but they apparently provide independent contributions to rewarding effects.* This appears to be particularly the case for the *acute* rewarding effects of opiates, which are thought to occur through a DA-independent system that is mediated through brainstem reward circuits, including the tegmental pedunculopontine nucleus (Laviolette, Gallegos, Henriksen, & van der Kogg, 2004).

Rewarding effects of opiates are also directly indicated by the fact that a range of μOR-agonists, when injected intracerebroventricularly or directly into the NAS, serve as unconditioned rewarding stimuli in a dose-dependent manner in producing a conditioned place preference, a behavioral measure of reward (Narita, Aoki, & Suzuki, 2000; Nelson & Panksepp, 1998; Shippenberg & Elmer, 1998). VTA-localized μORs particularly in the rostral zone of the VTA (Carlezon et al., 2000) mediate (1) rewarding effects such as self-administration behavior and conditioned place preference (Carlezon et al., 2000; Shippenberg & Elmer, 1998; Wise, 1998), (2) increased sexual activity and maternal behaviors (Callahan, Baumann, &

Rail, 1996; Leyton & Stewart, 1992; van Furth & van Ree, 1996), and (3) the persistently increased play behavior, social grooming, and social approach of rats subjected to morphine *in utero* (Hol, Niesink, van Ree, & Spruijt, 1996). Indeed, microinjections of morphine or a selective μOR-agonist into the VTA produced marked place preferences, whereas selective antagonism of μORs prevented morphine-induced conditioned place preference (Olmstead & Franklin, 1997). Indeed, transgenic mice lacking the μOR gene show no morphine-induced place preferences or physical dependence from morphine consumption, whereas morphine induces both of these behaviors in wild-type mice (Matthes et al., 1996; Simonin et al., 1998). Most importantly, such mice also fail to develop an affiliative bond to their mothers (Moles, Kieffer, & D'Amato, 2004). And, significantly, opiate but not oxytocin antagonists block the development of partner preference that is induced specifically by *repeated* exposure and *repeated* sexual activity in rodents (Carter, Lederhendler, & Kirkpatrick, 1997).

An *interaction* of DA and μ-opiates in the experience of reward throughout appetitive and consummatory phases of *affiliative* engagement appears to involve two processes: During the anticipatory phase of goal acquisition, μOR activation in the VTA can increase DA release in the NAS and hence the experience of reward (Marinelli & White, 2000). Subsequently, the firing rate of VTA neurons decreases following delivery and consumption of appetitive reinforcers (e.g., food, sex, and liquid) (Schultz et al., 1997). At the same time, μOR activation in the NAS (perhaps by opiate release from higher-threshold NAS terminals that colocalize DA and opiates [Le Moal & Simon, 1991]) decreases NAS DA release, creating an opiate-mediated experience of reward associated with consummation that is independent of DA. Thus, in contrast to the incentive motivational effects of DA during the anticipation of reward, opiates may subsequently induce calm pleasure and bring consummatory behavior to a gratifying conclusion. This may explain the fact that higher doses of μOR-agonists administered into the NAS can block the self-administration of certain psychostimulant drugs of abuse in animals and reduce appetitive behaviors (Hyztia & Kiiannaa, 2001; Johnson & Ait-Daoud, 2000; Kranzler, 2000).

In sum, as illustrated in Figure 8.1, distal affiliative cues (e.g., friendly smiles and gestures and sexual features) serve as incentive stimuli that activate DA-facilitated incentive-reward motivation, desire, wanting, and approach to affiliative objects. As these objects are reached, more proximal affiliative stimuli (e.g., pleasant touch) strongly activate μ-opiate release which promotes an intense state of pleasant reward, warmth, affection, and physiological quiescence and brings approach behavior to a gratifying conclusion. Throughout this entire sequence of goal acquisition, the contextual cues associated with approach to the goal, and the cues specifically related to the goal, are all associated with the experience of reward. It is beyond the scope of this chapter, but it is worth noting that DA and μ-opiates play a critical role in strengthening the association between these contextual cues and reward (Depue & Morrone-Strupinsky, in press). Thus, these two neuromodulators are critical to establishing our preferences and memories for particular contexts and affiliative cues predictive of reward.

Individual Differences in DA–Incentive and μOR–Reward Processes

Individual differences in agentic extraversion and affiliation are subject to strong genetic influence (Tellegen et al., 1988). If personality disturbance occurs in the region located at the extreme tails of individual difference distributions in the traits of agentic extraversion and affiliation, it is important to show that the neuromodulators associated with incentive motivation and affiliative reward are sources of individual differences in these behavioral systems. Animal research demonstrates that individual differences in DA functioning contribute significantly to variation in incentive-motivated behavior, as does much human work (Depue & Collins, 1999; Depue, Luciana, Arbisi, Collins, & Leon, 1994). Inbred mouse and rat strains with variation in the number of neurons in the VTA DA cell group or in several indicators of enhanced DA transmission show marked differences in behaviors dependent on DA transmission in the VTA–NAS pathway, including levels of spontaneous exploratory activity and DA agonist-induced locomotor activity, and increased acquisition of self-administration of psychostimulants (Depue & Collins, 1999).

Similar findings for μ-opiates exist (Depue & Morrone-Strupinsky, in press). Individual differences in humans and rodents have been demonstrated in levels of μOR expression and binding that are associated with a preference for μOR-agonists such as morphine (Uhl et al., 1999; Zubieta et al., 2001). In humans, individual differences in central nervous system μOR densities show a range of up to 75% between lower and upper thirds of the distribution (Uhl et al., 1999), differences that appear to be related to variation in the rewarding effects of alcohol in humans and rodents (Berrettini, Hoehe, Ferraro, DeMaria, & Gottheil, 1997; Olson et al., 1997).

Differences of this magnitude in the *expressive* properties of the μOR gene could contribute substantially to individual variation in μOR-induced *behavioral* expression via an effect on beta-endorphin functional potency. For instance, one source of this individual variation is different single nucleotide polymorphisms (SNPs) in the μOR gene, OPRM1 (Berrettini et al., 1997; Bond et al., 1998; Gelernter, Kranzler, & Cubells, 1999). The most prevalent of these is A118G, which is characterized by a substitution of the amino acid Asn by Asp at codon 40, with an allelic frequency of 10% in a mixed sample of former heroin abusers and normal controls

(Bond et al., 1998). Although this SNP did not bind all opiate peptides more strongly than other SNPs or the normal nucleotide sequence, it did bind beta-endorphin three times more tightly than the most common allelic form of the receptor (Bond et al., 1998). Furthermore, beta-endorphin is three times more effective in agonist-induced activation of G-protein-coupled potassium channels at the A118G variant receptor compared to the most common allelic form (Bond et al., 1998).

Genetic variation in μOR properties is related to response to rewarding drugs, such as morphine, alcohol, and cocaine, and to opiate self-administration behavior in animals (Berrettini et al., 1997). For instance, when transgenic insertion was used to increase μOR density specifically in mesolimbic areas thought to mediate substance abuse via VTA DA neurons, transgenic mice showed increased self-administration of morphine compared to wild-type mice, even when the amount of behavior required to maintain drug intake increased tenfold (Elmer, Pieper, Goldberg, & George, 1995). Thus, the efficacy of morphine as a reinforcer was substantially enhanced in transgenic mice. Conversely, μOR knockout mice do not develop conditioned place preference and physical dependence on morphine, whereas morphine induces both of these behaviors in wild-type mice (Matthes et al., 1996).

Taken together, these studies suggest that genetic variation in DA and μOR properties in humans and rodents is (1) substantial, (2) an essential element in the variation in the rewarding value of DA and opiate agonists, and (3) critical in accounting for variation in the Pavlovian learning that underlies the association between contextual cues and reward, as occurs in partner and place preferences (Elmer et al., 1995; Matthes et al., 1996).

Anxiety or Neuroticism

Anxiety and Fear as Two Distinct Behavioral Systems

Adaptation to aversive environmental conditions is crucial for species survival, and at least two distinct behavioral systems have evolved to promote such adaptation. One system is fear (often labeled "harm avoidance" in the trait literature, but this is different than Cloninger, Svrakic, and Przybeck's, 1993, harm avoidance, which actually assesses anxiety), which is a very specific behavioral system that evolved as a means of escaping unconditioned aversive stimuli that are inherently dangerous to survival, such as tactile pain, injury contexts, snakes, spiders, heights, approaching strangers, and sudden sounds. These stimuli are specific, discrete, and explicit, and in turn elicit specific, short-latency, high-magnitude phasic responses of autonomic arousal, subjective feelings of panic, and behavioral escape. Specific, discrete neutral stimuli associated with these unconditioned events elicit conditioned fear. Such conditioned stimuli (CSs) elicit a different behavioral profile than unconditioned stimuli (UCSs) in that freezing and suppression of operant behavior (i.e., behavioral inhibition), as opposed to active escape, characterize the former, though both response systems involve autonomic arousal, pain inhibition, and reflex potentiation.

There are, however, many aversive circumstances that do not involve specific, discrete, explicit stimuli that evolutionarily have been neurobiologically linked to subjective fear and escape. That is, there are many situations in which specific aversive cues do not exist, but rather the stimulus conditions are associated with an elevated *potential* risk of danger or aversive consequences. In such cases, no explicit aversive stimuli are present to inherently activate escape circuitries. Nevertheless, the stimuli can be unconditioned in nature, as in darkness, open spaces, unfamiliarity, and predator odors, or they can be conditioned contextual cues (general textures, colors, relative spatial locations, sounds) that have been associated with previous exposure to specific aversive stimuli (Davis, Walker, & Lee, 1997; Davis & Shi, 1999; Fendt, Endres, & Apfelback, 2003). Conceptually, these stimuli are characterized in common by unpredictability and uncontrollability—or, more simply, uncertainty.

To reduce the risk of danger in such circumstances, a second behavioral system evolved, *anxiety*. Anxiety is characterized by negative emotion or affect (anxiety, depression, hostility, suspiciousness, distress) that serves the purpose of informing the individual that although no explicit, specific aversive stimuli are present, conditions are potentially threatening (White & Depue, 1999). This affective state, and the physiological arousal that accompanies it, continues or reverberates until the uncertainty is resolved. Associated responses, which may functionally help to resolve the uncertainty, are heightened attentional scanning of the uncertain environment and cognitive worrying and rumination over possible response–outcome scenarios. An important point is that no specific motor response is linked to anxiety, because no motor response is specified under stimulus conditions of uncertainty. Caution and locomotor modulation are necessary, but behavioral inhibition will not allow the individual to explore the environment to discover if danger is indeed lurking. An example is a deer entering an open meadow: Caution, slow approach, heightened attentional scanning, and enhanced cognitive activity are optimal, not freezing. This is in direct contradiction to Gray's (1973) theory that the best marker for anxiety is behavioral inhibition; rather, CS fear is associated with such inhibition. Thus, Davis et al. (1997) and Barlow (2002) suggest that the stimulus conditions and behavioral characteristics of fear and anxiety are different, although a similar state of intense autonomic arousal is associated with both emotional states, rendering them similar at the subjective level. The prolonged negative subjective state of anxiety, however, distinguishes its subjective state from the rapid, brief state of panic associated with the presence of a specific fear stimulus.

There is another important difference between fear and anxiety at the trait level of analysis. In personality inventories, fear typically is represented as a primary or facet level scale, not a higher-order factor (Tellegen & Waller, in press). Fear usually also is associated with a higher-order trait of constraint. In contrast, anxiety, which is typically referred to as neuroticism, is one of the most reliably identified higher-order traits and does not load highly on a constraint higher-order factor. This higher-order nature of anxiety but not fear is related to the fact that, just like agentic extraversion, the eliciting stimuli for anxiety occur frequently in a civilized society, whereas the specific stimuli that elicit fear do not. This means that anxiety represents a general behavioral system that is activated by a broad *class* of stimulus, whereas fear represents a more specific behavioral system that evolved to respond to specific stimuli critical for survival.

The trait literature supports the *independence* of anxiety and fear, which as personality traits are subject to distinct sources of genetic variation (Tellegen et al., 1988). As the averaged correlations derived from numerous studies in Tables 8.1, 8.2, and 8.3 show, the relation between neuroticism (anxiety) and harm avoidance (fear) is essentially zero (White & Depue, 1999). As shown in Tables 8.2 and 8.3, the magnitude of emotional distress and autonomic arousal elicited by discrete stimuli associated with physical harm (Table 8.2) is significantly related to harm avoidance but not neuroticism, whereas conditions of uncertainty associated with external evaluations of the self (Table 8.3) are significantly related to neuroticism but not harm avoidance (White & Depue, 1999). Furthermore, Table 8.2 shows that in contrast to Gray's (1973, 1992) and Cloninger's (Cloninger et al., 1993) theoretical position that anxiety is associated with behavioral inhibition, it is harm avoidance rather than neuroticism that

TABLE 8.1 Correlation between Trait Measures of Fear and Anxiety

Fear	Anxiety		
	Tellegen NEM	Eysenck N	STAI
Tellegen Harm Avoidance	−.03	−.02	
Jackson Harm Avoidance			.05
Lykken Physical Activity		−.01	.05
Hodges Physical Danger			.02
Zuckerman SSS (reversed)	.08	.04	

Note. From Depue and Lenzenweger (2001). Copyright 2001 by The Guilford Press. Reprinted by permission.

TABLE 8.2. Correlation of Emotional Distress, Behavioral Inhibition, and Heart Rate and Electrodermal Responses to Aversive Stimuli with Trait Measures of Fear and Anxiety

| | Emotional distress | | | | Behavioral inhibition | | | | Threatened shock | | |
| | | | | | | | | | | Electrodermal | |
Trait	Heights	Rat	Snake	Shock	Heights	Rat	Snake	Cockroach	Heart rate	Specific	Nonspecific
Fear	.43	.54	.62	.64	.44	.35	.51	.46	.48	.43	.53
Anxiety	.17	.20	.14	.04	.15		.07		.09	.14	.17

Note. From Depue and Lenzenweger (2001). Copyright 2001 by The Guilford Press. Reprinted by permission.

409

TABLE 8.3. Correlation of Emotional Distress to Contexts Associated with Threats to the Self with Trait Measures of Fear and Anxiety

Trait	Emotional distress			
	Exam	Intelligence test	Public speaking	Failure feedback
Fear	.11	.09	.05	.08
Anxiety	.48	.47	.57	.52

Note. From Depue and Lenzenweger (2001). Copyright 2001 by The Guilford Press. Reprinted by permission.

correlates significantly with indices of behavioral inhibition in contexts of physical danger. Indeed, one of the most reliable indices of conditioned fear in animals is behavioral inhibition (Davis et al., 1997; Le Doux, 1998; Panksepp, 1998), which is not the case for stimulus-induced anxiety (Davis et al., 1997). Thus, these various findings suggest that anxiety and fear are distinctly different traits, and analysis of clinical anxiety disorders reached equivalent conclusions (Barlow, 2002).

Neurobiology of Anxiety

The psychometric independence of fear and anxiety is mirrored in their dissociable neuroanatomy. Species-specific UCSs having an evolutionary history of danger elicit fear and defensive motor escape, facial and vocal signs, autonomic activation, and antinociception specifically from the lateral longitudinal cell column in the midbrain periaquiductal gray (PAG; see Figure 8.2) (Bandler & Keay, 1996). In turn, PAG efferents converge on the ventromedial and rostral ventrolateral regions of the medulla, where somatic–motor and autonomic information, respectively, is integrated and transmitted to the spinal cord (Guyenet et al., 1996; Holstege, 1996). Although these processes can occur without cortex (Panksepp, 1998), association of discrete, explicit neutral stimuli (fear CS) with a UCS and primary negative reinforcement occurs via cortical uni- and polymodal sensory efferents that converge on the basolateral complex of the amygdala (although crude representations of external stimuli can rapidly reach the basolateral amygdala subcortically from the thalamus) (Aggleton, 1992; Davis et al., 1997; LeDoux, 1998). Fear CSs elicit a host of behavioral, neuropeptide, and autonomic responses via output from the basolateral amygdala to the central amygdala, which in turn sends functionally *separable* efferents to many hypothalamic and brainstem targets (Aggleton, 1992; LeDoux, Cicchetti, Xagoraris, & Romanski, 1990). In the case of fear CS, as noted previously, the motor response is not escape but rather freezing or *behavioral inhibi-*

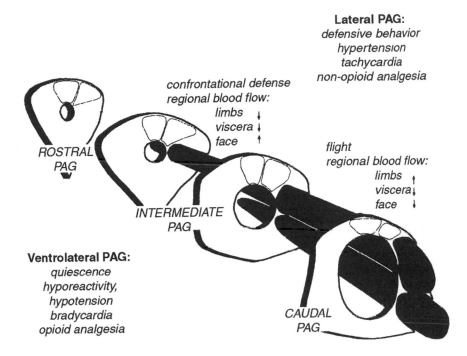

Lateral PAG:
defensive behavior
hypertension
tachycardia
non-opioid analgesia

confrontational defense
regional blood flow:
limbs ↓
viscera ↓
face ↑

flight
regional blood flow:
limbs ↑
viscera ↓
face ↓

ROSTRAL
PAG

INTERMEDIATE
PAG

Ventrolateral PAG:
quiescence
hyporeactivity,
hypotension
bradycardia
opioid analgesia

CAUDAL
PAG

FIGURE 8.2. Schematic illustration of the lateral and ventrolateral neuronal columns within (from left to right) the rostral midbrain periacquiductal gray (PAG), the intermediate PAG (two sections) and the caudal PAG. Injections of excitatory amino acids (EAA) within the lateral and ventrolateral PAG column evoke fundamentally opposite alterations in sensory responsiveness, and somatic and autonomic adjustments. EAA injections made within the intermediate, lateral PAG evoke a confrontational defensive reaction, tachycardia, and hypertension associated with decreased blood flow to limbs and viscera and increased blood flow to extracranial vascular beds. EAA injections make within the caudal, lateral PAG evoke flight, tachycardia and hypertension associated with decreased blood flow to visceral and extracranial vascular beds and increased blood flow to limbs. In contrast, EAA injections made within the ventrolateral PAG evoke cessation of all spontanious activity (i.e., quiescence), a decreased responsiveness to the environment, hypotension and bradycardia. The lateral and ventrolateral PAG also mediate different types of analgesia. Adapted from Bandler and Keay (1996). Copyright 1996 by Elsevier Science. Adapted by permission.

tion, which involves activation of the caudal ventrolateral cell column of the PAG shown in Figure 8.2 (LeDoux, 1998).

The neuroanatomic distinction between fear and anxiety has been delineated by use of the fear-potentiated auditory-induced startle paradigm. In this paradigm, an established, explicit light CS activates a cell assembly representing the association between CS, UCS (e.g., shock), and tactile pain located in the basolateral amygdala. Excitation of this assembly by the CS activates efferents to the central amygdala, which in turn monosynaptically potentiates startle reflex circuitry in the reticular nucleus of the caudal pons that is activated simultaneously by, for example, a loud, sudden noise. This potentiation of the startle reflex by a fear CS is *phasic* in nature, occurring almost immediately after light onset but returning to baseline amplitude shortly after light offset (Davis et al., 1997). Lesions of the central amygdala reliably block explicit fear CS-potentiated startle and behavioral inhibition. In contrast, nondiscrete, contextually related aversive stimulation (e.g., prolonged *bright light* in an *unfamiliar* environment, which are aversive UCS's for nocturnal rats) elicits robust startle potentiation that endures *tonically* as long as the aversive conditions are present, even when the central amygdala is lesioned. These findings suggest that these types of stimulus conditions, which are typically associated with the elicitation of anxiety, rely on a different neuroanatomical foundation in generating an enduring potentiation of the startle reflex (Davis et al., 1997).

The enduring potentiating effects of nondiscrete, contextually related aversive stimuli on the startle reflex is dependent on a group of structures collectively referred to as the *extended amygdala*, which receives massive projections from basolateral and olfactory amygdala complexes, and which represents a macrostructure that is characterized by two divisions, central and medial (Heimer, 2003; McGinty, 1999). As shown in Figure 8.3, these two divisions originate from the central and medial nuclei of the amygdala and consist of cell groups that are distributed throughout the sublenticular area, bed nucleus of the stria terminalis (BNST), around striatal and pallidal structures, and back to merge specifically with the caudomedial region of the NAS. Contextual stimuli are conveyed to the BNST and other central extended amygdala regions via perirhinal + basolateral amygdala (e.g., bright light) and parahippocampal + entorhinal + hippocampal (contextual stimuli) glutamatergic efferents (Annett, McGregor, & Robins, 1989; Bechara et al., 1995; Everitt & Robbins, 1992; Gaffan, 1992; Heimer, 2003; LeDoux, 1998; Selden, Everitts, Jarrard, & Robbins, 1991; Sutherland & McDonald, 1990). Viewing the sublenticular area and lateral BNST as a foundation for anxiety processes is supported in part by the fact that, in contrast to the central amygdala, (1) neurons in the sublenticular area show maximal prolonged responsiveness specifically to unfamiliar stimuli (Rolls, 1999), and (2) electrical stimulation or lesions of the BNST

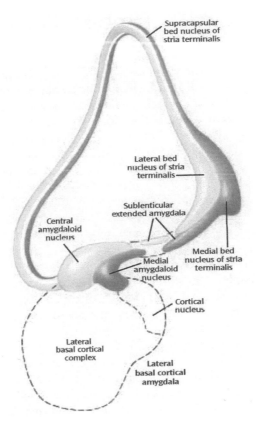

FIGURE 8.3. The central and medial divisions of the extended amygdala, shown in isolation from the rest of the brain. From Heimer (2003). Copyright 2003 by American Psychiatric Association. Reprinted by permission.

did not initiate or block, respectively, the behavioral inhibition elicited by an explicit fear CS (LeDoux et al., 1990), which mirrors the lack of association of behavioral inhibition with trait anxiety discussed earlier.

Similar to the outputs from the central nucleus of the amygdala, most structures of the central division of the extended amygdala can transmit this motivationally relevant information to some or all hypothalamic and brainstem structures related to emotional expression (Heimer, 2003; Holstege, 1996). Whereas the basolateral complex of the amygdala is involved in pairing positive and negative reinforcement with stimuli that are discrete and explicit and that have been analyzed for their specific characteristics, at least the central division of the extended amygdala appears to associate *general contextual features and nonexplicit, nondiscrete* conditioned and unconditioned stimuli with reinforcement (e.g., light conditions, physical features, and spatial relations) (Davis et al., 1997; Davis & Shi, 1999; McDonald, Shammah-Iagnado, Shi, & Davis, 1999). Thus, two emotional learning systems may have evolved: the basolateral amygdala to associate reinforcement with explicit, specific characteristics of objects (i.e., for fear), and the BNST to associate reinforcement with nonexplicit spatial and contextual stimulus aspects (i.e., for anxiety).

A major finding of importance in understanding the association between anxiety and the central extended amygdala is that injection of corticotropin-releasing hormone (CRH) into the BNST potentiates startle in a dose-dependent manner for up to 2 hours' duration (Davis et al., 1997). It is not surprising then that lesions of the BNST, or injection of a CRH antagonist in the BNST, significantly attenuate both bright light- or CRH-enhanced startle without having any effect on discrete fear CS-potentiated startle (Davis et al., 1997). In contrast, lesions of the central amygdala eliminate the discrete fear CS-potentiated startle but have no effect on CRH-enhanced startle. Prolonged bright light-induced startle potentiation is also blocked by (1) lesions of the fornix, which carries hippocampal efferents conveying salient context to the BNST (Amaral & Witter 1995), (2) glutamatergic antagonists injected into the BNST that block hippocampal efferent input, and (3) buspirone, a potent anxiolytic (Davis et al., 1997). Conversely, lesions of, or glutamate antagonists injected in, the central amygdala blocked fear CS-potentiated startle but had no effect on startle elicited by bright light conditions or on anxiolytic effects in the elevated plus maze, where benzodiazepines have a robust anxiolytic effect (Davis et al., 1997; Treit, Pesold, & Rotzinger, 1993). The basolateral amygdala is involved in both bright light- and CS-potentiated startle due to processing of visual information, but not in CRH-enhanced startle.

Thus, with respect to potentiation of the startle reflex, there is a multivariate double dissociation of the central amygdala and the BNST. As summarized in Figure 8.4 (Davis et al., 1997), the nature of the different stimulus conditions that activate these two structures suggests that the amygdala connects explicit phasic stimuli that predict aversive UCSs with rapidly activated evasive responses and subjective fear. In contrast, prolonged contextual and/or unfamiliar stimuli that connote uncertainty about expected outcome are associated with a neurobehavioral response system that coordinates activation of (1) the negative affective state of anxiety to inform the individual that the current context is uncertain and potentially dangerous, (2) autonomic arousal to mobilize energy for potential action, (3) selective attention in order to maximize sensory input at specified locations in the visual field, and (4) cognition in order to derive a response strategy. Nevertheless, as shown in Figure 8.4, efferents from the BNST

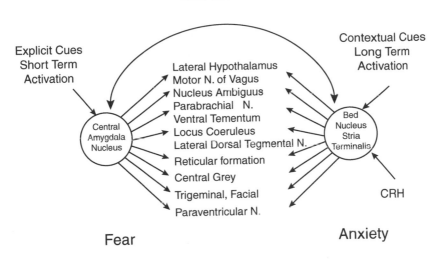

FIGURE 8.4. Hypothetical schematic suggesting that the central nucleus of the amygdala and the bed nucleus of the stria terminalis may be differentially involved in fear versus anxiety, repsectively. Both brain areas have highly similar hypothalamic and brainstem targets known to be involved in specific signs and symptoms of fear and anxiety. However, the stress peptide corticotropin-releasing hormone (CRH) appears to act on receptors in the bed nucleus of the stria terminalis rather than the amygdala, at least in terms of an increase in the startle reflex. Futhermore, the bed nucleus of the stria terminalis seems to be involved in the anxiogenic effects of a very bright light presented for a long time but not when that very same light was previously paired with a shock. Just the opposite is the case for the central nucleus of the amygdala, which is critical for fear conditioning using explicit cues such as a light or tone paired with aversive stimulation (i.e., conditioned fear). Adapted from Davis, Walker, and Lee (1997). Copyright 1997 by the New York Academy of Sciences. Adapted by permission.

and sublenticular area innervate many of the same hypothalamic and brainstem regions as the central amygdala (Heimer, 2003), suggesting that fear and anxiety derive their somewhat similar subjective nature from common neuroendocrine and autonomic response systems (Davis et al., 1997; LeDoux, 1998; Rolls, 1999).

The significance of the prolonged startle-potentiation effects of CRH in the BNST is that CRH and the BNST appear to be integrators of behavioral, neuroendocrine, and autonomic responses to stressful circumstances (Leri, Flores, Rodaros, & Stewart, 2002; Pacak, McCarty, Palkovits, Kopin, & Goldstein, 1995; Shaham, Erb, & Stewart, 2000). This integration is accomplished by the activity of both the peripheral and central CRH systems. The peripheral system involves CRH neurons located in the paraventricular nucleus of the hypothalamus, which when activated initiate the series of events that ends in the release of cortisol from the adrenal cortex (Strand, 1999). Cortisol then circulates in the bloodstream and increases energy reserves (gluconeogenesis) and, if not excessive in quantity, can enhance neurotransmitters involved in modulating emotion and memory (Kim & Diamond, 2002).

In contrast, the central CRH system is composed of CRH neurons located in many different subcortical brain regions that modulate emotion, memory, and central nervous system arousal (Strand, 1999). Whereas the majority of CRH neurons in the central nervous system do not mediate the effects of stress, some of the CRH-containing regions that are important in mediating stress effects are illustrated in Figure 8.5. For instance, the basolateral amygdala detects discrete aversive stimuli associated with the stressful circumstances and activates the extensive array of CRH neurons located in the central amygdala. These CRH neurons project to many brain regions that modulate emotion, memory, and arousal, including the peripheral CRH neurons in the paraventricular nucleus in the hypothalamus (Strand, 1999). Stress variables associated with context and uncertainty activate CRH neurons in the BNST, which have similar projection targets as the central amygdala (Erb, Salmaso, Rodaros, & Stewart, 2001; Macey, Smith, Nader, & Porrino, 2003; Shaham et al., 2000). Both the central amygdala and the BNST can activate CRH neurons in the lateral hypothalamus, a region that integrates central nervous system arousal. In turn, the lateral hypothalamic CRH projections modulate autonomic nervous system activity. Importantly, as illustrated in Figure 8.5, all three sources of CRH projections—the central amygdala, BNST, and lateral hypothalamus—innervate CRH neurons in the paragiganticocellularis (PGi) (Aston-Jones et al., 1996), which is located in the rostral ventrolateral area of the medulla in the brainstem. The PGi is a massive nucleus that provides major integration of central and autonomic arousal and, in turn, coordinates and triggers arousal responses to urgent stimuli via two main pathways eminating from its own population of CRH neurons, which make up 10% of PGi neurons (Aston-Jones et al., 1996). One CRH pathway modulates the autonomic nervous system and hence peripheral arousal effects via projections to the intermediolateral cell column of the spinal cord, activating sympathetic preganglionic autonomic neurons.

The other CRH pathway modulates central arousal effects via activation of the locus coeruleus (LC), where PGi CRH innervation of the LC in humans and monkeys is dense (Aston-Jones et al., 1996). The LC, which is composed of ~20,000 neurons that provide the major source of norepin-

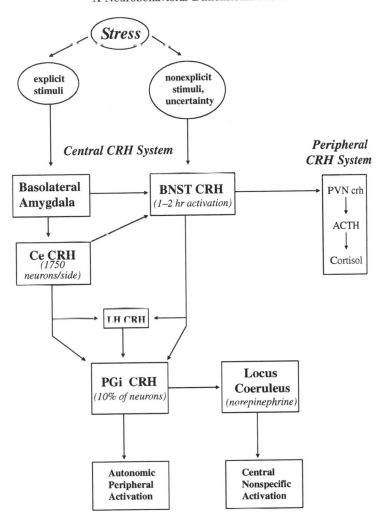

FIGURE 8.5. Components of the central and peripheral corticotrophin re-leasing-hormone (CRH) systems. Ce, central amygdala nucleus; BNST, bed nucleus of the stria terminalis; LH, lateral hypothalamus; Pgi, paragiganticocellularis; PVN, paraventricular nucleus of the hypothalamus; ACTH, corticotropic hormone from the anterior pituitary.

ephrine (NE) in the brain, innervates the entire brain (Oades, 1985). LC neurons that release NE onto beta-adrenergic receptors are responsible for producing a nonspecific emotional activation via broadly collateralizing axons to the central nervous system (Aston-Jones et al., 1996), and this NE release to chronic stress is increased in inbred rat strains with high anxiety (Blizzard, 1988) and in posttraumatic stress disorder patients (Charney, Grillon, & Bremner, 1998). This nonspecific emotional activation pattern comprises a global urgent response system that responds to unpredicted events and hence facilitates behavioral readiness alerting (enhanced sensory processing) and attention (enhanced selection of stimuli) (Aston-Jones et al., 1996), which are characteristic of states of anxiety in highly stress-reactive rodents and monkeys (Blizzard, 1988; Redmond, 1987). And this central arousal can be enduring: PGi CRH activation of LC neurons endures and peaks 40 minutes after stimulation of the PGi (Aston-Jones et al., 1996). This persistent activation of spontaneous activity in the LC renders the effects of short-lived, nonsalient stimuli of little effect on the LC, such that salient stimuli have an inordinate effect on LC activity and hence, in turn, on central activation. Thus, taken together, the central CRH neuron system is capable of activating a vast array of behaviorally relevant processes during stressful conditions, including activation of the peripheral CRH system.

CRH administration in rodents, as well as in transgenic mice that have an overproduction of CRH centrally (but not peripherally), generates specifically via CRH2 receptors anxiogenic effects, including reduced exploration of unfamiliarity and of the elevated T-maze, reduced sleep, reduced food intake and sexual activity, and increased sympathetic and behavioral signs of anxiety (Nie et al., 2004; Strand, 1999).

These findings taken together suggest that anxiety is essentially a stress response system that relies on a network of CRH neuron populations to modulate behaviorally relevant responses to the stressor. The most potent factors in determining the magnitude of a stressor are the very psychological factors that are eliciting stimuli of the anxiety system: uncontrollability, unpredictability, unfamiliarity, unavoidability, and uncertainty. For example, an animal that can control shock shows little evidence of stress, while the animal that is yoked to the first animal and receives shock without control shows severe behavioral and physiological effects of stress. Thus, it is not the physical nature of the shock that is stressful but, rather, the psychological factor of uncontrollability and unpredictability. Furthermore, from the standpoint of trait anxiety or neuroticism, the strongest primary or facet scale in the higher-order factor of anxiety in Tellegen's personality questionnaire is termed "stress reactivity" due to the stress-related content of items loading on the scale (Tellegen & Waller, in press).

Nonaffective Constraint or Impulsivity

Delimiting the Heterogeneity of Impulsivity/Constraint

Impulsivity comprises a heterogeneous cluster of lower-order traits that includes sensation seeking, risk taking, novelty seeking, boldness, adventuresomeness, boredom susceptibility, unreliability, and unorderliness. This lack of specificity is reflected in the fact that the content of the measures of impulsivity is heterogeneous, and that not all these measures are highly interrelated. We (Depue & Collins, 1999) demonstrated elsewhere that at least three different neurobehavioral systems may underlie this trait complex:

1. *Positive incentive motivation*, associated with exploratoration of novel stimulus conditions.
2. *Low fear*, as indicated in risk taking, attraction to physically dangerous activities, and lack of fear of physical harm.
3. *Low levels of a nonaffective form of impulsivity*, which results in disinhibition of the foregoing neurobehavioral systems, as suggested by several researchers (Depue, 1995, 1996; Depue & Spoont, 1986; Panksepp, 1998; Spoont, 1992; Zuckerman, 1994).

As a means of disentangling and clarifying this complexity (see Figure 8.6), we plotted the trait loadings derived in 11 studies (see Appendix 8.1) in which two or more multidimensional personality questionnaires were jointly factor analyzed in order to derive general, higher-order traits of personality. All studies identified a higher-order trait of impulsivity that *lacks affective content*, which in Figure 8.6 was labeled "constraint" following Tellegen (Tellegen & Waller, in press), who introduced the term to emphasize its independence from emotional traits such as extraversion and neuroticism. All studies also found constraint to be orthogonal to a general, higher-order extraversion trait. Figure 8.6 shows a continuous distribution of traits within the two intersecting orthogonal dimensions of extraversion and constraint. Nevertheless, three relatively homogeneous clusterings of traits can be delineated on the basis of the position and content of traits, relative to extraversion and constraint. First, lower-order traits associated with agentic extraversion (sociability, dominance, achievement, positive emotions, activity, energy) cluster at the high end of the extraversion dimension without substantial association with constraint. A tight clustering of most of these traits to extraversion is evident. Second, various traits of impulsivity that *do not incorporate strong positive affect* (e.g., conscientiousness) cluster tightly around the high end of the constraint dimension without substantial association with extraversion; Eysenck's psychoticism

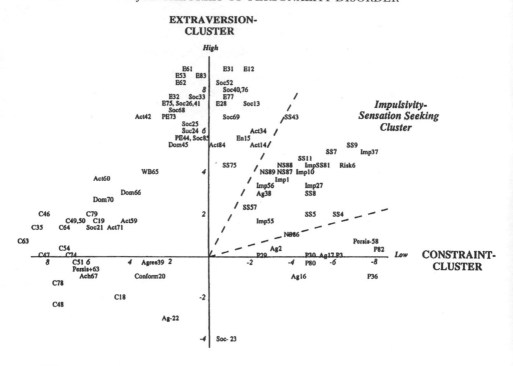

FIGURE 8.6. A plotting of loadings of personality traits derived in 11 studies in which more than one multidimensional personality questionnaire was jointly factor analyzed as a means of deriving general traits of personality. All of these studies defined a general nonaffective impulsivity trait, referred to as constraint (horizontal dimension in the figure), that was separate from the general extraversion trait (vertical dimension in the figure). The figure illustrates three clusterings of traits: an extraversion cluster at the high end of the extraversion dimension; conscientiousness and psychoticism–aggression clusters at the high and low end of the constraint dimension, respectively; and an impulsivity–sensation-seeking cluster within the dashed lines. The figure illustrates that extraversion and *non*affective constraint dimensions are generally identified and found to be orthogonal, and that impulsivity-sensation seeking traits *associated with strong positive affective* arise as a joint function of the interaction of extraversion and constraint. See Appendix 8.1 for the identity of the trait measure abbreviations with numbers, the questionnaires to which the abbreviations correspond, and the studies providing the trait loadings. From Depue and Collins (1999).

trait and various aggression measures are located at the low end of constraint and show little association with extraversion. Third, all but one trait measure of impulsivity *that incorporate positive affect* (sensation seeking, novelty seeking, risk taking) are located within the dashed lines in Figure 8.6, and are moderately associated with both extraversion and constraint. Thus, currently most trait models of personality separate a nonaffective form of impulsivity and extraversion into distinct traits, although the terms used for the former vary from "conscientiousness" (Costa & McCrae, 1992; Goldberg & Rosolack, 1994) to constraint (Tellegen & Waller, in press) and impulsivity–unsocialized sensation seeking (Zuckerman, 1994).

Conceptually, the complexity of impulsivity can be clarified by hypothesizing that *nonaffective* constraint lacks ties to a specific motivational–emotional system (Depue & Collins, 1999). As discussed later, a vast body of animal and human literature demonstrates that constraint so conceived functions as a central nervous system variable that modulates the threshold of stimulus elicitation of motor behavior, both positive and negative emotions, and cognition (Coccaro & Siever, 1991; Depue, 1995, 1996; Depue & Spoont, 1986; Panksepp, 1998; Spoont, 1992; Zald & Depue, 2001; Zuckerman, 1994). This formulation is consistent with findings that low constraint is associated in both animals and humans with a generalized motor–cognitive–affective impulsivity but is not preferentially associated with any specific motivational system (Depue & Spoont, 1986; Spoont, 1992; Zald & Depue, 2001). Alternatively, *affective* impulsivity emerges from the interaction of nonaffective constraint with other distinct affective–motivational systems, such as positive incentive motivation–agentic extraversion (as in Figure 8.6) or anxiety–neuroticism.

Elicitation of behavior can be modeled neurobiologically by use of a minimum threshold construct, which represents a central nervous system weighting of the external and internal factors that contribute to the probability of response expression (Depue & Collins, 1999). External factors are characteristics of environmental stimulation, including magnitude, duration, and psychological salience. Internal factors consist of both state (e.g., stress-induced endocrine levels) and trait biological variation. We propose that nonaffective constraint is the personality trait that reflects the greatest central nervous system weight on the construct of a minimum response threshold. As such, constraint exerts a general influence over the elicitation of any emotional behavior, and hence constraint is not preferentially associated with any specific neurobehavioral–motivational system. In this model, other higher-order personality traits would thus reflect the influence of neurobiological variables that strongly contribute to the threshold for responding, such as DA in the facilitation of incentive motivated behavior, μ-opiates in the experience of affiliative reward, and CRH in the potentiation of anxiety.

Neurobiology of Nonaffective Constraint

The important question is what type of central nervous system variables could provide a major weighting of behavioral elicitation thresholds. Functional levels of neurotransmitters that provide a strong, relatively generalized *tonic inhibitory* influence on behavioral responding would be good candidates as significant modulators of a response elicitation threshold, and hence would likely account for a large proportion of the variance in the trait of nonaffective constraint. We and others previously (Coccaro & Siever, 1991; Depue, 1995, 1996; Depue & Spoont, 1986; Panksepp, 1998; Spoont, 1992; Zald & Depue, 2001; Zuckerman, 1994) and Lesch (1998) most recently suggested that serotonin (5-HT), acting at multiple receptor sites in most brain regions, is such a modulator (Azmitia & Whitaker-Azmitia, 1997; Tork, 1990). As reviewed many times in animal and human literatures (Coccaro et al., 1989; Coccaro & Siever, 1991; Depue, 1995, 1996; Depue & Spoont, 1986; Lesch, 1998; Spoont, 1992; Zald & Depue, 2001; Zuckerman, 1994), 5-HT modulates a diverse set of functions— including emotion, motivation, motor, affiliation, cognition, food intake, sleep, sexual activity, and sensory reactivity—such as nociception, sensitization to auditory and tactile startle stimuli, and escape latencies following PAG stimulation—and is associated with many clinical conditions, including violent suicide across several types of disorder, obsessive–compulsive disorder, disorders of impulse control, aggression, depression, anxiety, arson, and substance abuse (Coccaro & Siever, 1991; Depue & Spoont, 1986; Lesch, 1998; Spoont, 1992). Furthermore, *reduced* 5-HT functioning in animals (Depue & Spoont, 1986; Spoont, 1992) and humans (Coccaro et al., 1989) is also accompanied by *irritability* and *hypersensitivity* to stimulation in most sensory modalities (Spoont, 1992), which may be due to the important role played by 5-HT in the inhibitory modulation of sensory input at several levels of the brain (Azmitia & Whitaker-Azmitia, 1997; Tork, 1990), as well as to significant 5-HT modulation of the lateral hypothalamic region that activates autonomic reactivity under stressful conditions (Azmitia & Whitaker-Azmitia, 1997). Thus, 5-HT plays a substantial modulatory role in general neurobiological functioning that affects many forms of motivated behavior. In this sense, nonaffective constraint might be viewed as reflecting the influence of the central nervous system variable of 5-HT, which we refer to later as *neural constraint*.

An important but difficult area of research is to determine which personality traits best assess the general modulatory role of 5-HT. As a beginning, we found that 5-HT agonist-induced increases in serum prolactin secretion were correlated significantly and specifically only with the Constraint/Impulsivity scale (−.44, $p < .01$) from Tellegen's personality questionnaire of 13 primary scales (Depue, 1995, 1996).

Conceptualizing Individual Differences Underlying Personality Traits

As discussed above, models of elicitation of behavioral processes often employ a minimum threshold that represents a central nervous system weighting of the external and internal factors that contribute to initiation of those processes (Depue & Collins, 1999). In addition to the effects of neural constraint (5-HT) (or nonaffective constraint at the behavioral level), the threshold is weighted most strongly by the joint function of two main variables: (1) magnitude of eliciting stimulation and (2) level of postsynaptic receptor activation of the neurobiological variable thought to contribute most variance to the behavioral process in question, such as DA to incentive motivation, μ-opiates to affiliative reward, and CRH to anxiety. The relation between these two variables is represented in Figure 8.7 as a trade-off function (White, 1986), where pairs of values (of stimulus magnitude and receptor activation) specify a diagonal representing the minimum threshold value for elicitation of a behavioral process. Findings reviewed previously show that agonist-induced *state* changes in DA, μOR, and CRH activation influence the threshold of incentive motivated behavior, affiliative reward, and anxiety, respectively. Because the two input variables (stimulus magnitude and receptor activation) are interactive, independent variation in either one not only modifies the probability of eliciting the behavioral process, but it also simultaneously modifies the value of the other variable that is required to reach a minimum threshold of elicitation. Finally, individual variation in variables that significantly modulate the threshold, especially 5-HT-related neural constraint (or nonaffective constraint), would serve as a source of modulation of the threshold of elicitation of *all* behavoral processes. This is shown for 5-HT in Figure 8.7.

A threshold model allows behavioral predictions that help to conceptualize the effects of individual differences in neurobiological functioning on personality traits. A *trait* dimension of postsynaptic receptor activation of *variable X* (e.g., DA, μ-opiate, or CRH) is represented on the horizontal axis of Figure 8.7, where two individuals with divergent trait levels are demarcated: A (low trait level) and B (high trait level). These two divergent individuals may be used to illustrate the effects of trait differences in variable X receptor activation on elicitation of behavioral processes (e.g., incentive motivated behavior, affiliative reward, or anxiety).

As Figure 8.7 indicates, for any given eliciting stimulus, the degree of variable X reactivity will, on average, be larger in individual B versus A.

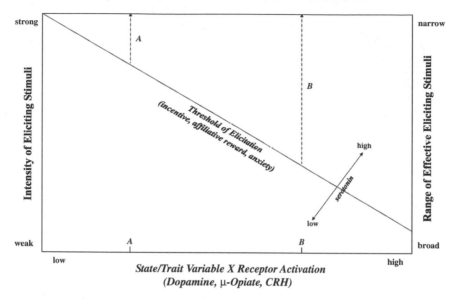

FIGURE 8.7. A minimum threshold for elicitation of a behavioral process (e.g., incentive motivation–positive affect, affiliative reward–affection, anxiety–negative affect) is illustrated as a trade-off function between eliciting stimulus magnitude (left vertical axis) and *variable X* (e.g., dopamine, μ-opiate, CRH) postsynaptic receptor activation (horizontal axis). Range of effective (eliciting) stimuli is illustrated on the right vertical axis as a function of level of receptor activation. Two hypothetical individuals with low and high *trait* postsynaptic receptor activation (demarcated on the horizontal axis as A and B, respectively) are shown to have narrow (A) and broad (B) ranges of effective stimuli, respectively. Threshold effects due to serotonin modulation are illustrated as well.

Hence, the subjective emotional and motivational experiences that are facilitated by variable X (e.g., incentive, affection, and anxiety) will also be more enhanced in B versus A (Depue & Collins, 1999; Depue & Morrone-Strupinsky, in press). In addition, the difference between individuals A and B in magnitude of subjective experience may contribute to variation in the contemporaneous encoding of a stimulus's intensity or salience (a form of state-dependent learning) and, hence, in the stimulus's encoded salience in subsequent memory consolidation. Accordingly, individuals A and B may develop differences in the capacity of mental representations of (incentive, affiliative, anxiety) contexts to activate the relevant motivational (incentive, affiliative, anxiety) processes, which is significant due to the predominant motivation of behavior in humans by symbolic representations of goals.

If individual differences in encoding apply across the full range of stimulus magnitudes, trait differences in the reactivity of variable X may have marked effects on the *range* of effective (i e , eliciting) stimuli. This is illustrated in Figure 8.7, where the right vertical axis represents the range of effective (eliciting) stimuli. Increasing trait levels of variable X (horizontal axis) are associated with an increasing efficacy of weaker stimuli (left vertical axis) and, thus, with an increasing range of effective stimuli (right vertical axis). In Figure 8.7 individuals A and B are shown to have a narrow versus broad range, respectively. Significantly, the broader range for individual B suggests that, on average, B will experience more frequent elicitation of subjective emotional experiences associated with variable X activity (incentive, affection, anxiety). This means that the probability at any point in time of being in a variable X-facilitated state for individual B is higher than for A. Therefore, when subsequent relevant stimuli are encountered, their subjectively evaluated magnitude will show a stronger positive bias for B than A. Thus, trait differences in variable X may *proactively* influence the evaluation and encoding of relevant stimuli and may not be restricted to *reactive* emotional processes. This raises the possibility of variation in the *dynamics* of behavioral engagement with the environment. A positive relation between *state* variable X activation and stimulus efficacy in the threshold model suggests that, as an initial stimulus enhances variable X activation, the efficacy of subsequently encountered stimuli may be increased proportional to the degree of the initial variable X activation. Under conditions of strong variable X activation, perhaps even previously subthreshold stimuli may come to elicit behavioral processes (incentive, affiliative reward, anxiety).

THE INTERACTIVE NATURE
OF EMOTIONAL TRAITS AND CONSTRAINT

Three of the higher-order personality traits discussed previously (agentic extraversion, affiliation, anxiety) provide the qualitative emotional content of comtemporaneous behavior, depending on which neurobehavioral–motivational system is being elicited at any point in time. The fourth trait, nonaffective constraint, modulates the probability of elicitation of all those systems. As the very construct of personality connotes, however, the affective or emotional *style* of an individual is determined by the interaction of all four higher-order traits. This means that differential strength between these personality traits, or differential reactivity of their underlying neurobehavioral systems, will determine the relative predominance of particular affective or emotional behavior in individuals. We now consider some of these relevant trait interactions as preparatory discussion for the model of personality disturbance which follows.

Agentic Extraversion × Anxiety

Differential relative strength of the traits of agentic extraversion and anxiety has a substantial influence on the predominant affective or emotional style of an individual. Agentic extraversion is associated with a highly positive affective state, whereas anxiety is associated with a negative affective state. Moreover, both traits are associated with *general* neurobehavioral systems, meaning that they both are subject to frequent elicitation by a broad class of stimulus (incentives and uncertainty, respectively). As illustrated in Figure 8.8, the interaction of these two traits leads to various types of affective style depending on the values of the two traits. The upper right (positive) and lower left (negative) quadrants manifest the greatest contrast and consistency in affective styles, whereas the affective style of individuals in the upper left quandrant is mixed, depending on the relative salience of the most recent incentive versus uncertainty context. The lower right quadrant is characterized by both low positive and negative affective activation and therefore manifests as impoverished affective–emotional behavior reminiscent of clinical descriptions of schizoid behavior.

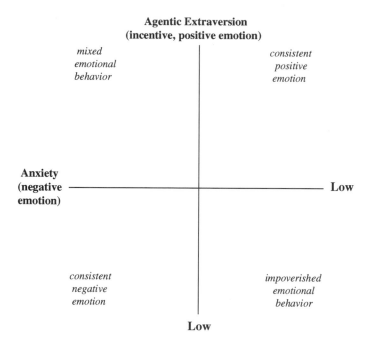

FIGURE 8.8. Interaction of the higher-order personality traits of agentic extraversion and anxiety. See text for details.

Agentic Extraversion × Affiliation

The nature of an individual's interpersonal behavior is dependent on the relative strength of agentic extraversion and affiliation. Agentic extraversion is associated with social engagement and dominance, whereas affiliation reflects the capacity to experience reward from affiliative interactions. As discussed in the Introduction, theories and research on interpersonal behavior have demonstrated that these two traits are independent and characterize most of the variance in interpersonal behavior. As illustrated in Figure 8.9, their interaction produces substantive differences in interpersonal style. Affiliation at the high end modulates the dominance and competitive aggression of agentic extraversion, creating an *amiable* interpersonal style ranging from follower to leader depending on the level of agentic extraversion. Perhaps more relevant to personality disturbance, the low end of affiliation manifests as aloof, cold, and uncaring, which ranges from isolated and submissive to manipulative and domineering with increasing levels of agentic extraversion. The left lower quadrant is reminiscent of clinical descriptions of schizoid behavior, whereas the lower right is more in keeping with antisocial behavior.

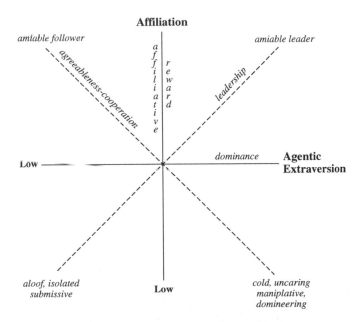

FIGURE 8.9. Interaction of the higher-order personality traits of agentic extraversion and affiliation. See text for details.

Affiliation × Separation Anxiety

An additional trait interaction would seem particularly relevant to characterizing interpersonal behavior in personality disturbance: an interaction between affiliation and separation anxiety or distress. The latter trait is rarely assessed in personality inventories, but it is a significant influence in most interpersonal relations at one time or another and becomes impairing at extreme levels. Although manifestation of separation anxiety or distress is correlated with the existence of an affiliative bond, we take the position with others (Insel, 1997; Nelson & Panksepp, 1998; Panksepp, 1998; Young, Wang, & Insel, 1998) that processes underlying affiliative bonding are not the same as those involved in social separation distress. Affectively, affiliation and separation are distinctly different and not two sides of a coin. Separation is characterized by the presence of frustration, protest, and anxiety and not just the absence of warmth and pleasure (and vice versa). In fact, there are data that support a bidimensional organization of affiliation and separation distress, because the neural pathways underlying affiliative engagement (e.g., maternal behavior) are different from those that allow for inhibition of separation distress (Eisenberger, Lieberman, & Williams, 2003; Insel, 1997; Nelson & Panksepp, 1998).

In behavioral terms, separation anxiety or distress may reflect the anxiety of *uncertainty* generated by removal of protective, supportive safety cues. From a broader evolutionary perspective, separation leading to social isolation can be characterized as unconditionally aversive, having *no discrete, explicit stimulus source*—similar to the human experience of being in the dark (Davis et al., 1997; Davis & Shi, 1999; White & Depue, 1999). In humans, social isolation, rejection, and/or ostracization generates a sense of anxiety, guilt, and apprehension. Put differently, separation anxiety or distress may in part reflect a very basic neurobehavioral anxiety system that serves to motivate attempts to reverse social isolation via reintegration into a social group (Barlow, 2002; White & Depue, 1999). It may be that separation anxiety or distress is associated to other related traits such as rejection sensitivity and dependency, both of which reflect anxiety over social isolation. This system would be associated with neural networks involved in recognition of social uncertainty and rejection, experience of psychic pain (Eisenberger et al., 2003), and expression of anxiety.

Future research needs to establish the extent to which separation anxiety and the higher-order trait of anxiety are related: Do they reflect the same underlying neurobehavioral system elicited by uncertainty, or do they reflect distinct systems. The answer to this question may help to clarify the fundamental distinctions, if they exist, between negative affect, rejection sensitivity, and separation anxiety that characterizes borderline-, dependent-, and avoidant-like personality disturbance.

As illustrated in Figure 8.10, the dimension of separation distress is portrayed as one of dependency. In interaction with affiliation, the four quadrants can be seen to represent four different social attachment styles frequently described in the literature: (1) *secure* (upper left, where the individual is affectively bonded and not overly distraught with anxiety about losing that bond, and is therefore socially gratified); (2) *ambivalent* (upper right, where the individual is adequately bonded but has intense anxiety about separation from the bond, thereby vascillating between the desire for closeness and protective interpersonal distance. It is in this quadrant that one might expect borderline-, avoidant-, and dependent-like interpersonal disturbance. Moreover, when this quadrant is accompanied by elevation on the higher-order trait of anxiety, the interpersonal disturbance will also be associated with alienation and suspicion of the motives of others, because interpersonal alienation is a strong marker of this trait [Tellegen & Waller, in press]); (3) *avoidant–anxious* (lower right, where the individual is not affectively bonded but is anxious about being isolated and alone and

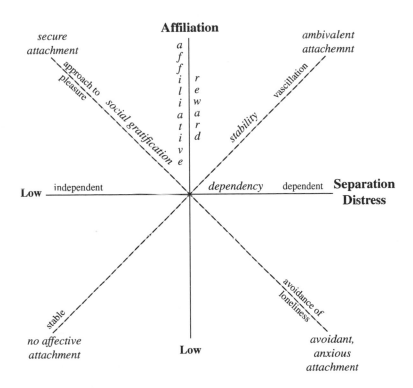

FIGURE 8.10. Interaction of the higher-order personality trait of affiliation and separation distress. See text for details.

thereby avoids loneliness through non-bonded interpersonal relations); and (4) *no affective attachment* (lower left, where there is an absence of affiliative bonding and little anxiety in being separated from social contact, resulting in a stable absence of social attachment that characterizes schizoid-like interpersonal disturbance).

Agentic Extraversion, Anxiety, Aggression, Affiliation × Nonaffective Constraint

A vast body of animal and human evidence consistently associates reduced functioning of 5-HT neurotransmission with *behavioral instability*. This instability is manifested as lability (i.e., a heightened probability of competing behavioral responses due to a reduced threshold of response elicitation) (Spoont, 1992). Therefore, instability or labilitiy will increase as a function of increasing stimulus influences on response elicitation of other behavioral systems (Depue & Spoont, 1986). This means that the effects of constraint depend on interactions with other personality traits that reflect activity in those behavioral systems. That is, the *qualitative content* of unstable behavior will depend on which neurobehavioral–motivational system, or *affective* personality trait, is being elicited at any point in time (Zald & Depue, 2001), although differential strength of various personality traits will obviously produce relative predominance of particular affective behaviors *within individuals*.

An example of the interaction of neurobiological variables associated with constraint (5-HT) and agentic extraversion (DA) helps to illustrate the behavioral instability resulting from low constraint. 5-HT is an inhibitory modulator of a host of DA-facilitated behaviors, including the reinforcing properties of psychostimulants, novelty-induced locomotor activity, the acquisition of self-administration of cocaine, and DA utilization in the NAS (Ashby, 1996; Depue & Spoont, 1986; Spoont, 1992). This modulatory influence arises in large part from the dense dorsal raphe efferents to the VTA and NAS, connections that are known to modulate DA activity (Ashby, 1966; Azmitia & Whitaker-Azmitia, 1997; Spoont, 1992). A 5-HT-related reduction in the threshold of DA facilitation of behavior results in an exaggerated response to incentive stimuli which is most apparent in reward–punishment conflict situations. In such situations, exaggerated responding to incentives results in (1) a greater weighting of immediate versus delayed future rewards, (2) increased reactivity to the reward of safety or relief associated with active avoidance (e.g., suicidal behavior), (3) impulsive behavior (i.e., a propensity to respond to reward when withholding or delaying a response may produce a more favorable long-term outcome), and (4) various attempts to experience the increased magnitude and frequency of incentive reward (e.g., self-administration of DA-active substances) (Babor, Hoffman, & Delboca, 1992; Coccaro & Siever, 1991; Depue & Iacono, 1989; Lesch, 1998). All these effects impair the ability to sustain long-term goal-directed behavior programs (such as obtaining a college degree) by mental representations of expected rewards that can be repeatedly accessed and held online in prefrontal cortex, and thereby symbolically motivate behavior (Depue & Collins, 1999; Goldman-Rakic, 1987).

A 5-HT–DA interaction is more formally illustrated in the threshold model of behavioral facilitation in Figure 8.7 above, where 5-HT values modulate the probability of DA facilitation (variable X) of incentive behavior across the entire range of incentive stimulus magnitude (Depue & Collins, 1999). This interaction is also modeled in Figure 8.11 within a personality framework, where the affectively unipolar dimension of agentic extraversion (DA facilitation) is seen in interaction with nonaffective constraint (5-HT inhibition) (Depue, 1996). The interaction of these two traits creates a diagonal dimension of *behavioral stability* that applies equally to affective, cognitive, interpersonal, motor, and incentive processes (Depue

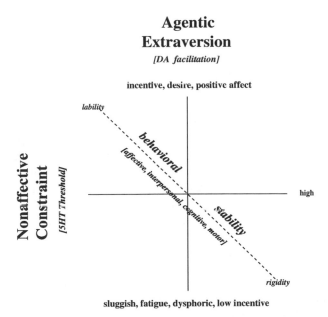

FIGURE 8.11. Interaction of the higher-order personality traits of agentic extraversion and nonaffective constraint. See text for details. From Depue and Lenzenweger (2001). Copyright 2001 by The Guilford Press. Reprinted by permission.

& Spoont, 1986; Spoont, 1992; Zald & Depue, 2001). The diagonal represents the line of greatest variance in stability, ranging from lability in the upper left quadrant of the two-space (low 5-HT, high DA) to rigidity in the lower right (high 5-HT, low DA).

It is important to note that the extent of lability is affected not only by a 5-HT influence, but also by DA's more general facilitatory effects on the flow of neural information, where increased DA activity promotes *switching* between response alternatives (i.e., behavioral flexibility) (Depue & Iacono, 1989; Oades, 1985; Spoont, 1992). Indeed, when DA transmission is very low, a problem in exceeding the response facilitation threshold occurs, whereas at very high DA transmission levels, a high rate of switching between response alternatives is seen, which can evolve into a low *variety* of responses when abnormally high (e.g., stereotypy) (Oades, 1985). Thus, DA's role in switching between response alternatives may explain several of the *non*affective manifestations of extraverted behavior, such as rapidity of attentional shifts and cognitive switching between ideas.

This conceptualization of the interaction of 5-HT and DA may be relevant to interpersonal behavior. Brothers and Ring (1992) and others (Adolphs, 2003) have argued that humans have an innate cognitive *alphabet* of ethologically significant behavioral signs that signal the emotional intention of others. This alphabet is integrated into its highest representation in human social cognition as a *person* with propensities and dispositions that have valence for the observer, a social construct akin to personality. Personality research has demonstrated that the representation of others exists in two independent, contrasted forms as the *familiar-good other* and the *unfamiliar-evil other*, and the representation of the self is similarly represented in two independent positive and negative forms (Tellegen & Waller, in press). This is consistent with the fact that most percepts and concepts are represented in the brain as separate unified entities (Squire & Kosslyn, 1998). Interestingly, increased DA activation results in a more rapid switching between contrasting percepts, such as two perceptual orientations of the Necker cube or of an ascending–descending staircase (Oades, 1985). Speculatively, we suggest that the frequent, sometimes rapid fluctuation between extreme mental representations of others and/or the self as *good* or *bad* that characterize several forms of personality disorders is related primarily to reduced 5-HT functioning (e.g., borderline-like interpersonal disturbance). Furthermore, this condition would be exaggerated when in interaction with increasing DA functioning (e.g., histrionic-like interpersonal disturbance).

As illustrated in Figure 8.12, interaction between constraint–5-HT and trait anxiety–CRH dimensions may create a range of anxious phenotypes that vary in their stability, ranging from most highly labile, episodic, and stress reactive in the upper left quadrant, to chronically anxious with per-

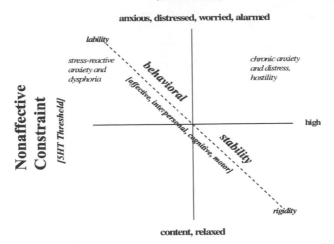

FIGURE 8.12. Interaction of the higher-order personality traits of anxiety and nonaffective constraint. See text for details.

sistent reverberating negative affect that creates an attitudinal hostility in the upper right quadrant (Zald & Depue, 2001). In support of this interaction, Goddard, Charney, and Germine (1995) recently demonstrated in normal subjects that, when combined with a 5-HT antagonist, activation by an NE agonist of LC norepinephrine projections (which is activated by stress-induced PGi CRH neurons) resulted in significantly *greater* (1) NE release in the brain, and (2) subjective feelings of anxiety, nervousness, and restlessness than when the NE agonist was administered without a 5-HT antagonist. Moreover, together with these findings, our model would account for the weak relation (accounting for 3–4% of the variance in behavior) between trait anxiety and a genotypical variant of the 5-HT uptake transporter, which may lead to reduced 5-HT functioning via negative feedback effects on 5-HT cells (Lesch, 1998). In this case, reduced 5-HT functioning may disinhibit the LC NE activity-induced autonomic arousal thought to contribute to subjective anxiety (Azmitia & Whitaker-Azmitia, 1997).

Affective aggression is a goal-oriented pattern of attack behavior that is strongly modulated by incentive motivational processes and is markedly disinhibited by conditions of reduced 5HT functioning (Coccaro & Siever 1991; Depue & Spoont, 1986; Lesch, 1998; Panksepp, 1998; Spoont 1992). This interaction is likely more complex in that behavioral expre

sion of affective aggression is relative to the strength of the separate but tightly linked neurobehavioral system of fear (Panksepp, 1998). Thus, in Figure 8.13, the vertical axis is represented as a ratio of the strength of affective aggression to fear, and this ratio is modulated by constraint–5-HT to produce heightened episodic, impulsive aggression in the upper left quadrant and more chronic aggression and attitudinal hostility in the upper right quadrant. The common finding that reduced 5-HT functioning is associated with increased affective aggression is thus expressed in Figure 8.13 but is seen as a function of fear as well.

   Finally, an interaction of 5-HT variation with affiliation was discussed previously, where reduced 5-HT functioning creates frequent, rapid fluctuations between extreme mental representations of others as *good* or *bad*. Such unstable evaluations of others greatly impairs interpersonal relations and may be aggravated in individuals with elevated trait anxiety levels (e.g., borderline-like interpersonal impairment). Another effect of reduced 5-HT on affiliation was observed by Higley, Mehlman, Taub, and Higley (1992), who demonstrated that monkeys with low 5-HT functioning are overly aggressive and socially rejected by peers. Such monkeys manifest appropriate sociosexual behavior, but its expressive features, in terms of timing and magnitude, appear to be poorly modulated, thereby negatively arousing

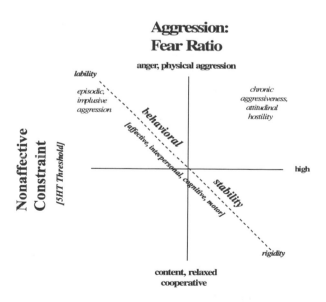

FIGURE 8.13. Interaction of the higher-order personality traits of anxiety and nonaffective constraint. See text for details.

peers (Higley et al., 1992). It may be that this effect is enhanced in individuals with elevated trait aggression levels.

Conclusion

Models of personality traits based on only one neurotransmitter are clearly simplistic and require other modifying factors (Ashby, 1996). In addition, individual differences of psychobiological origin in lower-order traits will represent error variance in predicting higher-order traits from any one variable alone (Livesley, Jang, & Vernon, 1998). Using agentic extraversion as an example, 5-HT will certainly not be the only tonic inhibitory modulator of an elicitation threshold. For instance, functional levels of gamma-aminobutyric acid (GABA) tonic inhibitory activity may also influence the threshold of behavioral facilitation as an inhibitor of substance P, a neuromodulator having excitatory effects on VTA DA neurons (Kalivas, Churchill, & Klitenick, 1993; Le Moal & Simon, 1991). Moreover, receptors for GABA, cholecystokinin (CCK), opiates, substance P, and neurotensin are found in the VTA, and their activation can markedly affect DA activity (Kalivas et al., 1993; LeMoal & Simon, 1991). Also, because monoamine oxidase (MAO) is responsible for presynaptic degradation of biogenic amines (DA, 5-HT, NE), it may be an important variable in interaction with DA functioning, particularly MAO-B which predominates in primates and has DA as a specific substrate (Mitra, Mohanakumar, & Ganguly, 1994).

Despite the complexity inherent in the interaction of neurotransmitters in emotional traits, there is good reason to start with one neurotransmitter of substantial effect within the neurobehavioral system underlying a trait, explore the details of its relation to that trait first, and then gradually build complexity by adding additional factors one at a time. This is particularly true of biogenic amines and neuropeptides, because they are phylogenetically old and modulate brain structures associated with behavioral processes relevant to personality, including emotions, motivation, motor propensity, and cognition (Depue & Collins, 1999; Lesch, 1998; Luciana, Depue, Arbiss, & Leon, 1992; Luciana, Collins, & Depue, 1998; Oades, 1985). Furthermore, considering their nonspecific modulatory influence and broad distribution patterns in the brain (Ashby, 1996; Aston-Jones et al., 1996; Oades & Halliday, 1987; Tork, 1990), variation in a single neuromodulator can have widespread effects on behavior and on the functioning of multifocal neural networks (Mesulam, 1990), as animal research on the behavioral effects of DA, CRH, μ-opiates, and 5-HT has clearly demonstrated. Therefore, variation in biogenic amines and neuropeptides may provide powerful predictors of human behavioral variation. Thus, such neuromodulators may serve as important building blocks for more complex models of personality traits.

A MODEL OF PERSONALITY DISTURBANCE

Illustration of the interactions of two traits taken at a time, as previously, is informative but of course underestimates the complexity of reality. The neurobehavioral systems underlying all of the higher-order traits interact. Therefore, we conceive of personality disturbance as *emergent* phenotypes arising from the interaction of the above neurobehavioral systems underlying major personality traits.

Our multidimensional model is illustrated in Figure 8.14. In the model, the axes are defined by neurobehavoral systems rather than by traits, because traits are only approximate, fallible estimates of these systems, and trait measures vary in content and underlying constructs. In Figure 8.14, behavioral approach based on positive *incentive motivation* (underlying agentic extraversion) and anxiety (underlying neuroticism or trait anxiety) are modeled as a ratio of their relative strength, because the opposing nature of their eliciting stimuli affects behavior in a reciprocal manner, such that the *elicitation* or *expression* of one system is influenced by the strength of the other (Gray, 1973). As discussed previously, the interaction of these two systems strongly influences the style of an individual's emotional behavior. The affiliative reward dimension (underlying trait affilia-

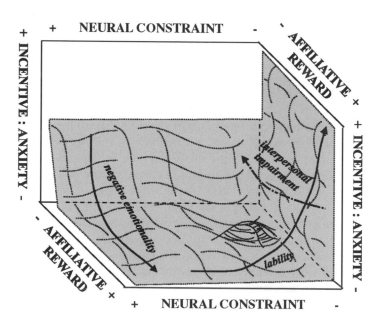

FIGURE 8.14. A multidimensional model of personality disturbance. See text for details.

tion) in the model largely influences the interpersonal domain, whereas the neural constraint (underlying the trait of nonaffective constraint) dimension modulates the expressive features of the other systems. Due to the limitation of graphing more than three dimensions, it should be noted that the model includes two other systems/traits that we suggest influence the manifestation of personality disturbance. As suggested in the earlier section on trait interactions, we believe a dimension of affective aggression:fear is necessary to account for the full range of antisocial (high aggression:low fear) behavior, and that a dimension of separation anxiety/rejection sensitivity strongly contributes to dependent-, avoidant-, and borderline-like disturbance (all high on this dimension). Taken together, then, the model proposes that the interaction of at least six neurobehavioral systems underlying dimensional personality traits are necessary to account for the emergent phenotypes observed in personality disturbance.

Three significant features of the model that are illustrated in the figure are worth emphasizing. First, the phenotypical expression of personality disturbance, represented by the gray-shaded *reaction* surface in the figure (accounting for ~10% of the population; Lenzenweger, Lorenger, Korfine, & Neff, 1997; Livesley, 2001; Torgersen, Kringlen, & Cramer, 2001), is continuous in nature, changing in character gradually but seamlessly across the surface in a manner that reflects the changing product of the mulitdimensional interactions. It may be that certain areas of the surface are associated with increased probability (risk) of certain features of personality disturbance, and this is represented in the right-back area of the figure as an elevation in the surface that is continous rather than distinct in contour. Thus, this representation is not meant to imply that a distinct disorder or category exists in that particular area of the surface. Second, the extent and positioning of the reaction surface is weighted most heavily by increasing anxiety, decreasing neural constraint, and decreasing affiliative reward. This weighting is also reflected in the lines with directional arrows overlaying the gray surface in the figure, which illustrate increasing negative emotionality, lability, and interpersonal impairment. These three factors were found to be the most common characteristics of all personality disorders in the meta-analysis of Saulsman and Page (2004), thereby empirically supporting their emphasis in our model. Third, viewing personality disturbance as a *reaction* surface implies that the magnitude of disturbance at any point on the surface is variable, waxing and waning with fluctuations in environmental circumstances, stressors, and interpersonal disruptions, both within and across persons over time. Indeed, we recently demonstrated in a longitudinal assessment of the stability of formally defined personality disorders that phenotypical intensity varied markedly over time, thereby affecting the presence/absence of diagnostic status as well as level of symptomatology (Lenzenweger, Johnson, & Willett, in press).

Implications of the Model

Several implications of the model can be outlined. First, the model may help to explain sex differences in some forms of personality disturbance. The increased prevalence of males with antisocial behavior may reflect the higher mean of males in the population on the trait of aggression:fear and a lower mean on nonaffective constraint (including 5-HT functioning; Spoont, 1992). In addition, the increased prevalence of females in clinical populations with borderline- and dependent-like personality disturbance may reflect a combination of (1) their higher mean on both trait anxiety (borderline) and separation distress (dependent), (2) their higher mean on affiliation, thereby increasing the need for social relationships whose loss is feared, (3) their lower mean on agentic extraversion, particularly social dominance, hence enhancing the predominance of high levels of trait anxiety, and (4) their lower mean on aggression:fear, hence decreasing the prevalence of antisocial behavior (Depue & Collins, 1999; Kohnstamm, 1989; Tellegen & Waller, in press).

Second, the model suggests that research on the lines of causal neurobiological influence within the structure of *normal* personality will need to be a primary focus if the neurobiological nature of personality disturbance is to be fully understood. At present, there is a paucity of systematic research in this domain (Depue & Collins, 1999; Depue & Morrone-Strupinsky, in press). Third, the multidimensional nature of the model indicates that univariate biological research in personality disturbance will inadequately discover the neurobiological nature of personality disturbance. Thus, not only is multivariate assessment suggested, but methods of *combinatorial* representation of those multiple variables—as in profile, finite mixture modeling, latent class, discriminant function, and multivariate taxonomic analyses—will need to be more fully integrated in this area of research. Finally, the trend in development of neurotransmitter-specific drugs may not fully complement the pharmocotherapy requirements of personality disturbance. If personality disturbance represents emergent phenotypes of multiple, interacting neurobehavioral systems, then (1) basic research on the pharmacological modulation of neurobehavioral systems and (2) clinical research on multiregiment pharmacotherapy is greatly needed.

APPENDIX 8.1. Personality Questionnaire Traits[a] Used in 11 Studies That Correspond to the Numbered Trait Abbreviations Illustrated in Figure 8.5

Study	Numbered trait abbreviation[b] (in numerical order)	Corresponding personality questionnaire trait[c]
Zuckerman et al. (1989)	Imp1	Buss–Plomin EASI, Inhibitory Control
	Ag2	Buss–Plomin EASI, Anger
	P3	Eysenck Personality Questionnaire, Psychoticism
	SS4	Sensation Seeking Scales, Boredom Susceptibility
	SS5	Sensation Seeking Scales, Experience Seeking
	Risk6	Jackson Personality Inventory, Risk Taking
	SS7	Buss–Plomin EASI, Sensation Seeking
	SS8	Sensation Seeking Scales, Disinhibition
	SS9	Karolinska Scale of Personality, Monotony Avoidance
	Imp10	Karolinska Scale of Personality, Impulsivity
	SS11	Sensation Seeking Scales, Thrill–Adventure Seeking
	E12	Eysenck Personality Questionnaire, Extraversion
	Soc13	California Personality Inventory, Sociability
	Act14	Buss–Plomin EASI, Activity
	En15	Jackson Personality Inventory, Energy Level
	Ag16	Buss–Durkee Hostility Inventory
	Ag17	Personality Research Form, Aggression
	C18	Strelau Temperament Inventory, Restraint
	C19	Jackson Personality Inventory, Responsibility
	Conform20	Jackson Personality Inventory, Conformity
	Soc21	California Personality Inventory, Socialization
	Ag-22	Karolinska Scale Personality, Inhibition of Aggression
	Soc-23	Karolinska Scale of Personality, Detachment
	Sco24	Buss–Plomin EASI, Sociability
	Soc25	Jackson Personality Inventory, Social Participation
	Soc26	Personality Research Form, Affiliation
	Imp27	Buss–Plomin EASI, Decision Time
Goldberg & Rosolack (1994)	E28	Eysenck Personality Questionnaire, Extraversion (with factors I and III)
	P29	Esysenck Personality Questionnaire, Psychoticism (with factors I and III)
	P30	Eysenck Personality Questionnaire, Psychoticism (with factors I and II)
Zuckerman et al. (1993) (four-factor solution with entire scales)	E31	Costa & McCrae NEO, Extraversion
	E32	Eysenck Personality Questionnaire, Extraversion
	Soc33	Zuckerman–Kuhlman Personality Questionnaire, Sociability
	Act34	Zuckerman–Kuhlman Personality Questionnaire, Activity
	C35	Costa & McCrae NEO, Conscientiousness
	P36	Eysenck Personality Questionnaire, Psychoticism
	Imp37	Zuckerman–Kuhlman Personality Questionnaire, Impulsive Sensation Seeking

Study	Numbered trait abbreviation[b] (in numerical order)	Corresponding personality questionnaire trait[c]
	Ag38	Zuckerman–Kuhlman Personality Questionnaire, Aggression
	Agree39	Costa & McCrae NEO, Agreeableness
Zuckerman et al. (1993) (five-factor solution with primary scales included)	Soc40	Costa & McCrae NEO, E2, Gregariousness
	Soc41	Costa & McCrae NEO, E1, Warmth
	Act42	Costa & McCrae NEO, E4, Activity
	SS43	Costa & McCrae NEO, E5, Excitement Seeking
	PE44	Costa & McCrae NEO, E6, Positive Emotions
	Dom45	Costa & McCrae NEO, E3, Assertiveness
	C46	Costa & McCrae NEO, C4, Achievement
	C47	Costa & McCrae NEO, C5, Self-Discipline
	C48	Costa & McCrae NEO, C6, Deliberation
	C49	Costa & McCrae NEO, C3, Dutiful
	C50	Costa & McCrae NEO, C1, Competence
	C51	Costa & McCrae NEO, C2, Order
Angleitner & Ostendorf (1994)[d]	Soc52	Buss–Plomin EASI III, Sociability I
	E53	Costa & McCrae NEO, Extraversion
	C54	Costa & McCrae NEO, Conscientiousness
	Imp55	Buss–Plomin EASI III, Noninhibition Control
	Imp56	Buss–Plomin EASI III, Short Decision Time
	SS57	Buss–Plomin EASI III, Sensation Seeking
	Persis-58	Buss–Plomin EASI III, Nonpersistence
	Act 59	Buss–Plomin EASI III, Activity–Tempo
	Act60	Buss–Plomin EASI III, Activity–Vigor
Panter, Tanaka, & Hoyle (1994)	E61	Goldberg Surgency
	E62	Costa & McCrae NEO, Extraversion
	C63	Goldberg Conscientiousness
	C64	Costa & McCrae NEO, Conscientiousness
Church (1994)	WB65	Tellegen Multidimensional Personality Questionnaire, Well-Being
	Dom66	Tellegen Multidimensional Personality Questionnaire, Social Potency
	Soc68	Costa & McCrae NEO, E1, Warmth
	Soc69	Costa & McCrae NEO, E2, Gregariousness
	Dom70	Costa & McCrae NEO, E3, Assertiveness
	Act71	Costa & McCrae NEO, E4, Activity
	SS72	Costa & McCrae NEO, E5, Excitement Seeking
	PE73	Costa & McCrae NEO, E6, Positive Emotions
	C74	Costa & McCrae NEO, Conscientiousness
Tellegen & Waller (1996)	E75	Tellegen Multidimensional Personality Questionnaire, Positive Emotionality
	Soc76	California Personality Inventory, Personal Orientation
	E77	Eysenck Personality Questionnaire, Extraversion

Study	Numbered trait abbreviation[b] (in numerical order)	Corresponding personality questionnaire trait[c]
	C78	Tellegen Multidimensional Personality Questionnaire, Constraint
	C79	California Personality Inventory, Rigidity
	P80	Eysenck Personality Questionnaire, Psychoticism
Zuckerman (1996)	ImpSS81	Zuckerman–Kuhlman Personality Questionnaire, Impulsive Sensation Seeking
	P82	Eysenck Personality Questionnaire, Psychoticism
	E83	Eysenck Personality Questionnaire, Extraversion
	Act84	Zuckerman–Kuhlman Personality Questionnaire, Activity
	Soc85	Zuckerman–Kuhlman Personality Questionnaire, Sociability
Waller et al. (1991) (interscale correlations, not factor loadings)	NS86	Cloninger Tridimensional Personality Questionnaire, Novelty Seeking (average of NS subscale correlations with Tellegen Multidimensional Personality Questionnaire, Well-Being [best E estimate] and Control [best Constraint estimate])
Stallings et al. (1996) (interscale correlations, not factor loadings)	NS87	Cloninger Tridimensional Personality Questionnaire, Novelty Seeking (NS correlated with Eysenck Personality Questionnaire)
	NS88	Cloninger Tridimensional Personality Questionnaire, Novelty Seeking (NS correlated with Eysenck Personality Questionnaire E and KSP Impulsivity)
	NS89	Cloninger Tridimensional Personality Questionnaire, Novelty Seeking (NS correlated with Eysenck Personality Questionnaire E and KSP Monotony Avoidance

[a] References for the trait measures may be found in the study that used them.
[b] A "minus" sign appearing after letters but before the number indicates the inverse of the abbreviated descriptor (e.g., Soc-23 is Detachment, the inverse of Sociability).
[c] EASI, Energy–Activity–Sociability–Impulsivity; Sensation Seeking Scales, of Zuckerman; NEO, Neuroticism–Extraversion–Openness; MPQ,= Multidimensional Personality Questionnaire; KSP, Karolinska Scale of Personality.
[d] Only established questionnaires used.

ACKNOWLEDGMENTS

This work was supported by Research Grant Nos. MH55347 awarded to Richard A. Depue and MH-45448 awarded to Mark F. Lenzenweger.

REFERENCES

Adolphs, R. (2003). Cognitive neuroscience of human social behavior. *Nature Reviews Neuroscience*, 4, 165–178.

Aggleton, J. (1992). *The amygdala: Neurobiological aspects of emotion, memory, and mental dysfunction.* New York: Wiley-Liss.

Aharon, I., Etcoff, N., Ariety, D., Chabris, C., O'Connor, E., & Breiter, H. (2001). Beautiful faces have variable reward value. *Neuron*, 32, 537–551.

American Psychiatric Association. (1994). *Diagnostic and statistical manual of mental disorders* (4th ed.). Washington, DC: Author.

Annett, L., McGregor, A., & Robbins, T. (1989). The effects of ibotenic acid lesions of the nucleus accumbens on spatial learning and extinction in the rat. *Behavioral and Brain Research*, 31, 231–242.

Ashby, C. (1996). *The modulation of dopaminergic neurotransmission by other neurotransmitters.* Boca Raton, FL: CRC Press.

Aston-Jones, G., Rajkowski, J., Kubiak, P, Valentino, R., & Shiptley, M. (1996). Role of the locus coeruleus in emotional activation. In G. Holstege, R. Bandler & C. Saper (Eds.), *The emotional motor system* (pp. 254–279). New York: Elsevier.

Azmitia, E., & Whitaker-Azmitia, P. (1997). Development and adult plasticity of serotonergic neurons and their target cells. In H. Baumgarten & M. Gothert (Eds.), *Handbook of experiential pharmacology: Vol. 129. Serotonergic neurons and 5-HT receptors in the CNS* (pp. 1–39). New York: Springer-Verlag.

Babor, T., Hofmann, M., & Delboca, F. (1992). Types of alcoholics: 1. Evidence for an empirically derived typology based on indicators of vulnerability and severity. *Archives of General Psychiatry*, 49, 599–608.

Bandler, R., & Keay, K. (1996). Columnar organization in the midbrain periaqueductal gray and the integration of emotional expression. In G. Holstege, R. Bandler, & C. Saper (Eds.), *The emotional motor system* (pp. 571–605). New York: Elsevier.

Barlow, D. H. (2002). *Anxiety and its disorders* (2nd ed.). New York: Guilford Press.

Bechara, A., Tranel, D., Damasio, H., Adolphs, R., Rockland, C., & Damasio, A. (1995). Double dissociation of conditioning and declarative knowledge relative to the amygdala and hippocampus in humans. *Science*, 269, 1115–1118.

Benjamin, J., Li, L., Patterson, C., Geenberg, B., Murphy, D., & Hamer, D. (1996). Population and familial association between the D4 dopamine receptor gene and measures of novelty seeking. *Nature Genetics*, 12, 81–84.

Berrettini, W. H., Hoehe, M., Ferraro, T. N. , DeMaria, P., & Gottheil, E. (1997). Human mu opioid receptor gene polymorpnhisms and vulnerability to substance abuse. *Addiction and Biology*, 2, 303–308.

Berridge, K. C. (1999). Pleasure, pain, desire, and dread: Hidden core processes of emotion. In D. Kahneman, E. Diener, & N. Schwarz (Eds.), *Well-being: The foundations of hedonic psychology* (pp. 525–557). New York. Russell Sage

Blizzard, D. A. (1988). The locus ceruleus: A possible neural focus for genetic differences in emotionality. *Experientia, 44,* 491–495.

Blackburn, J. R., Phillips, A. G., Jakubovic, A., & Fibiger, H. C. (1989). Dopamine and preparatory behavior: II. A neurochemical analysis. *Behavioral Neuroscience, 103,* 15–23.

Block, J. (2001). Millennial contrarianism: The five-factor approach to personality description 5 years later. *Journal of Personality, 69,* 98–107.

Bond, C., LaForge, K. S., Tian, M., Melia, D., Zhang, S., Borg, L., Gong, J., Schluger, J., Strong, J. A., Leal, S. M., Tischfield, J. A., Kreek., M. J., & Yu, L. (1998). Single-nucleotide polymorphism in the human mu opioid receptor gene alters b-endorphin binding and activity: Possible implications for opiate addiction. *Proceedings of the National Academy of Sciences, 95,* 9608–9613.

Breiter, H., Aharon, I., Kahneman, D., Dale, A., & Shizgal, P. (2001). Functional imaging of neural responses to expectancy and experience of monetary gains and losses. *Neuron, 30,* 619–639.

Breiter, H. C., Gollub, R. L., Weisskoff, R. M., Kennedy, D. N., Makris, N., Berke, J. D., Goodman, J. M., Kantor, H. L., Gastfriend, D. R., Riorden, J. P., Mathew, R. T., Rosen, B. R., & Hyman, S. E. (1997). Acute effects of cocaine on human brain activity and emotion. *Neuron, 19,* 591–611.

Brothers, L., & Ring, B. (1992). A neuroethological framework for the representation of minds. *Journal of Cognitive Neuroscience, 4*(2), 107–118.

Cador, M., Taylor, J., & Robbins, T. (1991). Potentiation of the effects of reward-related stimuli by dopaminergic-dependent mechanisms in the nucleus accumbens. *Psychopharmacology, 104,* 377–385.

Carlezon, W., Haile, C., Coopersmith, R., Hayashi, Y., Malinow, R., Neve, R., & Nestler, E. (2000). Distinct sites of opiate reward and aversion within the midbrain identified using a herpes simplex virus vector expressing GluR1. *Journal of Neuroscience, 20*(RC62), 1–5.

Carter, S., Lederhendler, I., & Kirkpatrick, B. (1997). *The integrative neurobiology of affiliation* (Vol. 807). New York: New York Academy of Sciences.

Charney, D. S., Grillon, C, & Bremner, D. (1998). The neurobiological basis of anxiety and fear: Circuits, mechanisms, and neurochemical interactions (Part I). *Neuroscientist, 4,* 35–44.

Church, A. T. (1994). Relating the Tellegen and five-factor models of personality structure. *Journal of Personality and Social Psychology, 67,* 898–909.

Church, T., & Burke, P. (1994). Exploratory and confirmatory tests of the big five and Tellegen's three- and four-dimensional models. *Journal of Personality and Social Psychology, 66,* 93–114.

Clark, L. A., & Livesley, W. J. (1994). Two approaches to identifying the dimensions of personality disorder. In P. T. Costa, Jr. & T. A. Widiger (Eds.), *Personaltiy disorders and the five factor model of personality* (pp. 302–331). Washington, DC: American Psychological Association.

Clark, L. A., Livesley, W. J., Schroeder, M. L., & Irish, S. L. (1996). Convergence of two systems for assessing personality disorder. *Psychological Assessment, 8,* 294–303.

Cloninger, C. R., Svrakic, D., & Przybeck, T. (1993). A psychobiological model of temperament and character. *Archives of General Psychiatry, 50,* 975–990.

Coccaro, E., & Siever, L. (1991). *Serotonin and psychiatric disorders.* Washington, DC: American Psychiatric Association Press.

Coccaro, E., Siever, L., Klar, H., Maurer, G., Cochrane, K., Cooper, T., Mohs, R., & Davis, K. (1989). Serotonergic studies in patients with affective and personality disorders. *Archives of General Psychiatry, 46,* 587–599.

Costa, P., & McCrae, R. (1992). *Revised NEO Personality Inventory (NEO-PI-R). and NEO Five-Factor Inventory (NEO-FFI) (professional manual).* Odessa, FL: Psychological Assessment Resourses.

Costa, P. T., Jr., & Widiger, T. A. (1994). *Personaltiy disorders and the five factor model of personality.* Washington, DC: American Psychological Association.

Damasio, D. (2003). *Looking for Spinoza.* New York: Harcourt.

David, V., & Cazala, P. (2000). Anatomical and pharmacological specificity of the rewarding effect elicited by microinjections of morphine into the nucleus accumbens of mice. *Psychopharmacology, 150,* 24–34.

Davis, M., & Shi, C. (1999). The extended amydala: Are the central nucleus of the amygdala and the bed nucleus of the stria terminalis differentially involved in fear versus anxiety. In J. F. McGinty (Ed.), Advancing from the ventral striatum to the extended amygdala. *Annals of New York Academy of Sciences, 877,* 281–291.

Davis, M., Walker, D., & Lee, Y. (1997). Roles of the amygdala and bed nucleus of the stria terminalis in fear and anxiety measured with the acoustic startle reflex. *Annals of the New York Academy of Sciences, 821,* 305–331.

Depue, R. (1995). Neurobiological factors in personality and depression. *European Journal of Personality, 9,* 413–439.

Depue, R. (1996). Neurobiology and the structure of personality: Implications for the personality disorders. In J. F. Clarkin & M. F. Lenzenweger (Eds), *Major theories of personality disorder* (pp. 149–163). New York: Guilford Press.

Depue, R. A., & Collins, P. F. (1999). Neurobiology of the structure of personality: Dopamine, facilitation of incentive motivation, and extraversion. *Behavioral and Brain Sciences, 22,* 491–569.

Depue, R., & Iacono, W. (1989). Neurobehavioral aspects of affective disorders. *Annual Review of Psychology, 40,* 457–492.

Depue, R. A., & Lenzenweger, M. F. (2001). A neurobehavioral dimensional model of personality disorders. In W. J. Livesley (Ed.), *Handbook of personality disorders* (pp. 136–176). New York: Guilford Press.

Depue, R., Luciana, M., Arbisi, P., Collins, P., & Leon, A. (1994). Dopamine and the structure of personality: Relation of agonist-induced dopamine activity to positive emotionality. *Journal of Personality and Social Psychology, 67,* 485–498.

Depue, R. A., & Morrone-Strupinsky, J. V. (in press). A neurobehavioral model of affiliative bonding: Implications for conceptualizing a human trait of affiliation. *Behavioral and Brain Sciences.*

Depue, R., & Spoont, M. (1986). Conceptualizing a serotonin trait: A behavioral dimension of constraint. *Annals of the New York Academy of Sciences, 487,* 47–62.

Di Chiara, G. (1995). The role of dopamine in drug abuse viewed from the perspective of its role in motivation. *Drug and Alcohol Dependence, 38,* 95–137.

Di Chiara, G., & North, R. A. (1992). Neurobiology of opiate abuse. *Trends in the Physiological Sciences, 13,* 185–193.

Digman, J. M. (1997). Higher-order factors of the big five. *Journal of Personality and Social Psychology, 73,* 1246–1256.

Domjan, M., Cusato, B., & Villarreal, R (2000). Pavlovian feed-forward mechanisms in the control of social behavior. *Behavioral and Brain Sciences, 23,* 1–29.

Drevets, W. C., Gautier, C., Price, J. C., Kupfer, D. J., Kinahan, P. E., Grace, A. A., Price, J. L., & Mathis, C. A. (2001). Amphetamine-induced dopamine release in human ventral striatum correlates with euphoria. *Biological Psychiatry, 49,* 81–96.

Dworkin, S., Guerin, G., Goeders, N., & Smith, J. (1988). Kainic acid lesions of the nucleus accumbens selectively attenuate morphine self-administration. *Pharmacology, Biochemistry and Behavior, 29,* 175–181.

Dyce, J. A., & Connor, B. P. (1998). Personality disorders and the five-factor model: A test of facet-level predictions. *Journal of Personality Disorders, 12,* 31–45.

Ebstein, R., Novick, O., Umansky, R., Priel, B., Osher, Y., Blaine, D., Bennett, E., Nemanov, L., Katz, M., & Belmaker, R. (1996). Dopamine D4 receptor (DRD4). Exon III polymorphism associated with the human personality trait of novelty seeking. *Nature Genetics, 12,* 78–80.

Eisenberger, N., Lieberman, M., & Williams, K. (2003). Does rejection hurt? An fMRI study of social exclusion. *Science, 302,* 290–292.

Ekselius, L., Lindstrom, E., von Knorring, L., Bodlund, O., & Kullgren, G. (1994). A principal component analysis of the DSM-III R axis II personality disorders. *Journal of Personality Disorders, 8,* 140–148.

Elmer, G. I., Pieper, J. O., Goldberg, S. R., & George, F. R. (1995). Opioid operant self-administration, analgesia, stimulation and respiratory depression in μ-deficient mice. *Psychopharmacology, 117,* 23–31.

Erb, S., Salmaso, N., Rodaros, D., & Stewart, J. (2001). A role for the CF-containing pathway from central nucleus of the amygdala to the bed nucleus of the stria terminalis in the stress-induced reinstatement of cocaine seeking in rats. *Psychopharmacology, 158,* 360–365.

Everitt, B., & Robbins, T. (1992). Amygdala-ventral striatal interactions and reward-related processes. In J. Aggleton (Ed.), *The amygdala: Neurobiological aspects of emotion, memory, and mental dysfunction* (pp. 145–159). New York: Wiley-Liss.

Fendt, M., Endres, T., & Apfelbach, R. (2003). Temporary inactivation of the bed nucleus of the stria terminalis but not of the amygdala blocks freezing induced by trimethylthiazoline, a component of fox feces. *Journal of Neuroscience, 23,* 23–28.

Fleming, A. S., Korsmit, M., & Deller, M. (1994). Rat pups are potent reinforcers to the maternal animal: Effects of experience, parity, hormones, and dopamine function. *Psychobiology*, 22(1), 44–53.

Fowles, D. C. (1987). Application of a behavioral theory of motivation to the concepts of anxiety and impulsivity. *Journal of Research in Personality*, 21, 417–435.

Gaffan, D. (1992). Amygdala and the memory of reward. In J. Aggleton (Ed.), *The amygdala: Neurobiological aspects of emotion, memory, and mental dysfunction* (pp. 201–242). New York: Wiley-Liss.

Gelernter, J., Kranzler, H., & Cubells, J. (1999). Genetics of two μ opioid receptor gene (OPRM1). Exon I polymorphisms: population studies, and allele frequencies in alcohol- and drug-dependent subjects. *Molecular Psychiatry*, 4, 476–483.

Gingrich, B., Liu, Y., Cascio, C., Wang, Z., & Insel, T. R. (2000). Dopamine D_2 receptors in the nucleus accumbens are important for social attachment in female prairie voles (*Microtus ochrogaster*). *Behavioral Neuroscience*, 114(1), 173–183.

Goddard, A., Charney, D., & Germine, M. (1995). Effects of tryptophan depletion on responses to yohimbine in healthy human subjects. *Biological Psychiatry*, 38, 74–85.

Goldberg, L., & Rosolack, T. (1994). The big five factor structure as an integrative framework. In C. Halverson, G. Kohnstamm, & R. Marten (Eds.), *The developing structure of temperament and personality from infancy to adulthood* (pp. 275–314). Hillside, NJ: Erlbaum.

Goldman-Rakic, P. S. (1987). Circuitry of the prefrontal cortex and the regulation of behavior by representational memory. In V. Mountcastle (Ed.), *Handbook of physiology* (pp. 373–417). Bethesda, MD: American Physiological Society.

Gottesman, I. I. (1997). Twins: En route to QTLs for cognition. *Science*, 276, 1522–1523.

Graves, F. C., Wallen, K., & Maestripieri, D. (2002). Opioids and attachment in rhesus macaque abusive mothers. *Behavioral Neuroscience*, 116, 489–493.

Gray, J. A. (1973). Causal theories of personality and how to test them. In J. R. Royce (Ed.), *Multivariate analysis and psychological theory* (pp. 302–354). New York: Academic Press.

Gray, J. (1992). Neural systems, emotion and personality. In J. Madden, S. Matthysee, & J. Barchas (Eds.), *Adaptation, learning and affect* (pp. 95–121). New York: Raven Press.

Guyenet, P., Koshiqa, N., Huangfu, D., Baraban, S., Stornetta, R., Li, Y-W. (1996). Role of medulla oblongata in generation of sympathetic and vagal outflows. In G. Holstege, R. Bandler, & C. Saper, *The emotional motor system* (pp. 510–552). New York: Elsevier.

Heimer, L. (2003). A new anatomical framework for neuropsychiatric disorders and drug abuse. *American Journal of Psychiatry*, 160, 1726–1739.

Herbert, J. (1993). Peptides in the limbic system: Neurochemical codes for coordinated adaptive responses to behavioural and physiological demand. *Progress in Neurobiology*, 41, 723–791.

Herz, A. (1998). Opioid reward mechanisms: A key role in drug abuse? *Canadian Journal of Physiology and Pharmacology, 76,* 252–258.

Higley, J., Mehlman, P., Taub, D., & Higley, S. (1992). Cerebrospinal fluid monoamine and adrenal correlates of agression in free-ranging rhesus monkeys. *Archives of General Psychiatry, 49,* 436–441.

Hilliard, S., Domjan, M., Nguyen, M., & Cusato, B. (1998). Dissociation of conditioned appetitive and consummatory sexual behavior: Satiation and extinction tests. *Animal Learning and Behavior, 26*(1), 20–33.

Hol, T., Niesink, M., van Ree, J., & Spruijt, B. (1996). Prenatal exposure to morphine affects juvenile play behavior and adult social behavior in rats. *Pharmacology, Biochemistry, and Behavior, 55,* 615–618.

Holstege, G. (1996). The somatic motor system. In G. Holstege, R. Bandler, & C. Saper (Eds.), *The emotional motor system* (pp. 56–78). New York: Elsevier.

Hyztia, P., & Kiianmaa, K. (2001). Suppression of ethanol responding by centrally administered CTOP and naltrindole in AA and Wistar rats. *Alcohol Clinical and Experimental Research, 25,* 25–33.

Ikemoto, W., & Panksepp, J. (1996). Dissociations between appetitive and consummatory responses by pharmacological manipulations of reward-relevant brain regions. *Behavioral Neuroscience, 110,* 331–345.

Insel, T. R. (1997). A neurobiological basis of social attachment. *American Journal of Psychiatry, 154*(6), 726–733.

Johnson, B., & Ait-Daoud, N. (2000). Neuropharmacological treatments for alcoholism: Scientific basis and clinical findings. *Psychopharmacology, 149,* 327–344.

Kalivas, P., Churchill, L., & Klitenick, M. (1993). The circuitry mediating the translation of motivational stimuli into adaptive motor responses. In P. Kalivas & C. Barnes (Eds.), *Limbic motor circuits and neuropsychiatry* (pp. 216–252). Boca Raton, FL: CRC Press.

Kendler, K. S., McGuire, M., Gruenberg, A. M., O'Hare, A., Spellman, M., & Walsh, D. (1993). The Roscommon Family Study: III. Schizophrenia-related personality disorders in relatives. *Archives of General Psychiatry, 50,* 781–788.

Keverne, E. B. (1996). Psychopharmacology of maternal behaviour. *Journal of Psychopharmacology, 10*(1), 16–22.

Kim, J., & Diamond, D. (2002). The stressed hippocampus, synaptic plasticity and lost memories. *Nature Reviews Neuroscience, 3,* 453–462.

Kohnstamm, G. (1989). Temperament in childhood: Cross-cultural and sex differences. In G. Kohnstamm, J. Bates, & M. Rothbart (Eds.), *Temperament in childhood* (pp. 317–365). New York: Wiley.

Korfine, L., & Lenzenweger, M. F. (1995). The taxonicity of schizotypy: A replication. *Journal of Abnormal Psychology, 104,* 26–31.

Kranzler, H. R. (2000). Pharmacotherapy of alcoholism: Gaps in knowledge and opportunities for research. *Acohol and Alcoholism, 35,* 537–547.

La Buda, C., Sora, I., Uhl, G., & Fuchs, D. (2000). Stress-induced analgesia in mu-opioid receptor knockout mice reveals normal function of the delta-opioid receptor system. *Brain Research, 869,* 1–10.

Laviolette, S. R., Gallegos, R. A., Henriksen, S. J., & van der Kooy, D. (2004). Opiate state controls bi-directional reward signaling via GABA-A receptors in the ventral tegmental area. *Nature Neuroscience, 10,* 160–169.

LeDoux, J. (1998). *The emotional brain.* New York: Simon & Schuster.

LeDoux, J., Cicchetti, P., Xagoraris, A., & Romanski L. (1990). The lateral amygdaloid nucleus: Sensory interface of the amygdala in fear conditioning. *Journal of Neuroscience, 10,* 1062–1069.

Le Moal, M., & Simon, H. (1991). Mesocorticolimbic dopaminergic network: Functional and regulatory roles. *Physiological Reviews, 71,* 155–234.

Lenzenweger, M. F. (1998). Schizotypy and schizotypic psychopathology: Mapping an alternative expression of schizophrenia liability. In M. F. Lenzenweger & R. H. Dworkin (Eds.), *Origins and development of schizophrenia: Advances in experimental psychopathology* (pp. 93–121). Washington, DC: American Psychological Association.

Lenzenweger, M. F., & Clarkin, J. F. (1996). The personality disorders: History, classification, and research issues. In J. F. Clarkin & M. F. Lenzenweger (Eds.), *Major theories of personality disorder* (pp. 1–35). New York: Guilford Press.

Lenzenweger, M. F., Johnson, M. D., & Willett, J. B. (in press). Individual growth curve analysis illuminates stability and change in personality disorder features: The Longitudinal Study of Personality Disorders. *Archives of General Psychiatry.*

Lenzenweger, M. F., & Korfine, L. (1992). Confirming the latent structure and base rate of schizotypy: A taxometric analysis. *Journal of Abnormal Psychology, 101,* 567–571.

Lenzenweger, M. F., & Loranger, A. W. (1989). Detection of familial schizophrenia using a psychometric measure of schizotypy. *Archives of General Psychiatry, 46,* 902–907.

Lenzenweger, M. F., Loranger, A. W., Korfine, L., & Neff, C. (1997). Detecting personality disorders in a nonclinical population: Application of a two-stage procedure for case identification. *Archives of General Psychiatry, 54,* 345–351.

Leri, F., Flores, J., Rodaros, D., & Stewart, J. (2002). Blockade of stress-induced but not cocaine-induced reinstatement by infusion of noradrenergic antagonists into the bed nucleus of the stria terminalis or the central nucleus of the amygdala. *Journal of Neuroscience, 22,* 5713–5718.

Lesch, K-P. (1998). Serotonin transporter and psychiatric disorders. *The Neuroscientist, 4,* 25–34.

Leyton, M., & Stewart, J. (1992). The stimulation of central kappa opioid receptors decreases male sexual behavior and locomotor activity. *Brain Research, 594,* 56–74.

Livesley, W. J. (2001). Commentary on reconceptualizing personality disorder categories using trait dimensions. *Journal of Personality, 69,* 277–286.

Livesley, W. J., Jackson, D. N., & Schroeder, M. L. (1992). Factorial structure of traits delineating personality disorders in clinical and general population samples. *Journal of Abnormal Psychology, 101,* 432–440.

Livesley, W., Jang, K., & Vernon, P. (1998). Phenotypic and genetic structure of traits delineating personality disorder. *Archives of General Psychiatry, 55,* 941–948.

Livesley, W. J., Schroeder, M. L., Jackson, D. N., & Jang, K. L. (1994). Categorical distinctions in the study of personality disorder: Implication for classification. *Journal of Abnormal Psychology, 103,* 6–17.

Luciana, M., Collins, P., & Depue, R. (1998). Opposing roles for dopamine and serotonin in the modulation of human spatial working memory functions. *Cerebral Cortex, 8,* 218–226.

Luciana, M., Depue, R. A., Arbisi, P., & Leon, A. (1992). Facilitation of working memory in humans by a D2 dopamine receptor agonist. *Journal of Cognitive Neuroscience, 4,* 58–68.

Macey, D., Smith, H., Nader, M., & Porrino, L. (2003). Chronic cocaine self-administration upregulates the norepinephrine transporter and alters functional activity in the bed nucleus of the stria terminalis of the Rhesus monkey. *Journal of Neuroscience, 23,* 12–16.

MacLean, P. (1986). Ictal symptoms relating to the nature of affects and their cerebral substrate. In E. Plutchik & H. Kellerman (Eds.), *Emotion: Theory, research, and experience. Vol. 3: Biological foundations of emotion* (pp. 283–328). New York: Academic Press.

Marinelli, M., & White, F. (2000). Enhanced vulnerability to cocaine self-administration is associated with elevated impulse activity of midbrain dopamine neurons. *Journal of Neuroscience, 20,* 8876–8885.

Martel, F., Nevison, C., Simpson, M., & Keverne, E. (1995). Effects of opioid receptor blockade on the social behavior of rhesus monkeys living in large family groups. *Developmental Psychobiology, 28,* 71–84.

Matheson, M. D., & Bernstein, I. S. (2000). Grooming, social bonding, and agonistic aiding in rhesus monkeys. *American Journal of Primatology, 51,* 177–186.

Matthes, H. W., Maldonado, R., Simonin, F., Valverde, O., Slowe, S., Kitchen, I., Befort, K., Dierich, A., Le Meur, M., Dolle, P., Tzavara, E., Hanoune, J., Roques, B. P., & Kieffer, B. L. (1996). Loss of morphine-induced analgesia, reward effect and withdrawal symptoms in mice lacking the μ-opioid-receptor gene. *Nature, 383,* 819–823.

McDonald, A., Shammah-lagnado, S., Shi, C., & Davis, M. (1999). Cortical afferents to the extended amygdala. In J. F. McGinty (Ed.), *Advancing from the ventral striatum to the extended amygdala* (pp. 309–338). New York: New York Academy of Sciences.

McGinty, J. F. (1999). Regulation of neurotransmitter interactions in the ventral striatum. In J. F. McGinty (Ed.), *Advancing from the ventral striatum to the extended amygdala amygdala* (pp. 129–139). New York: New York Academy of Sciences.

Mesulam, M. (1990). Large-scale neurocognitive networks and distributed processing for attention, language, and memory. *Annals of Neurology, 28,* 597–613.

Millon, T. (1997). *The Millon inventories: Clinical and personality assessment.* New York: Guilford Press.

Mitra, N., Mohanakumar, K., & Ganguly, D. (1994). Resistance of golden hamster: Relationship to MAO-B. *Journal of Neurochemistry, 62,* 1906–1912.

Moles, A., Kieffer, B. L., & D'Amato, F. R. (2004). Deficit in attachment behavior in mice lacking the m-opioid receptor gene. *Science, 304,* 1983–1986.

Morrone, J., Depue, R., Sherer, N., & White, T. (2000). Film-induced incentive motivation and positive affect in relation to agentic and affiliative components of extraversion. *Personality and Individual Differences, 29,* 199–216.

Morrone-Strupinsky, J. V., & Depue, R. A. (2004). Differential relation of two distinct, film-induced positive emotional states to affiliative and agentic extraversion. *Personality and Individual Differences, 36,* 1109–1126.

Narita, M., Aoki, T., & Suzuki, T. (2000). Molecular evidence for the involvement of NR2B subunit containing N-methyl-D-aspartate receptors in the development of morphine-induced place preference. *Neuroscience, 101,* 601–606.

Nelson, E. E., & Panksepp, J. (1998). Brain substrates of infant–mother attachment: Contributions of opioids, oxytocin, and norepinephrine. *Neuroscience and Biobehavioral Reviews, 22*(3), 437–452.

Nie, Z., Schweitzer, P., Roberts, A., Madamba, S., Moore, S., & Siggins, G. (2004). Ethanol augments GABA-ergic transmission in the central amygdala via CRF1 receptors. *Science, 303,* 1512–1514

Niesink, R. J. M., Vanderschuen, L. J. M. J., & van Ree, J. M. (1996). Social play in juvenile rats in utero exposure to morphine. *NeuroToxicology, 17*(3–4), 905–912.

Oades, R. (1985). The role of noradrenaline in tuning and dopamine in switching between signals in the CNS. *Neuroscience and Biobehavioral Reviews, 9,* 261–282.

Oades, R., & Halliday, G. (1987). Ventral tegmental (A10). system: Neurobiology. 1. Anatomy and connectivity. *Brain Research Review, 12,* 117–165.

Olausson, H., Lamarre, Y., Backlund, H., Morin, C., Wallin, B. G., Starck, G., Ekholm, S., Strigo, I., Worsley, K., Vallbo, A. B., & Bushnell, M. C. (2002). Unmyelinated tactile afferents signal touch and project to insular cortex. *Nature Neuroscience, 5,* 900–904.

Olive, M., Koenig, H., Nannini, M., & Hodge, C. (2001). Stimulation of endorphin neurotransmission in the nucleus accumbens by ethanol, cocaine, and amphetamine. *Journal of Neuroscience, 21*(RC184), 1–5.

Olmstead, M., & Franklin, K. (1997). The development of a conditioned place preference to morphine. *Behavioral Neuroscience, 111,* 1324–1334.

Olson, G., Olson, R., & Kastin, A. (1997). Endogenous opiates: 1996. *Peptides, 18,* 1651–1688.

Ostrowski, N. L. (1998). Oxytocin receptor mRNA expression in rat brain: Implications for behavioral integration and reproductive success. *Psychoneuroendocrinology, 23*(8), 989–1004.

Pacak, K., McCarty, R., Palkovits, M., Kopin, I., & Goldstein, D. (1995). Effects of immobilization on in vivo release of norepinephrine in the bed nucleus of the stria terminalis in conscious rats. *Brain Research, 688,* 242–246.

Panksepp, J. (1998). *Affective neuroscience: The foundations of human and animal emotions.* New York: Oxford University Press.

Pfaus, J. G., Smith, W. J., & Coopersmith, C. B. (1999). Appetitive and consummatory sexual behaviors of female rats in bilevel chambers: I. A correlational and factor analysis and the effects of ovarian hormones. *Hormones and Behavior, 35,* 224–240.

Pich, E., Pagliusi, S., Tessari, M., Talabot-Ayer, D., van Huijsduijnen, R., & Chiamulera, C. (1997). Common neural substrates for the addictive properties of nicotine and cocaine. *Science, 275,* 83–86.

Polan, H. J., & Hofer, M. A. (1998). Olfactory preference for mother over home nest shavings by newborn rats. *Developmental Psychobiology, 33,* 5–20.

Porges, S. (1998). Love: An emergent property of the mammalian autonomic nervous system. *Psychoneuroendocrinology, 23,* 837–861.

Porges, S. (2001). The polyvagal theory: Phylogenetic substrates of a social nervous system. *International Journal of Psychophysiology, 42,* 123–146.

Redmond, D. E. (1987). Studies of the nucleus locus coeruleus in monkeys and hypotheses for neuropsychopharmacology. In J. Y. Meltzer (Ed.), *Psychopharacology: The third generation of progress* (pp. 967–975). New York: Raven Press.

Reynolds, S. K., & Clark, L. A. (2001). Predicting dimensions of personality disorder from domains and facets of the five-factor model. *Journal of Personality, 69,* 199–222.

Robbins, T., Cador, M, Taylor, J., & Everitt, B. (1989). Limbic–striatal interactions in reward-related processes. *Neuroscience and Biobehavioral Reviews, 13,* 155–162.

Rolls, E. T. (1999). *The brain and emotion.* New York: Oxford University Press.

Saulsman, L. M., & Page, A. C. (2004). The five-factor model and personality disorder empirical literature: A meta-analytic review. *Clinical Psychology Review, 23,* 1055–1085.

Schlaepfer, T. E., Strain, E. C., Greenberg, B. D., Preston, K. L., Lancaster, E., Bigelow, G. E., Barta, P. E., & Pearlson, G. D. (1998). Site of opioid action in the human brain: Mu and kappa agonists' subjective and cerebral blood flow effects. *American Journal of Psychiatry, 155*(4), 470–473.

Schneirla, T. (1959). An evolutionary and developmental theory of biphasic processes underlying approach and withdrawal. In M. Jones (Ed.), *Nebraska Symposium on Motivation* (pp. 144–171). Lincoln: University of Nebraska Press.

Schultz, W., Dayan, P., & Montague, P. (1997). A neural substrate of prediction and reward. *Science, 275,* 1593–1595.

Selden, N., Everitt, B., Jarrard, L., & Robbins, T. (1991). Complementary roles of the amygdala and hippocampus in aversive conditioning to explicit and contextual cues. *Neuroscience, 42,* 335–350.

Shaham, Y., Erb, S., & Stewart, J. (2000). Stress-induced relapse to heroin and cocaine seeking in rats: A review. *Brain Research Reviews, 33,* 13–33.

Shippenberg, T. S., & Elmer, G. I. (1998). The neurobiology of opiate reinforcement. *Critical Reviews in Neurobiology, 12*(4), 267–303.

Silk, J. B., Alberts, S. C., & Altmann, J. (2003). Social bonds of female baboons enhance infant survival. *Science, 302,* 1231–1234.

Spoont, M. (1992). Modulatory role of serotonin in neural information processing: Implications for human psychopathology. *Psychological Bulletin, 112,* 330–350.

Squire, L., & Kosslyn, S. (1998). *Findings and current opinion in cognitive neuroscience*. Cambridge, MA: MIT Press.

Stefano, G., Goumon, Y., Casares, F., Cadet, P., Fricchione, G., Rialas, C., Peter, D., Sonetti, D., Guarna, M., Welters, I., & Bianchi, E. (2000). Endogenous morphine. *Trends in Neuroscience, 23*, 436–442.

Strand, F. L. (1999). *Neuropeptides: Regulators of physiological processes*. Cambridge, MA: MIT Press.

Sutherland, R., & McDonald, R. (1990). Hippocampus, amygdala and memory deficits in rats. *Behavioral and Brain Research, 37*, 57–79.

Tellegen, A., Lykken, D. T., Bouchard, T. J., Wilcox, K. J., Segal, N. L., & Rich, S. (1988). Personality similarity in twins reared apart and together. *Journal of Personality and Social Psychology, 54*, 1031–1039.

Tellegen, A., & Waller, N. G. (in press). Exploring personality through test construction: Development of the multidimensional personality questionnaire. In S. Briggs & J. Cheek (Eds.), *Personality measures: Development and evaluation* (Vol. 1). New York: JAI Press.

Timberlake, W., & Silva, K. (1995). Appetitive behavior in ethology, psychology, and behavior systems. In N. Thompson (Ed.), *Perspectives in ethology: Vol 11. Behavioral design* (pp. 211–253). New York: Plenum Press.

Torgersen, S., Kringlen, E., & Cramer, V. (2001). The prevalence of personality disorders in a community sample. *Archives of General Psychiatry, 58*, 590–596.

Tork, I. (1990). Anatomy of the seroonergic system. *Annals of the New York Academy of Science, 600*, 9–32.

Treit, D., Pesold, C., & Rotzinger, S. (1993). Dissociating the anti-fear effects of septal and amygdaloid lesions using two pharmacologically validated models of rat anxiety. *Behavioral Neuroscience, 107*, 770–785.

Uhl, G. R., Sora, I., & Wang, Z. (1999). The μ opiate receptor as a candidate gene for pain: Polymorphisms, variations in expression, nociception, and opiate responses. *Proceedings of the National Academy of Sciences, 96*, 7752–7755.

van Furth, W., & van Ree, J. (1996). Sexual motivation: Involvement of endogenous opioids in the ventral tegmental area. *Brain Research, 729*, 20–28.

Volkow, N., Wang, G., Fischman, M., Foltin, R., Fowler, J.,Abumrad, N., Vitkun, S., Logan J., Gatley, S., Pappas, N., Hitzemann, R., & Shea, C. (1997). Relationship between subjective effects of cocaine and dopamine transporter occupancy. *Nature, 386*, 827–829.

Wang, Z., Yu, G., Cascio, C., Liu, Y., Gingrich, B., & Insel, T.R. (1999). Dopamine D_2 receptor-mediated regulation of partner preferences in female prairie voles (*Microtus ochrogaster*): A mechanism for pair bonding? *Behavioral Neuroscience, 113*(3), 602–611.

Watson, C., & Clark, L. (1997). Extraversion and its positive emotional core. In S. Briggs, W. Jones, & R. Hogan (Eds.), *Handbook of personality psychology* (pp. 72–96). New York: Academic Press.

Watson, D., & Tellegen, A. (1985). Towards a consensual structure of mood. *Psychological Bulletin, 98*, 219–235.

White, N. (1986). Control of sensorimotor function by dopaminergic nigrostriatal neurons: Influence on eating and drinking. *Neuroscience and Biobehavioral Reviews, 10*, 15–36.

White, T. L., & Depue, R. A. (1999). Differential association of traits of fear and anxiety with norepinephrine- and dark-induced pupil reactivity. *Journal of Personality and Social Psychology, 77*(4), 863–877.

Widiger, T. A., Trull, T. J., Clarkin, J. F., Sanderson, C., & Costa, P. T., Jr. (1994). A description of the DSM-III-R and DSM-IV personality disorders with the Five Factor Model of personality. In P. T. Costa, Jr. & T. A. Widiger (Eds.), *Personality disorders and the five factor model of personality* (pp. 41–56). Washington, DC: American Psychological Association.

Wiedenmayer, C., & Barr, G. (2000). Provide title. *Behavioral Neuroscience, 114,* 125–138.

Wiggins, J. (1991). Agency and communion as conceptual coordinates for the understanding and measurement of interpersonal behavior. In D. Cicchetti & W. Grove (Eds.), *Thinking clearly about psychology: Essays in honor of Paul Everett Meehl* (pp. 89–113). Minneapolis: University of Minnesota Press.

Wise, R. (1998). Drug-activation of brain reward pathways. *Drug and Alcolhol Dependence, 51,* 13–22.

Wolterink, G., Cador, M., Wolterink, I., Robbins, T., & Everitt, B. (1989). Involvement of D_1 and D_2 receptor mechanisms in the processing of reward-related stimuli in the ventral striatum. *Society of Neuroscience, 15,* 490.

Wynell, C. L., & Berridge, K. C. (2000). Intra-accumbens amphelamine increases the conditioned incentive salience of sucrose reward: Enhancement of reward "wanting" without enhanced "liking" on response reinforcement. *Journal of Neuroscience, 20,* 8122–8130.

Young, L. J., Wang, Z., & Insel, T. R. (1998). Neuroendocrine bases of monogamy. *Trends in the Neurosciences, 21,* 71–75.

Zald, D., & Depue, R. (2001). Serotonergic modulation of positive and negative affect in psychiatrically healthy males. *Personality and Individual Differences, 30,* 71–86.

Zubieta, J-K., Smith, Y., Bueller, J., Xu, Y., Kilbourn, M., Jewett, D., Meyer, C., Koeppe, R., & Stohler, C. (2001). Regional mu opioid receptor regulation of sensory and affective dimensions of pain. *Science, 293,* 311–315.

Zuckerman, M. (1994). An alternative five-factor model for personality. In C. Halverson, G. Kohnstamm, & R. Marten (Eds.), *The developing structure of temperament and personality from infancy to adulthood* (pp. 114–137). Mahwah, NJ: Erlbaum.

Index